I1018875

Special Diet
Diet
Celebrations

NO WHEAT, GLUTEN, DAIRY, OR EGGS

Other books by Carol Fenster, Ph.D.

Wheat-Free Recipes & Menus:
Delicious Dining without Wheat or Gluten

Special Diet Solutions:
Healthy Cooking without Wheat, Gluten, Dairy, Eggs, Yeast, or Sugar

Special
Diet
Celebrations

NO WHEAT, GLUTEN, DAIRY, OR EGGS

Savory Palate, Inc.
8174 South Holly, Suite 404
Littleton, CO 80122-4004

Special Diet Celebrations
No Wheat, Gluten, Dairy, or Eggs

SUMMARY
1. Wheat-free, gluten-free, celiac, diabetes, cookbook
2. Wheat intolerance, gluten intolerance, food sensitivity, food allergy

Edited by Mary Bonner
Cover design by Shaeffer Reagan Design
Illustrations by Jeanne VonWyl
Author photo by R.S. Little Studio

For orders and information, contact:
Savory Palate, Inc.
8174 South Holly, Suite 404
Littleton, CO, 80122-4004
(800) 741-5418   (303) 741-5408

CONTENTS

To husband Larry, son Brett, and . . .
the newest member of our family—daughter-in-law Helke

ACKNOWLEDGEMENTS

Celebrations are special times—regardless of what is being celebrated. This cookbook was a joy to write because I know it will be used to make special occasions memorable. I am deeply indebted to the following people who gave so generously of their time so you could celebrate with your favorite food.

To those who helped with testing recipes and providing excellent feedback, I truly appreciate your input—and please extend my thanks to the family and friends who lent their taste buds to the tasting process: Jane Dennison-Bauer, Julie Cary, Mary Courtney; Sandy Dempsey; Terri Ditmer; Laura Dolson; Donna Franz; Caroline Herdle; Jane Holcomb; Ruth Horelica; Janene Lenard; Alicia Pitzer; Janet Rinehart; Debbie Roth; Lynn Samuel, L.P.N.; Judy Sarver; Chris Silker; Jenny View; Peggy Wagener; Anne Washburn; Cecile Weed; and Sue Weilgopolan.

To those who helped with reviewing the manuscript and providing extremely valuable feedback, I sincerely appreciate your help: Rosanne G. Ainscough, R.D., C.D.E., Diabetes Dietitian Educator; Mary Lou Bonner; Gail Bright, R.D., Colorado Allergy & Asthma Centers; Sheila E. Crowe, M.D., Associate Professor, Department of Internal Medicine, University of Texas Medical Branch, Galveston, TX; Kathy Gibbons, Ph.D., nutritional counseling and biochemist Leon Greos, M.D., Colorado Allergy & Asthma Centers, P.C.; Dianna S. Hayton, R.N., Patient Educator, Colorado Allergy and Asthma Centers, P.C.; Cynthia Kupper, C.R.D., CEO & President, Gluten Intolerance Group of North America; Anne Munoz-Furlong, Founder, The Food Allergy Network, Fairfax, VA; Janet Y. Rinehart, Chairman, Houston Celiac Sprue Support Group and Past President, CSA/USA, Inc.; Nancy Carol Sanker, OTR, Education and Support Group Project Director, Asthma and Allergy Foundation of America; Ellen Speare, B.S., Clinical Nutritionist, Wild Oats Markets; Gail Spiegel, M.S., R.D., CDE ; Joanne M. Vitanza, M.D., Colorado Allergy and Asthma Centers, P.C.; Peggy A. Wagener, publisher of Sully's Living Without magazine; Ann Whelan, publisher of Gluten-Free Living newsletter; and Maura Zazenski.

What People Are Saying About

Special Diet*Celebrations*

Lots of tips, simple instructions. You take the fear out of making these foods.
-Cynthia Kupper, CRD, CDE - CEO & President
Gluten Intolerance Group of North America

Well written, informative, appealing, unique.
-Sheila E. Crowe, M.D., Associate Professor
Department of Internal Medicine,
University of Texas Medical Branch, Galveston, TX

I like the idea of targeting dietary needs for special occasions.
-Joanne M. Vitanza, M.D.
Colorado Allergy & Asthma Centers, P.C.

A great source of information. Much needed by our patients.
-Dianna S. Hayton, R.N., Patient Educator
Colorado Allergy & Asthma Centers, P.C.

*It will shorten the amount of time I have to spend educating clients about
recipes and substitutes. You made another wonderfully great and useful book
that can fix any "special" dietary needs.*
-Ellen Speare, B.S., Clinical Nutritionist
Wild Oats Markets

I think it's great. Thanks for including nutritional values.
-Janet Rinehart, Chairman
Houston Celiac Sprue Support Group
and Past President, CSA/USA, Inc.

A normal cookbook for special people.

-Ann Whelan, publisher
Gluten-Free Living newsletter

Special Diet Philosophy

Birthdays, anniversaries, parties—celebrations of any kind. This is the good stuff, the stuff life is made of. These are the occasions we use to the mark significant stages in our lives, to bond with our family, to connect with friends, and to re-affirm our connections to treasured rituals, traditions, and customs. Inevitably, food takes center stage.

And, yet for those of us with food sensitivities, these joyous occasions can be downright dangerous. The foods we once ate—and that everyone expects us to continue eating—are now off-limits. But the good news is that you can continue to eat these foods—if they're prepared with appropriate substitutes for the problem ingredients.

I have wanted to write this book for a long time. Why? Because I live on a special diet—just like you. And I know from personal experience that it is the special occasions that can be most challenging. For example, it's not easy to say "no" when someone puts a piece of cake (containing forbidden ingredients) in front of you saying "*Happy Birthday, I baked your favorite cake!*

Food Plays a Symbolic Role in Our Lives
Perhaps I am more aware than others of the symbolic role that food plays in our lives. In addition to being a culinary professional, my sociological background keeps me aware of how we use food to communicate with others. It is the celebrations, the holidays, the special occasions in our lives where food becomes the celebratory medium. Rituals associated with food become the memories of a lifetime. Fortunately, my training as a home economist gives me the technical ability to transform recipes into dishes that are safe, delicious to eat, and appropriate for any celebratory occasion.

If you've purchased my earlier books, you know my story. I suffered from chronic sinusitis most of my life until I learned to avoid my own particular food villains—especially wheat and certain wheat-related grains. For someone raised on a farm in Nebraska and who married into a wheat-farming family, this was unsettling to say the least! But, enough about that.

Today, I am an expert in helping people with special diet needs manage a healthy diet. Once they identify their own particular food villains (with the help of a health professional), I help them eat the foods they love—without the ingredients they don't want.

There is almost always an appropriate substitute for a particular problem ingredient—the secret lies in knowing what the substitute is and how to use it. I've created this cookbook so you can cook for those special occasions without wheat or gluten—and, also—without dairy, eggs, or refined sugar. You can also avoid corn or soy if you're careful to read ingredient labels.

Special Diet—Not Limited, Restrictive, or Alternative

You'll notice I don't refer to my diet as restricted, limited, or alternative. Instead, I refer to it as a "special" diet because it is tailored to suit my body and its needs. I'm very aware of the psychological aspects of adjusting to this diet. However, it is very important to refer to our diets with positive, rather than negative words. Our bodies hear what our brains are thinking, so I try to keep my thoughts and actions positive at all times. To me, "special" is a positive term.

And, I constantly remind myself to rejoice in what I *can* eat, rather than what I *can't* eat. I've learned to indulge my passion for food and still enjoy the dishes I ate before I had food sensitivities. Whenever I'm tempted, I say to myself— *Nothing tastes as good as feeling good feels.* All it takes is to imagine how I will feel if I eat the forbidden food, and that's enough to make me realize it isn't worth it.

Getting in Touch with Your Inner Chef

Some people love to cook. However, many others tell me they don't like to cook, don't have time to prepare meals, or feel inadequate in the kitchen. Despite the growing availability of mixes and ready-made foods, you will need to prepare some dishes yourself.

Yes, this usually requires preparing most dishes from scratch. But, as I remind my students in cooking classes—there are two major benefits when you cook from scratch: (1) you gain control over what you eat, and (2) you control the standards under which that food is prepared. And remember the psychological aspects—it's very rewarding to create a tasty dish that you, your family, and your guests enjoy.

Cooking Is Like Producing a Play

A creative way to think about meal preparation is to imagine the cook(s) as the producer(s) of a play. Your kitchen is the theater and the different dishes in the meal play different roles. For example, the entrée plays the main role, while the side dishes are the supporting roles. Desserts are the grand finale, breads are the rising stars, and so on. The audience is family or guests and the producer's job is to create a safe, healthy, delicious meal for them. When you do a good job, the audience is appreciative—just like in a play.

Inside each of us is the capacity to create healthy, nutritious meals for ourselves and our families. On those days when I resent the constant demand for three meals a day, I remind myself that I'm fortunate to be healthy. Eating nutritious food that is right for my body is the best way to maintain that health.

I hope you, your family, and your guests truly enjoy these dishes at your celebrations. Bon Appetit! Celebrate everything with food!

INTRODUCTION

How to Use This Book
This book is a resource for people on special diets. It is meant to help you eat the dishes you want—after your health professional tells you which ingredients to avoid. Specifically, this book is for people who *know* they must avoid wheat, gluten, dairy, eggs, and refined sugar.

This book should not be used to "self-diagnose" yourself or others, to determine whether you have a particular condition that warrants a special diet, or to determine the particular ingredients you should avoid. Let a health professional guide you in this process.

Can This Book Help You?
If you belong to any of the following groups of people, then the recipes in this book are appropriate for your diet:

(1) People who <u>must</u> avoid gluten in their diets. This includes persons with celiac disease (also known as celiac sprue, gluten intolerance, gluten sensitive enteropathy, and dermatitis herpetiformis). In addition, 5% of people with insulin-dependent (Type 1) diabetes have celiac disease, so the recipes include nutrient values and food exchanges for managing this particular diet.

(2) People who must avoid wheat and all wheat-related grains because of wheat allergies or intolerances or other special dietary considerations. For those with additional sensitivities, substitutes may be used for dairy, eggs, and sugar.

(3) Vegetarians and vegans who want baked goods without dairy and eggs.

Why People Must Avoid Certain Ingredients
Celiac Disease
Celiac disease (also called celiac sprue and related forms of gluten intolerance or gluten-sensitive enteropathy) is a genetically transmitted condition in which gluten (a protein in certain grains) destroys the small intestine's ability to absorb nutrients from food. Another form of the disease is dermatitis herpetiformis (DH) with symptoms of skin rashes and blisterlike spots. Some celiac associations believe about 1 in every 2,500-3,000 persons in the United States has celiac disease. However, that number may be just the tip of the iceberg because Great Britain, Ireland, and Northern Europe report a much higher incidence—1:300 in the general population. Currently, research is underway to determine if the U.S. incidence rates actually approach those of European countries.

Persons with celiac disease must avoid all forms of gluten, which is present in wheat and wheat-related grains such as barley, rye, spelt, oats and the lesser known grains of kamut and triticale. All recipes in this book avoid these grains by using gluten-free flours and by specifying gluten-free substitutes for other ingredients as well.

The recipes are designed so you can make them without gluten—plus instructions for omitting additional problem ingredients—dairy, eggs, or refined sugar— if necessary.

Celiac disease is a lifelong condition which requires strict adherence to a gluten-free diet. This condition must be managed with the help of a gastroenterologist, who performs a series of tests before a final diagnosis can be made.

A particularly useful resource for this group is the Cooperative Gluten-Free Commercial Products Listing published by the Celiac Sprue Association. This publication lists products and ingredients that are gluten-free. Many other national associations provide beneficial information as well. (See Associations in Appendix.)

Celiac Disease and Diabetes
Approximately 1 in every 20 (or 5%) of people with insulin-dependent (Type 1) diabetes also have celiac disease. And some celiacs have Type 2 diabetes. Both groups must avoid all forms of gluten—while monitoring the rest of their diets, as well.

How can celiacs with diabetes use this book? Each gluten-free recipe contains nutrient values and food exchanges for monitoring daily nutrient intake. (See Food Exchanges in Appendix.) Each recipe offers guidelines for using alternative sweeteners in place of refined sugar. Non-calorie sweeteners may be used where appropriate.

The combination of celiac disease and diabetes demands a very careful diet. Persons using these recipes are urged to work closely with a health professional to assure a balanced diet. See Appendix for associations that provide information on diabetes.

Food Allergies and Intolerances
Although there is not one official national statistic, food allergies are thought to affect anywhere from 1 to 5% of the general population. The Food Allergy Network says 1 to 2% of adults have true food allergies. Others estimate that nearly 50% of Americans suffer from food intolerances and sensitivities. Whether you are allergic (your reaction is usually sudden and more pronounced) or intolerant (your reaction may be delayed and more subtle), these recipes show you how to cook without the problem ingredients.

The ingredients most likely involved in allergies or intolerances include wheat, dairy, eggs, and refined sugar (although many other foods can cause problems). Some people avoid dairy products because they are allergic to milk proteins, while others are unable to digest the milk sugar, lactose. Some people are also bothered by corn or soy. Most recipes in this book contain substitutes that are soy and corn-free. But, you must read labels to avoid corn and soy. (See the Appendix for Hidden Sources of Corn and Soy.)

Diagnosis of a food allergy or intolerance should be made by a board-certified allergist or other health professional who specializes in this area. There are a variety of tests and procedures used to confirm a diagnosis; not all experts agree on a single approach. There are also many associations dedicated to helping people with these conditions. See the Appendix for a list of these associations.

Peanuts—A Special Type of Food Allergy

Allergy to peanuts is one of the most prevalent—and serious—food allergies. All recipes in this book avoid the use of peanuts, peanut oil, and peanut-containing ingredients. However, read all labels to make sure ingredients are peanut-free.

Vegetarians

Vegetarians do not eat meat, fish, and poultry. Vegans are vegetarians who abstain from eating all animal products, including eggs, milk, cheese, and other dairy items. If this is your lifestyle, you'll be pleased to know that most recipes in this book contain dairy-free and egg-free versions of baked goods. In addition, non-animal substitutes may be used such as a vegetable-based gelatin, instead of animal-based gelatin such as Knox brand.

Additives

A book on special diets isn't complete without mentioning food additives. All recipes in this book are intended to be as free of additives as possible because the recipes use mostly fresh, wholesome, unprocessed ingredients. However, you must carefully read labels to make sure the ingredients you choose are additive-free. In addition, choose organic ingredients, if possible.

Labels

Reading labels is very important when shopping for special diets. Learn to recognize the various names used for certain ingredients. For example, all-purpose flour, unbleached flour, semolina, and durum indicate the presence of wheat in prepared foods. Other words are used for eggs and dairy products, as well. See Appendix for a list of hidden sources of problem ingredients.

Also, *continue* to read labels on all ingredients—even the ones you've used for a long time. Manufacturers may change the contents of an ingredient—perhaps adding a substance. They may change the manner in which it was prepared, such as dusting the item with wheat flour to prevent sticking. Or the manufacturing process may introduce cross contamination with other problem ingredients. Call the manufacturer if you have concerns. Phrase your questions as clearly and concisely as possible and be sure to thank them for responding to your questions.

Nutritional Content and Food Exchanges

Managing a healthy diet is important to all of us, so nutrient values are offered as an aid to managing your nutritional intake. These values are based on the United States Department of Agriculture (USDA) guidelines and are only approximate. Exact nutrient values may vary according to serving sizes or brands used.

Also, some of these values are rounded according to the Food and Drug Administration (FDA) guidelines. For example, if there are fewer than 5 grams of fat, values are rounded to the nearest 1/2 gram. If there are more than 5 grams of fat, values are rounded to the nearest whole number. Carbohydrates and proteins are rounded to the nearest whole number. Calories are rounded to the nearest 5 calories.

Food Processor by ESHA is the software program used to calculate nutritional data and food exchanges. Exchange data for additional substitutions in each recipe are offered only if the exchanges are significantly altered by that substitution. Although these nutrient values and food exchanges tell you what is in each individual dish, it's wise to enlist the advice of a dietitian or nutritionist to assure your daily nutrient intake meets recommended levels. As with the nutrient data, food exchanges are only approximate and should be used as general guidelines. See Food Exchanges in the Appendix for additional information.

Serving Size

Serving sizes recommended by the American Diabetes Association are used in the calculation of nutrient values and food exchanges. Because we Americans are accustomed to eating very large portions, these serving sizes may seem quite small. In fact, the recommended serving size of meat equals the dimensions of an ordinary deck of playing cards. Bear in mind that it may take more than a single serving to fill you up so adjust your calculations accordingly. Make sure the diet guidelines outlined by your health care provider allow for any extra servings.

Why is Customizing Recipes Important?

Chances are, you've looked at cookbooks that either omit only a few of the ingredients you must avoid—or omit far more than you want to. This book is designed to help you customize dishes to exclude *only* the problem ingredients you and your family must avoid, while allowing you to leave in the ingredients you don't want to give up.

I often hear people in my cooking classes talk about having to prepare multiple versions of the same dish to suit their family's individual food concerns. This is not only time-consuming, but frustrating and inefficient—especially when one version can please everybody. In addition, when meal preparation becomes overwhelmingly difficult, it is tempting to stray from your recommended diet. This means that the symptoms you or your family wish to avoid will most likely return.

Here is some additional information about how these recipes allow you to customize dishes when one or more of the following is a problem ingredient.

Flour

Instead of wheat and gluten flours, the recipes in this book use a combination of flours —rice, bean, potato starch, and tapioca. Why these flours? This combination is safest for the largest number of people, the flours are least likely to compete with the flavors of the dish, and combinations of these flours produce the most pleasing results.

In place of rice flour, many recipes use garbfava flour (see Authentic Foods in Mail-Order Sources). It is made from a combination of garbanzo (chickpea) and fava (broad) beans. This flour is ideal for people who want to increase their protein intake, provided they're not allergic to or intolerant of legumes. The flour does not alter the dish's flavor, but does impart a slightly sweeter taste than rice flour. For people who are allergic to rice, this flour might be a welcome alternative. See Baking with Wheat-Free Flours in the Appendix for more information about this flour. (One caution: avoid this flour if you have a condition called glucose-6-phosphate dehydrogenase (G6PD) deficiency in which fava beans cause digestive problems.)

In place of potato starch, cornstarch can be substituted in a 1:1 ratio—provided you can eat corn. And 1 cup of tapioca flour can be replaced with 7/8 cup sweet rice flour. See Wheat-Flour Equivalents chart in the Appendix to customize your own recipes.

Some cooks prefer to use gluten-free flour mixes that they've mixed themselves or purchased pre-mixed. I prefer to tailor my flour combinations to produce the unique characteristics required in different baked goods. For example, cakes have a different texture from muffins and both are quite unlike pizza crust. Therefore, it makes sense to use different flour combinations for different types of dishes so you can better control the results. Also, persons with multiple food sensitivities often make substitutions for one or more components of a flour mix. Listing the ingredients separately allows them to customize the flours themselves.

Eggs

People avoid eggs for three main reasons: 1) allergies, 2) vegan diets, and 3) reducing cholesterol. Liquid egg substitutes (such as Egg-Beaters®) still contain eggs, so they're not appropriate for the allergic or vegan diet but they are low in cholesterol. Some *may* also contain wheat or cornstarch. Most of the baked goods in this book can be made without eggs. Just look for the words "without eggs" after the recipe name. Of course, using eggs produces a "lighter" baked item. See the Appendix for Baking with Egg Substitutes.

Dairy

People avoid dairy products for three reasons: 1) allergies, 2) lactose intolerance or 3) vegan diets. If lactose intolerance is your concern, you may use lactose-reduced milk in place of regular milk in these recipes. (Some celiacs cannot tolerate lactose-reduced products.) If, however, you are allergic to dairy products or just want to avoid all dairy products for personal reasons, there are suggestions for using milk substitutes made from rice, soy, or nut milk.

According to the Food Allergy Network newsletter (Vol. 5, #4, April-May, 1996), goat milk, goat yogurt, or goat cheeses are not recommended for those with milk allergies since the proteins are believed to be similar. Some people with lactose intolerance say they can tolerate goat products, but ask your physician about this. Be sure to read the label on these milk substitutes to make sure no other offending ingredients are present. For example, some "dairy-free" items contain casein, a milk protein that must be avoided by milk-allergic persons. And, celiacs should avoid oat milk.

There are also dairy-free yogurts and sour cream, but make sure they don't contain additional problem ingredients. See the Appendix for additional information on Baking with Dairy Substitutes and Hidden Sources of Dairy in prepared foods.

Refined Sugar

The recipes in this book are delicious—whether you use refined sugar (also known as white sugar or table sugar) or a sweetener appropriate for that particular dish. See Baking with Alternative Sweeteners in the Appendix for guidelines about using alternative sweeteners in place of refined sugar. Experts disagree about the degree of refinement in some alternative sweeteners. You may use your favorite non-calorie sweetener in dishes where it is appropriate, but you will need to experiment to find the right combinations.

Corn

Corn is one of those ingredients that mysteriously appears in ingredient lists on commercial products—often as a filler, emulsifier, or as a sweetener (as in corn syrup). If you read labels carefully, you can make most recipes in this book without corn and you can even make your own corn-free baking powder. (See chapter on Ingredients & Condiments.) See the Appendix for Hidden Sources of Corn.

Soy
There is considerable discussion these days about the health benefits of soy. Aside from those benefits, soy is used in this book for the beneficial properties it brings to cooking —namely, creaminess, moisture, and improved texture in baked goods. Many of the egg-free recipes in this book use soft silken tofu made from soy as a replacement for the binding qualities of eggs. Soy beverage can be used as a substitute for cow's milk. Some recipes use soy flour. However, many people must avoid soy for a variety of reasons. Check with your health professional about whether soy is appropriate for you. Read labels to see which products contain soy and see the Appendix for Hidden Sources of Soy.

Baking Without Conventional Ingredients
All conventional baked goods usually contain wheat, eggs, milk, sugar, and a leavening agent, and each ingredient plays a unique role in producing tasty, pleasingly textured results. What happens when we omit these ingredients? Let's take each separately.

Baking without wheat flour produces a somewhat heavier and denser product because the missing gluten can't establish a cell structure in which the leavening agent does its job. However, using xanthan gum helps alleviate this situation to the extent that many people can't distinguish between the same cake made with and without wheat flour.

Eliminating eggs has as dramatic an impact on baking as omitting wheat flour. In fact, eliminating wheat flour and eggs are the two biggest challenges to allergy-free baking. Eggs not only bind ingredients together and provide moisture, they are also leavening agents. This is the function we miss the most in baking. Several other ingredients can bind and moisturize a recipe, but eliminating eggs produces baked goods that are decidedly heavier and denser. For example, a cake that is light and airy when made *with* eggs becomes more like pound cake when made *without* eggs—but is still delicious!

Using milk substitutes is quite easy and usually has a minimal impact on the final product. In fact, most non-dairy milks can be used interchangeably with cow's milk in baking. Each type of milk has subtle taste differences and may produce slight color variations in the finished product (for example, soy milk may darken the product during baking). Decide which type of milk you prefer and stick with it. Be sure it doesn't contain problem ingredients such as casein (a milk protein) or barley malt extract (which is wheat-related).

Baking without refined sugar is uniquely challenging because the sugar substitutes can be solids or liquids and they change the chemical balance in a recipe. Also, the various sugar alternatives produce unique taste sensations and somewhat different color hues. Finally, some sugar alternatives produce decidedly less sweetness. But all sweeteners produce delicious results.

So, what does all this mean? Cooking without conventional ingredients is not harder —it's just slightly different. While there are a few more ingredients in each recipe, these ingredients are essential and require only a few more seconds of measuring. Also, certain ingredients cost somewhat more than conventional versions—a small price to pay for being able to resume eating your favorite dishes and maintaining a healthy diet.

Principles of Cooking without Wheat Or Gluten
Although cooking without conventional baking ingredients requires unique cooking techniques, omitting wheat and gluten present special challenges. Here are some guidelines for successful baking which have been incorporated into each recipe:

- Substitute rice, bean, potato starch, milo, and tapioca flours for wheat flour

- Mixture of flours (2-3) works better than single flour

- Extra ingredients such as xanthan gum, soy lecithin, and gelatin as well as different preparation techniques restore texture and appearance

- More leavening helps raise the dough and more flavorings restore flavor

- Dough is softer, moister, and stickier than traditional dough so bread machines and heavy-duty electric mixers are efficient aids for handling the dough

In addition to these guidelines, I find it useful to sift the ingredients *after* measuring to remove unmilled grains or foreign particles. To measure dry ingredients, use dry measuring cups or spoons and level the top off with a straight-edged knife. Don't pack the flour into the cup or spoon. Use liquid measuring cups for liquids. And, use standardized measuring cups and spoons from a reputable manufacturer for consistent results.

Tips For Altitude Adjustments
These recipes were developed at 5,000 feet altitude, but are not necessarily altitude-sensitive. If you're baking above 7,500 feet, no changes are usually required. At sea level, you *may* need to adjust recipes using these guidelines. It's best to follow the recipe the first time, then make adjustments (if necessary) next time.

- Increase baking powder or baking soda by 1/4 to 1/2. (If using acidic
- ingredients such as sour milk or buttermilk, no adjustments are needed.)
- Increase rising times for yeast breads by 30 minutes
- Increase each cup of sugar by 2-3 tablespoons
- Decrease liquid by 3-4 tablespoons per cup of liquid
- Decrease oven temperature by 25 degrees

Source: Colorado State University Cooperative Extension Bulletin 530A, 1985, and my personal baking experiences with wheat-free flours.

How to Read and Use These Recipes
In order to conserve space, some abbreviations are used throughout the book. The letters "gf" precede all ingredients that should be selected on the basis of their gluten-free status. The letters "df" precede all ingredients that should be selected on the basis of their dairy-free status. For example, chocolate chips are preceded by "gf/df" to indicate that chocolate chips without gluten or dairy should be used (if you have those sensitivities). The term oleo is used rather than margarine simply to conserve space.

Each recipe uses wheat-free, gluten-free flours. If wheat or gluten are your only sensitivities, follow the recipe using the dairy products, eggs, and sugar—as listed.

If, however, you must cook with substitutes for dairy . . . or eggs . . . or sugar—or all three—then use the substitute suggested. This substitute will either be printed on the same line as the original ingredient or noted with an asterisk and explained at the bottom of the page. Let's use the following example to clarify.

1 cup brown rice flour	1 cup milk (cow, rice, soy, nut)
2 eggs or 1/2 cup soft silken tofu	1 cup brown sugar or maple sugar

Someone with wheat or gluten-sensitivities only will make the recipe as listed, with no substitutes for the eggs, milk, or brown sugar. Another person—perhaps a wheat-sensitive person who also has dairy allergies will choose rice, soy, or nut milk—but use the eggs or brown sugar. A third person—perhaps with sensitivities to wheat, eggs, milk, and sugar—will use the tofu, perhaps soy milk, and the maple sugar. The directions explain what to do with the substitute ingredient(s).

Read through the recipe entirely before proceeding to make sure you know which substitutes, if any, you'll use. In order to know which ingredients are appropriate for your diet, be sure to read the Glossary, beginning on the next page. The Appendix provides additional information.

GLOSSARY OF INGREDIENTS

Read this section carefully before using this cookbook so you know what the ingredient is, what it looks like, and where to find it. No endorsement of products is intended, but certain brands are mentioned to help you find the ingredient. This information pertains to the United States only since brands and manufacturing processes vary by country.

Read labels carefully to make sure you know what you're eating. Continue to read labels since manufacturers can change the ingredients and the processes under which the ingredient is handled. And remember . . . *if in doubt about any ingredient, leave it out!*

Agave Nectar: Honey-like liquid from agave plant; 90% fructose. Brand name is Cucamonga. Found in baking aisle of natural food store.

Ascorbic Acid: Also called Vitamin C crystals or powder. Choose unbuffered version for maximum boost of leavening in baked goods. Found near supplements in natural food stores. (See **Vitamin C** in this section.)

Applesauce: Sold in supermarkets and natural food stores. Also available as baby food, but choose those (e.g., Gerber First) without extra fillers such as rice or tapioca. Organic versions are usually darker in color and will cause baked goods to be some-what darker. Used as binder and sweetener. (See Applesauce recipe on page 210.)

Arrowroot: Flour made from a West Indies root. Excellent thickener for fruit sauces or other sauces that do not require high heat. Adds glossy sheen to foods, making them appear to contain more fat than they actually do. Found in natural food stores.

Baking Powder: Ener-G® makes a gluten-free version. See page 211 for a recipe to make your own corn-free, gluten-free version.

Brown Rice Syrup: A syrup made from brown rice. Be sure to use Lundberg's gluten-free version. Found in baking aisle of natural food store.

Brown Sugar: Generally made from cane sugar, this is white refined sugar to which a little molasses has been added. Found in baking aisle of grocery or natural food stores.

Butter: If cow's milk butter is unsuitable, use oleo. Or use canola oil spread (Spectrum™), vegetable shortening, or same amount (may need to reduce by 1 tablespoon) of your favorite cooking oil. (See also **Canola Oil Spread, Oleo,** and **Oil** below.) If you're using butter, be sure to use unsalted butter.

Butter Flavored Salt or Sprinkles: Durkee makes a gluten-free version and Butter Buds are gluten-free, but both may contain dairy. Found in baking section. Butter-flavored (gluten-free) extracts may be used instead (see Mail-Order Sources).

Cane Sugar: Found in two forms: 1) white sugar which is highly refined, and 2) unbleached cane sugar which has more nutrients. Find unbleached cane sugar in baking aisle of natural food stores. See **Sucanat®**, which is also cane sugar. Or, use beet sugar instead of cane sugar.

Canola Oil: One of the most heart-healthy oils, it has a very low smoking point which means it won't cause baked goods to brown too quickly. Some celiacs *may* react to canola oil, which is made from the rape seed. You may substitute other oils, such as safflower or corn—or your favorite vegetable oil. Found in the baking aisle.

Canola Oil Spread: Sold under the brand name Spectrum™ from Spectrum Naturals, this 100% canola oil spread looks and tastes like butter with the consistency of mayonnaise. Non-hydrogenated, it bakes quite well but does not melt or blend into sauces cooked on the stovetop. Its fat is mostly mono-unsaturated, so it is a healthy substitute for vegetable shortening, oleo (margarine), or butter—which you may use instead. Contains soy protein. Found in refrigerated section near the butter in natural food stores and some supermarkets.

Cheese: See **Parmesan Cheese** below and also see Baking with Dairy Substitutes in Appendix for more information on related dairy products.

Chipotle Chiles: Dried jalapeno peppers. Found on Mexican shelf in supermarket or from The Chile Shop, 109 E. Water St., Santa Fe, NM, 87501.

Chocolate and Chocolate Chips: "Dairy-free" chocolate chips and bars are available in natural food stores, but may actually be processed on dairy equipment. Carob chips may be used instead of chocolate chips, but they may be sweetened with barley malt.

Cocoa Powder: Use unsweetened cocoa powder (Ghirardelli is a good brand). Carob powder may be substituted, but with significant loss of flavor and color.

Coffee Powder: Taster's Choice® makes a gluten-free instant coffee powder. Espresso powder (Medaglia D'Oro) may be used instead of coffee powder for fuller flavor.

Cooking Spray: Read labels carefully to select a spray that doesn't contain problem ingredients (such as wheat flour or soy). There are non-aerosol versions as well. Or, put your favorite oil in a non-aerosol pump-spray bottle, available at kitchen stores. Vegetable shortening or oil may be used to coat baking pans instead of cooking spray.

Cornstarch: Made from corn, this white powder is the same ingredient used to thicken sauces and puddings. Can be used as a flour in wheat-free cooking, but it is not the same as corn flour (which is yellow and has a heavier texture). Found in baking aisle of super-markets and natural food stores. See Wheat-Free Flours in Appendix.

Dried Cane Juice: Choose organic version. See **Sucanat®**.

Dry Milk Powder: A white milk powder that adds sugar and protein in baked goods. Found in natural food stores near flours or in baking section. Carnation® instant milk is not the same because it is granular and doesn't measure the same as dry milk powder. Use twice as much of the granules if that's all you have. Non-dairy versions available, but make sure they're casein-free if you're allergic to milk. See Baking with Dairy Substitutes in Appendix.

Eggs: Be sure to use large eggs. Egg whites may be used in place of whole eggs. Liquid egg substitutes may be used if they do not contain problem ingredients.

Egg Replacer: White powder made of various starches and a little leavening. May be used in addition to eggs in certain recipes or in place of eggs in others. Helps stabilize baked goods. Packaged in Ener-G® box and found in baking aisle of natural food store. See Baking with Egg Substitutes in Appendix.

Extracts or Flavorings: Flavorings restore flavor to baked goods when certain ingredients are omitted. Look for gluten-free brands including Frontier® (bottles labeled alcohol-free), or Spicery Shoppe available in natural food stores or Bickford Laboratories, available through mail-order. (See Mail-Order Sources in Appendix.)

Flaxseed or Flaxseed Meal: Seeds or meal (partially ground seeds) which can be used as egg substitute in certain recipes. Found in natural food stores. See Baking with Egg Substitutes in Appendix.

FOS: (Fructooligosaccharides). White, low-caloric powdered sweetener derived from fruit and vegetable carbohydrates. Found in supplement section of natural food stores. See Baking with Alternative Sweeteners in Appendix.

Fruit Juice Concentrate (frozen): Found in frozen food section. Look for pure fruit juices, where possible.

Garlic Powder or Garlic Salt: Look for gluten-free versions. Or use fresh garlic instead.

Gelatin Powder: Available in regular version (common brand name is Knox®) or kosher, which is made from vegetable sources. Adds moisture and helps bind ingredients together. Found in baking aisle of supermarkets and natural food stores. Kosher versions are at some natural food stores and may be marked "pareve". Or, use agar powder (not flakes), a vegetarian gelatin from seaweed. Found in natural food stores.

Granulated Fruit Sweetener (brand name Fruit Source™): Peach-colored granules. Made from dehydrated fruit juices and rice syrup (which is usually off-limits for celiacs). However, according to the manufacturer, FruitSource™ brand is gluten-free. Found in baking aisle of natural food stores.

Guar Gum: Plant-derived gum used to provide structure to baked goods so leavening can do its job. Also gives creamy texture to ice cream. Contains fiber so could be irritating to sensitive intestines. Can be used in place of xanthan gum, but use half again as much guar gum. Found in baking aisle or near bulk herbs of natural food stores.

Honey: Probably one of the most common substitutes for refined sugar in baking. Different varieties are available, each imparting a distinctive flavor and color to baked goods. Avoid giving honey to children under age 2 because of possible botulism. For safety, avoid unrefined honey.

Italian (Herb) Seasoning: A blend of spices and herbs, found in the spice section of all grocery stores and natural food stores. Choose gluten-free or make your own (page 221).

Jowar Flour: Made from sorghum (milo) plant. Available from Jowar Foods (See Mail-Order Sources in Appendix).

Ketchup: May contain distilled vinegar, which may be grain-based. Del Monte®, Heinz®, and Muir Glen® claim to be gluten-free. You can make your own using the recipe on page 218 or try the Apricot Ketchup on page 216.

Lecithin Granules or Liquid: Made from soy, lecithin emulsifies, stabilizes and texturizes baked goods (especially bread). Granular and liquid versions found in the supplement section of natural food stores (sometimes in the refrigerated sections.) Usually light or beige-yellow in color, the limited amount required (about 1/4 tea-spoon) does not change the flavor or appearance of the dish, but does enhance the texture and makes the dish seem to have more fat. Buy only pure soy lecithin.

Lemon Peel (Rind): Outermost portion of lemon. Adds flavor to baked goods. Use potato peeler to remove outermost peel from lemon, avoiding white pith. Chop with sharp knife or pulverize in small coffee grinder (reserved for spices) to desired con-sistency. Or, use zester or grater to remove peel from lemon. Use organic produce to avoid pesticides.

Maple Sugar: Maple syrup that has been dried into crystals. May lend a slight maple taste to baked goods. Available at natural food stores in baking aisle.

Maple Syrup: Made from maple tree sap and available at supermarkets and natural food stores. Most flavorful version for baking is Grade B, which is often sold in bulk in natural food stores. Choose organic maple syrup to avoid formaldehyde.

Milk: People with dairy allergies or lactose-intolerance should use alternatives such as rice, soy, or nut milk (called beverages). Choose casein-free substitutes if you're allergic to dairy or lactose-free products if you're lactose-intolerant. The Food Allergy Network newsletter (Vol. 5, #4, April-May, 1996) does not recommend goat's milk if you are truly dairy-allergic. Lactose-intolerant people often use goat's milk, but there is concern about this as well. Check with your physician.

Celiacs should avoid milk substitutes with barley malt or modified food starch, unless the starch source is known to be safe. Read labels to choose the milk appropriate for your condition. You may replace the milk with juice or water, but the flavor and texture of the baked item may be affected slightly since many recipes depend on the protein in milk. Choose low-sugar milks for savory dishes. See Baking with Dairy Substitutes in Appendix.

Molasses: Made from cane sugar and often used as a sweetener in baking. Use regular (unsulphured) molasses, not blackstrap molasses. Arrowhead Mills makes a sorghum-based pure syrup that can be used instead of cane molasses. Found in natural food stores.

Mustard: For dry mustard, use gluten-free brands or grind mustard seeds to a fine powder with coffee grinder. Dijonnaise (which is gluten-free) can be substituted for Dijon mustard.

Oil: Choose 100% pure oil. The heart-healthiest for baking are canola, safflower, and corn oil—and they work well in baked desserts because they're less likely to burn. Read labels to choose one best for you. See Cooking Oils in the Appendix.

Oleo: Also called oleo-margarine or margarine. An alternative for those who can't use dairy products, vegetable shortening, or other oils in baking. Make sure oleo is gluten-free (and dairy-free, if necessary) and suitable for baking (soft versions have too much water.)

Onion Powder, Onion Salt, and Minced Onion: Sold in baking section, along with liquid onion. Look for gluten-free versions or use freshly grated onion, instead.

Parmesan Cheese: Often from cow's milk, but may be made from goat or sheep's milk (check with your physician—milk-allergic and certain lactose-intolerant persons should avoid). Found in the refrigerated sections of natural food stores. Soyco® makes a brown rice version that contains casein (a milk protein) and another made of soy, labeled 100% dairy free and casein-free, and it contains texturized soy vegetable protein (TVP). Store on pantry shelf until opened, then refrigerate.

Potato Starch: Also called potato starch flour. Fine, white powder made from the starch of potatoes. Adds light, airy texture to baked goods. Found in flour section of natural food stores. Don't confuse with the heavy, dense potato flour made from potatoes and their skins.

Prune baby food: Prune baby food is the simplest way to use prunes as a replacement for some of the fat in baked goods or as a binder in place of eggs. Choose brands such as Gerber 1st® that have prunes only, without additional fillers or thickeners. Puréed prunes are also in the baking aisle of supermarkets or natural food stores. See the Appendix for suggestions on baking with prune puree as an alternative sweetener or binder. (Also see **Puréed Fruit** below.)

Puréed Fruit: Several fruits work nicely to help bind ingredients, add sweetness and moisture, and replace fat. Puréed pears impart little flavor or color. Puréed apples (applesauce or apple butter) impart a slight apple flavor, especially if the apple butter is spiced. The darker color and flavor of puréed prunes or dates make them useful only in darker, more strongly flavored dishes such as spice cakes or chocolate items.

Rice Bran: This is the outside layer of the rice kernel which is removed to make brown rice. Contains the bran and part of the rice germ. Found in natural food stores by Ener-G®, near the flours or in the baking aisle. Adds fiber to baked goods. Refrigerate after opening.

Rice Flakes: Also called rolled rice or rolled rice flakes. Similar to rice cereal, but with a larger grain that looks more like oatmeal. Found in natural food stores, often in bulk.

Rice Flour: Most common flour used in wheat and gluten-free baking. White rice flour is the rice kernel stripped of most of its nutrients. Brown rice flour contains more layers of the rice kernel—and more nutrients. Store brown rice flour in the refrigerator or freezer to extend shelf life and avoid rancidity. Found in the baking aisle or bulk sections of natural food stores and some supermarkets. See Wheat-Free Flours in Appendix.

Rice Milk: (Also called rice beverage.) Made from rice, this milk is an effective substitute for cow's milk. Available at natural food stores or supermarkets in liquid or powdered form (which must be reconstituted with water before using). Refrigerate liquid version after opening or reconstituting. Choose enriched or fortified versions. Celiacs must avoid those with barley-based brown rice syrup or malted cereal extract (which may contain barley). See Baking with Dairy Substitutes in Appendix.

Rice Polish: Portion of brown rice kernel removed in the process of making white rice. Contains part of the rice germ and bran—high in fiber. Refrigerate after opening. Found in Ener-G® box in the baking aisles of natural food stores.

Rolled Rice: See **Rice Flakes**.

Safflower Oil: Made from the safflower plant, this oil works well in baking or sautéing because of its relatively high smoke point (it won't burn as quickly). Found in baking aisle of supermarkets and natural food stores.

Salt: Use your favorite salt, but check the fillers that make them free-flowing. I prefer sea salt because it has no fillers—but it is more expensive. You may reduce salt in recipes to suit your individual taste and dietary needs, but overall flavor is affected.

Sour Cream Alternative: Made from soy and performs like real sour cream. Found in dairy section of natural food stores. Some brands contain casein or other ingredients that may be problematic, so read labels carefully.

Soy Flour: Derived from soy beans, this yellowish-tan flour is found in regular and lower-fat form—usually in the flour section of natural food stores. Refrigerate to avoid rancidity due to fat content. Works best in baked goods with fruit such as carrot cakes. Persons who are allergic to legumes should avoid this flour. See Wheat-Free Flours in Appendix.

Soy Margarine or Oleo: Available at natural food stores. Contains partially hydro-genated soybean oil and must be refrigerated. Legume-allergic persons should avoid. Soy margarine may be used in place of vegetable shortening, butter, or canola oil spread in baking.

Soy Milk: (Also called soy beverage.) Available at natural food stores or super-markets in liquid or powdered form (which must be reconstituted with water before using and is somewhat lighter in color). Liquid form must be refrigerated after open-ing or reconstituting. Read labels to avoid problem ingredients. See Baking with Dairy Substitutes in Appendix for guidelines on using soy milk to replace cow's milk.

Soy Sauce: Look for wheat-free tamari versions. May use Bragg's Amino Acids, which is non-fermented soy sauce without wheat and yeast.

Stevia: A sweet-leafed herb from Paraguay. Sold in powder (green or white), liquid, or leaf form. Slight licorice-like flavor that is perceptible in bland foods, but less noticeable in more strongly flavored dishes such as spice cakes.

Sucanat®: Dried cane juice with water removed. Coarse amber granules impart a mild molasses taste. Available in natural food stores in pre-packaged form in the baking aisle or in bulk form. See Baking with Alternative Sweeteners in Appendix for more information.

Sugar: Bleached or unbleached cane sugar may be used. Beet sugar may also be used. See Baking with Alternative Sweeteners in the Appendix.

Sun-Dried Tomatoes: Dehydrated tomatoes which are packaged dry or packed in oil. Choose the dry packaged version if the source of the oil is uncertain or inappropriate. Or, make your own using the recipe on page 214.

Sweet Rice Flour: Derived from short grain rice, this white powder produces baked goods that are more moist and firm than if "long-grain" rice flour is used. Sometimes called "sticky" or "glutinous" rice, it *does not* contain wheat gluten. Sold in boxes by Ener-G® in baking aisle or near flours in natural food stores. See Wheat-Free Flours in Appendix.

Tapioca Flour: Made from the cassava plant, this is a fine, white flour that adds chewiness and elasticity to baked goods. Sold in natural food stores in packages or bulk form. See Wheat-Free Flours in Appendix.

Tofu: Be sure to use the soft silken version (made by Mori-Nu®) in baked goods (unless otherwise specified). Store the aseptic (shelf-stable) packages on pantry shelf until opened. Then refrigerate in closed container and use within two days. Found in natural food stores in refrigerated section or in displays near the baking aisle.

Tomato Paste and Tomato Sauce: Use gluten-free versions of both. However, tomato sauce may contain corn syrup. Make your own (see page 216).

Vanilla Extract: Many brands contain alcohol (which may be wheat or gluten-based). Look for those that are alcohol-free, e.g., Frontier®. See **Extracts or Flavorings** in this chapter. See Mail Order Sources in Appendix.

Vanilla Powder: Derived from vanilla beans, this white powder may also have sugar added. Powdered vanilla bean is dark brown in color. Both are available by mail order from companies that sell flavorings and extracts. Powders may be used interchangeably with liquid vanilla extract, but may need to add a teaspoon of water to restore moisture to the batter or dough. See Mail Order Sources in Appendix.

Vinegar: Be sure to use cider or wine vinegar, which are wheat and gluten-free. Distilled vinegar may be grain-based. Make sure the cider vinegar is not just distilled vinegar with apple flavoring. Use Ener-G® yeast-free/gluten-free vinegar if yeast and fermentation are problems. This powder must be reconstituted with water before using and then refrigerated. Made from acetic acid and maltodextrin from corn.

Vitamin C Crystals or Powder: Derived from the fermentation of corn, this powder adds acid to yeast dough and strengthens the protein structure. Also acts as acid leavening component in quick breads which are baked in the oven, not in a bread machine. Sold in supplement sections of natural food stores. Make sure label says wheat and gluten-free. Choose unbuffered Vitamin C or it will not add acid to the bread.

Vegetable Oil: The best oils for baking are canola, safflower, and sunflower oil due to their higher smoking points, which means they won't burn as quickly (see page 248). Canola oil is one of the more heart-healthy oils, but you may use your favorite oil. Avoid using olive oil in baking unless specified in the recipe. Most oils are found in baking aisle of supermarkets and natural food stores.

Yeast: Choose gluten-free yeast such as Red Star® or SAF®. In this book, dry yeast is the term used to indicate regular yeast.

Yogurt: If you can use cow's milk, look for yogurts with no tapioca or modified food starch and that have good acidophilus content. Look for lactose-reduced yogurt. Milk-allergic people should not use goat's milk yogurt, but many lactose-intolerant people seem to do fine with it. Check with your physician about whether goat products are appropriate for you. Soy yogurt does not work in baking. See Baking with Dairy Substitutes in Appendix.

Xanthan gum: Derived from bacteria in corn sugar, this gum lends structure and texture to baked goods and thickens sauces. Probably the most indispensable ingredient when baking without wheat or gluten. Found in the baking aisle or near flours in natural food stores. Seems expensive, but lasts a long time since only a tiny amount is used in recipes.

Water: Some cooks insist that using filtered water instead of tap water produces a sweeter, fuller flavor in baked goods. Feel free to use the water of your choice.

Celebration Menus

These menus are designed to help you plan and execute the perfect special occasion. Each menu contains a main dish, side dish(es), bread, dessert, and suggested beverages. And each menu is designed to provide a balance of flavor, color, texture, and overall appearance so that the food you serve will look and taste wonderful.

For each menu, page numbers are listed beside the dish to show you where the recipe is located in this book. No page number means the dish does not require a recipe.

Afternoon Tea

Miniature Focaccia Sandwiches • 193
with
Focaccia Fillings • 194

Scones with Citrus Butter • 79

Ginger Pound Cake with
Cardamom Glaze • 109

Assorted Teas

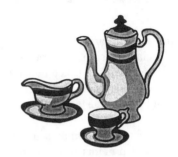

Brewing Tea: Start with a kettle of fresh water. Bring the water to a boil. While the water is heating, warm the teapot by pouring some hot water into it and let it stand for about 1 minute. Then pour the water out and dry the pot. (Heating the pot ensures that the water you boil will remain at the appropriate temperature to brew the tea leaves properly.)

In the teapot, place 1 heaping teaspoon of loose tea leaves per cup (plus one for the pot). Let leaves steep for 3 to 5 minutes. Stir once, allow the leaves to resettle, and then pour the tea through a strainer into the cups.

What kind of tea should you serve? Why, your favorite of course. Some people prefer Earl Grey (sweet, citrusy with bergamot), Darjeeling (fine, delicate), and Ceylon (pale, malty). But you could use Orange Pekoe and Pekoe (the old standby) or your favorite herbal tea—or perhaps green tea. Whatever you like! And, if you choose to serve iced tea, then follow your palate's desire.

Anniversary Dinner for Two

Salmon in Parchment • 40

Brown Rice Pilaf • 174

Steamed Asparagus

Mixed Greens with Basic Vinaigrette • 164

Heart Cake
with Chocolate Covered Strawberries • 110

Coffee & Tea

Anniversary Buffet Dinner

Chicken Breasts with Mango Chutney • 22
Pork Tenderloins with Ginger Sauce • 36
Lamb Chops with Rosemary Marinade • 46

Cooked White Long-Grain Rice

Mixed Greens with Basic Vinaigrette • 164

Italian Breadsticks • 63

Steamed Broccoli, Baby Carrots, &
Asparagus

Wedding Cake • 113-119

Birthday Cakes

Butterfly Cake • 121

Candle Cake • 123

Down on the Farm Cake • 127

Halloween Spider Web Cake • 128

Indy 500 Race Track Cake • 131

How Old Are You? Cake • 129

Choice of Frostings • 136-140

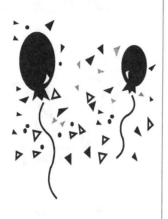

Bridal Shower Luncheon

Walnut Shrimp Salad • 46
or
Pasta Salad • 52

Italian Breadsticks • 63

Steamed Asparagus Spears

Chocolate Dipped, Filled Strawberries • 144

Coffee Tea, & Assorted Fruit Juices

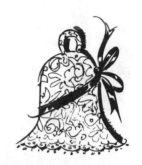

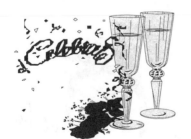

Bridal Shower Brunch

Breakfast Fruit Pizza • 83

Breakfast Sausage • 90

Brown Rice Pilaf • 174

Fruit Bowl

Lemon Poppy Seed Raspberry Cake • 85

Coffee, Tea, & Assorted Fruit Juices

Chinese Take-Out

Chinese Hot-Sour Soup • 56

Pork Fried Rice • 34

Sweet-and-Sour Pork • 38

Pad Thai • 51

Cantaloupe with Cinnamon • 142

Tea

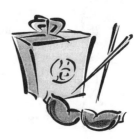

CHINESE

Cinco de Mayo

Green Chile Stew • 57

Cornbread with Green Chiles • 67

Tomatillo Rice • 178

*Platter of Fresh Vegetables
with
Avocado Bean Salsa • 197*

Mexican Chocolate Cake • 100

Coffee or Tea

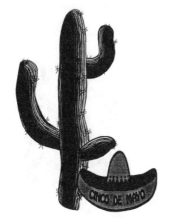

Congratulatory Dinner

Paella • 42

Mixed Greens with Basic Vinaigrette • 164

*Italian Breadsticks • 63
or
French Bread • 62*

Chocolate Mocha Fudge Trifle • 145

Coffee or Tea

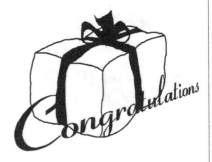

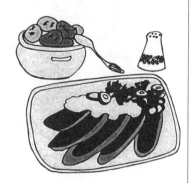

Small, Intimate Dinner Party

Oven-Baked Crab Cakes • 196

Potatoes Anna • 188

Caesar Salad without Eggs • 166

French Bread • 62

Steamed Broccoli

Chocolate Macaroon Tunnel Cake • 107

Coffee & Tea

Contemporary Dinner Party

Cornish Game Hens with Fruit Glaze • 20

Potatoes Anna • 188

French Bread • 62

Lettuce Salad, Pears & Feta Cheese • 169

Steamed Green Peas

Double Chocolate Cherry Torte • 108

Coffee & Tea

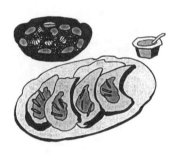

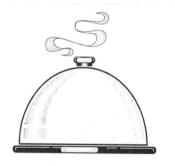

Elegant Dinner Party

Pork Medallions with Cherry Sauce • 35

Brown Rice Pilaf • 174

Spinach Salad with Strawberries • 170

Steamed Vegetables

Baked Alaska • 141 or Frozen Tiramisu • 147

Coffee & Tea

Comfort-Food Dinner Party

Chicken Earl Grey • 21

Garlic Mashed Potatoes • 186

French Bread • 62

Roasted Asparagus • 181

Cherry Cobbler • 143

Coffee & Tea

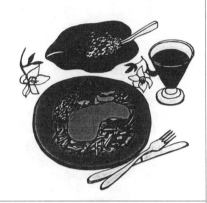

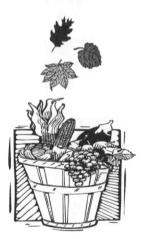

Fall Dinner

Pork Chops with Apple-Dijon Sauce • 33

Roasted Potatoes • 187

French Bread • 62

Mixed Greens with Basic Vinaigrette • 164

Sautéed Brussels Sprouts • 184

Applesauce Spice Cake • 97

Coffee & Tea

Father's Day

Grilled Pork, Orange-Rosemary Sauce • 32

Garlic Mashed Potatoes • 186

Waldorf Salad • 170

Corn-on-the-Cob
or
Steamed Green Peas

Rocky Road Brownies • 156

Coffee & Tea

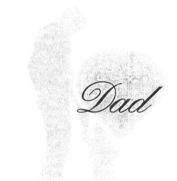

HAPPY DAD'S DAY

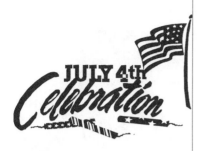

Fireworks on the Fourth

Barbecued Chicken • 20

Roasted (Grilled) Vegetables • 182

Garlic French Bread • 62

Chocolate Ice Cream Sandwiches • 153
Rocky Road Brownies • 156

Coffee, Tea, & Assorted Cold Beverages

Aprés Golf Party

Barbecued Ribs
with 19th Hole Barbecue Sauce • 31

Cabbage Coleslaw • 174

Potato Salad • 169

Fruit-Sweetened Gelatin Salad • 171

Garlic French Bread • 62

Double Chocolate Cherry Torte • 108

Coffee, Tea, & Assorted Cold Beverages

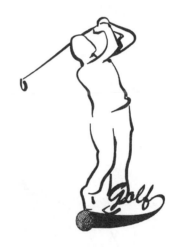

Fireside Candlelight Dinner

Coq Au Vin • 27

Pasta (Homemade Egg Pasta) • 176

Roasted Fennel • 181

Italian Breadsticks • 63

Mixed Greens with Basic Vinaigrette • 164

Chocolate Cherry Cake • 106

Coffee & Tea

Graduation Day

Tuna Burgers (or Hamburgers)
With Grilled Pineapple Slices • 45

Roasted Potatoes • 187

Fruit-Sweetened Gelatin Salad • 171

Italian Breadsticks • 63

Celebration Cookies • 152
Chocolate Cappuccino Ice Cream • 158

Coffee, Tea, & Assorted Cold Beverages

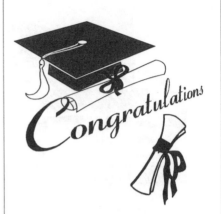

Halloween

Cakes
Basic Cake • 98-99

Basic Chocolate Cake • 100-101

Halloween Spider Web Cake • 128

Cookies, Bars, Muffins, Etc.
Bug Cookies • 150

Colorado Chocolate Chip Cookies • 154

Cookie Monsters • 150

Flower Pot Treats • 146

Granola Bars • 93

Pumpkin Muffins • 75

Snake Cookies • 150

Basic (Cut-Out) Cookies • 157

Beverages • 204-207

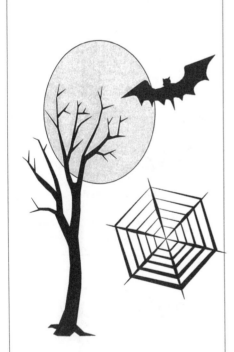

Mardi Gras

Bayou Red Beans & Rice • 37

Cornbread with Green Chiles • 67

*Platter of Fresh, Bite-Size Vegetables with
Chutney Appetizer Spread • 198*

*Pecan Nut Torte with Chocolate Ganache •
112*

Coffee (Chicory) & Tea

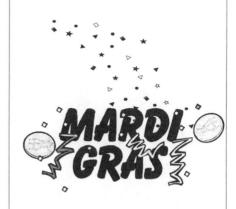

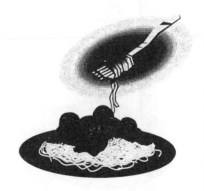

Mother's Day Breakfast

Blueberry Muffins with Lemon Curd• 72-73
or
Scones • 79-81
or
Gourmet Granola • 92

Fresh Fruit

Coffee, Tea, & Fruit Juice

O Sole Mio Supper

Spaghetti Sauce & Meatballs • 50

*Mixed Greens
with Tomato-Basil Vinaigrette • 165*

Roasted Fennel (on salad)• 181

Italian Breadsticks • 63

Frozen Tiramisu • 147

Coffee & Tea

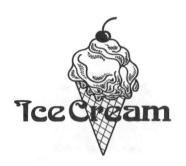

Ice Cream Social

Chocolate Sorbet • 158

Raspberry Sherbet • 160

Strawberry Sherbet • 160

Vanilla Ice Cream or Frozen Yogurt • 161

Cookies of Choice • 151-157

Caramel Sauce • 134
Chocolate Syrup • 136

Pasta Party

Fresh Tomato Basil Sauce with Pasta • 50

Spicy Fettuccini with Basil • 54

Spicy Shrimp & Pasta • 44

Mixed Greens
with Tomato-Basil Vinaigrette • 165

Focaccia • 61

Chocolate Mocha Fudge Trifle • 145

Coffee & Tea

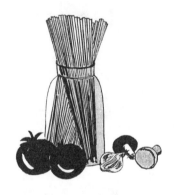

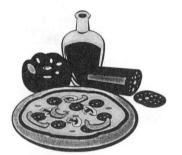

Pizza with Panache

Pizza with Pizza Sauce • 53
Toppings: Sausage • 47
Pineapple & Ham or Vegetarian

Mixed Greens with Basic Vinaigrette • 164

Chocolate Cherry Cookies • 152

Coffee & Tea

Portable Feasts
(Picnic, Tailgate Party)

Barbecued Chicken • 20

❧

Couscous Salad • 174
Potato Salad • 169
Jicama & Mandarin Orange Salad • 168
Fruit Salad with Balsamic Vinegar • 167

❧

Focaccia • 61

❧

Celebration Cookies • 152

❧

Coffee, Tea, & Assorted Cold Beverages

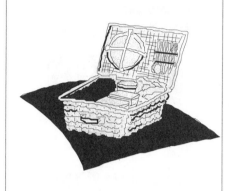

Rites of Spring Dinner

Lamb Chops with Rosemary Marinade • 46

❧

New Potatoes & Peas with Lemon & Dill • 187

❧

French Bread • 62

❧

Strawberries & Kiwi in Orange Juice

❧

Lemon Sorbet • 159
Basic (Cut-Out) Cookies • 157

❧

Coffee & Tea

Spring Luncheon

Asparagus Soup • 55

❧

Spinach Salad with Strawberries • 170

❧

Scones with Ham • 78

❧

Strawberry Sherbet • 160
"Oatmeal" Cookies • 155

❧

Coffee & Tea

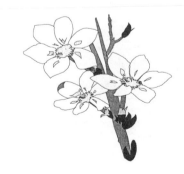

Hot Summer Days

Pasta Salad • 52

French Bread • 62
or
Italian Breadsticks • 63

Raspberry Sherbet • 160
Chocolate Cherry Cookies • 152

Assorted Cold Beverages

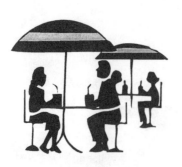

Hot Summer Nights

Grilled Chicken
with Mango/Black Bean Salsa • 23

Jicama & Mandarin Orange Salad • 168

Italian Breadsticks • 63

Roasted Potatoes • 187

Steamed Green Beans or
Corn on the Cob

Peach Melba Ice Cream Pie • 149

Assorted Cold Beverages

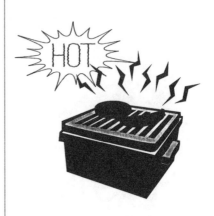

Sunday Dinner

Baked Ham • 30

Duchesse Potatoes • 185

French Bread • 62

Minted Peas

Fruit-Sweetened Gelatin Salad • 171

Chocolate Macaroon Tunnel Cake • 107

Coffee & Tea

Super Bowl Party

Colorado Chili • 57

Corn Bread with Green Chiles • 67

Platter of Ready-to-Eat Fresh Vegetables
(baby carrots, celery, broccoli, radishes)

Corn Chips & Mexican Tomato Salsa Dip •
200
or
Avocado Bean Salsa • 197

Celebration Cookies • 152

Coffee, Tea, & Assorted Cold Beverages

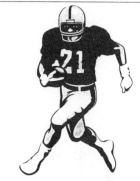

St. Patrick's Day

Corned Beef & Cabbage • 48

Colcannon • 184

Irish Soda Bread with Dried Cherries • 69

Steamed Broccoli or Green Peas

Irish Apple Cake • 111

Coffee & Tea

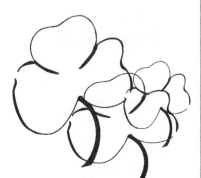

Valentine's Day Dinner

Red Snapper in Parchment • 40

Mixed Greens with Basic Vinaigrette • 164

Steamed Broccoli

French Bread • 62

Heart Cake & Chocolate Strawberries • 110

Coffee & Tea

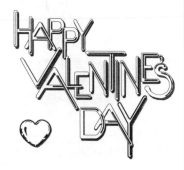

Wedding Reception Dinner

Raspberry-Basil Chicken • 25

Brown Rice Pilaf • 174

Steamed Vegetables of Choice

Spinach Salad with Strawberries • 170

French Bread • 62

Wedding Cake • 113-119
Coffee, Tea, & Assorted Beverages

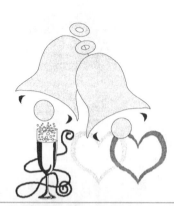

Wedding Breakfast

Blueberry Muffins with Lemon Curd • 72-73

Cappuccino Chocolate Chip Muffins • 74

Bran Muffins • 75

Gourmet Granola • 92

Bowl of Fresh Fruit

Coffee, Tea, & Assorted Fruit Juices

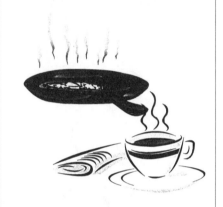

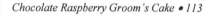

Wedding Cakes

Chocolate Raspberry Groom's Cake • 113

Coconut Wedding Cake • 114

Lemon Wedding Cake • 115

Spice Wedding Cake • 116-117

Yellow Tiered Wedding Cake • 119

White Wedding Cake With Fruit Filling • 118
Frostings • 136-140

Coffee, Tea, & Assorted Beverages

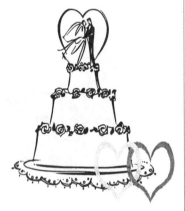

Wedding Reception Buffet

Miniature Focaccia Sandwiches • 193

Grilled Shrimp with Wraps • 195

Herbed Rice Salad • 177

Couscous Salad • 175

Grilled (Roasted) Vegetables • 182

Platter of Ready-to-eat Vegetables
(carrots, celery, radishes, broccoli, bell pepper)
Tuscan Bean Dip • 198

Platter of Ready-to-eat Fruits
(pineapple, melon, strawberries, kiwi, berries)

Wedding Cake • 113-119

Coffee, Tea, & Assorted Beverages

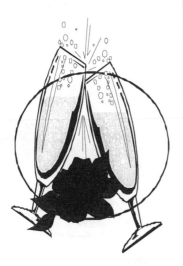

Buffet Tips

1. Allow at least 8 hors d'oeuvres per person if you're not serving a meal afterwards.

2. Choose a few make-ahead dishes to reduce preparation on the day of the event.

3. Balance the menu. Include hot dishes next to room-temperature salsas; crunchy vegetables next to creamy dips; decadent dishes next to low-calorie options. Use bright colors in food and some serving platters, balanced by neutral tones in others.

The idea is to provide variety in many ways so your guests enjoy the food from a visual, tactile, and aromatic perspective. Also, by providing variety your guests can pick and choose the food that work for them. And, the various textures, shapes, and sizes make the table visually appealing.

4. Envision the traffic flow up to and around a buffet table. Place plates, utensils, etc. at the most convenient, obvious location so guests aren't leaning over or around dishes or backtracking to pick up things they missed.

5. If you won't always be near the table to answer questions, put miniature place cards beside each food listing the contents. Food-sensitive guests will be grateful.

6. Use attractive garnishes, but make sure they're edible . . . or clearly marked as inedible. For example, Scotch bonnet peppers make beautiful garnishes but are terribly hot.

7. If you're serving outdoors, consider covers for the food to thwart bugs and pests.

8. Centerpieces add visual drama and help carry out the theme of the special occasion.

9. Introduce your guests to a new flavor or dish each time you entertain. Many people like to experiment with their taste buds. With a buffet, those who don't like to experiment aren't forced to eat something they know they won't like.

Breakfast

Gourmet Granola • 92

Breakfast Trifle • 90

Fresh Fruit

Cappuccino Chocolate Chip Muffins • 74

Coffee, Tea, & Assorted Fruit Juices

Brunch

Banana Pecan Waffles
with Maple Raisin Syrup • 86

Breakfast Sausage • 90
with
Brown Rice Pilaf • 174

Fruit Bowl

Coffee, Tea, & Assorted Fruit Juices

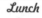

Lunch

Pizza Crust • 55
with
Pizza Sauce • 55

Mixed Greens with Basic Vinaigrette • 164

Platter of Fresh Ready-to-eat Vegetables
with
Sunny Tomato-Basil Dip • 201

Colorado Chocolate Chip Cookies • 154
Chocolate Cappuccino Ice Cream • 158
Coffee, Tea, & Assorted Beverages

Dinner

Veal (or Pork) Scaloppini • 52

Pineapple Coconut Rice • 180

French Bread • 62

Mixed Greens with Basic Vinaigrette • 164

Sautéed Brussels Sprouts • 184

Double Chocolate Cherry Torte • 108

Coffee & Tea

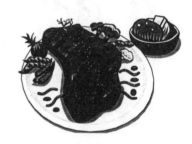

Secret Anniversaries of the Heart

For some of us, the most precious times are not the holidays on the calendar, but rather those we observe silently, in private. Let's call them "secret anniversaries of the heart." These special times are evoked by our senses and, of these, scent is one of the most powerful emissaries.

For example, the smell of roses makes me think of my maternal grandmother who used a rose-scented hand lotion. When I think of her I inevitably recall the cookies she always had waiting for her visiting grandchildren. (Her 12 children produced lots of visitors). To this day, I associate those cookies with her and her warm, unconditional love.

Think back over your life and your secret anniversaries. For many of us, certain memories trigger thoughts of food and celebratory times. Perhaps it is winning the coveted part in a school play . . . or the music that played on your first date or . . . when you found out you were pregnant with your first child. Maybe it's a sad memory such as the loss of a parent . . . or the day you learned about a job transfer that took you thousands of miles away from your friends and loved ones.

If these memories, whether they're happy or sad, evoke thoughts of food . . . then let those foods be markers for those anniversaries. Though she's been dead for nearly 20 years, I still have fond, warm thoughts as I prepare some of my Mother's favorite recipes. And, sometimes I prepare those dishes simply because I have that longing to reconnect with her using food as the medium. You don't have to explain why you're serving a particular dish. If it makes you happy or arouses melancholy thoughts that allow you to indulge your feelings, that's your secret.

Perhaps it is my training in sociology that enables me to see the symbolism in food. I prefer to use food in a way that celebrates life and the rituals we embrace. So my motto is "Celebrate anything and everything—with food".

Use the next page to record secret anniversaries of <u>your</u> heart. Encourage your family to think of foods (or aromas) that evoke pleasant memories and prepare those foods for them as a tribute. They'll be grateful.

Notes

Main Dishes

Whether you're entertaining in grand style, hosting a small, informal dinner party, or just fixing a special meal for your family . . . you'll find plenty of flavorful dishes in this chapter to take center stage for those special occasions.

Today's food trends include influences from Asian, Mediterranean, Southwestern, and Latin cuisine—so you'll find wonderfully flavored dishes here that incorporate those tastes, along with typically American main dishes as well. I've included a wide variety of different meats (beef, chicken, pork, fish) prepared in a variety of different methods (baked, grilled, roasted, simmered), with a variety of different sauces ranging from mildly flavored to bold and brash. In other words, there's something for everyone! Bon Appetit!

Beef & Lamb
Chorizo 47
Corned Beef & Cabbage 48
Lamb Chops with Rosemary Marinade 46
Orange Beef Stir-Fry 49
Sausage 47
Spaghetti Sauce & Meatballs 50
Veal (Pork) Scaloppini 52

Pork & Ham
Baked Ham 30
Bayou Red Beans & Rice 37
Barbecued Ribs with 19th Hole Sauce 31
Grilled Pork
with Orange-Rosemary Sauce 32
Pork Chops with Anise-Prune Sauce 30
Pork Chops with Apple-Dijon Sauce 33
Pork Fried Rice 34
Pork Medallions with Cherry Sauce 35
Pork Tenderloin with Ginger Sauce 36
Sweet-and-Sour Pork 38
Thai Pork Noodle Bowl 35

Pasta, Pizza, & Miscellaneous
Fresh Tomato Basil Sauce with Pasta 50
Pad Thai 51
Pasta Salad 52
Pizza Crust & Pizza Sauce 53
Spaghetti Sauce & Meatballs 50
Spice Rub for Meat 54
Spicy Fettuccini with Basil 54
Spicy Shrimp & Pasta 44

Fish & Shellfish
Coconut Shrimp
with Orange Marmalade 39
Red Snapper in Parchment 40
Paella 42
Poached Salmon 43
Salmon in Parchment 40
Shrimp Creole 41
Spicy Shrimp & Pasta 44
Tuna Burgers with
Grilled Pineapple Slices 45
Walnut Shrimp Salad 46

Soups & Stews
Asparagus Soup 55
Chinese Hot-Sour Soup 56
Colorado Chili 57
Green Chile Stew 57

Chicken & Poultry
Barbecued Chicken 20
Chicken Breasts with Mango Chutney 22
Grilled Chicken with
Mango/Black Bean Salsa 23
Chicken Cacciatore 26
Chicken Earl Grey 21
Coq Au Vin 27
Cornish Game Hens with Fruit Glaze 20
Southwestern Chicken
with Grilled Peaches 24
Raspberry-Basil Chicken 25
Stir-Fry Lemon Chicken 28
Stir-Fry Orange Chicken 29

Barbecued Chicken

(can be made without wheat, gluten, dairy, eggs, or sugar - see page xi about ingredients)

This sauce is so simple and easy, yet your guests will love it. You can make it the day before, chill, and it is ready to use when you are.

1 small can (5.5 oz) tomato juice	1 teaspoon gf Worcestershire sauce
1 garlic clove, minced	1/4 cup fresh lemon juice
1/2 teaspoon onion powder	1 tablespoon butter or oleo
1 teaspoon grated lemon peel	1/4 teaspoon cayenne pepper
1/4 teaspoon black pepper	1 pound chicken pieces

Combine all sauce ingredients in small, heavy saucepan. Simmer over low-medium heat for 10-15 minutes. Brush on chicken as it grills. Serves 4.

								Exchanges		
Calories	Fat	% Fat Cal	Protein	Carb	Chol	Sodium	Fiber	Carb	Meat	Fat
190	9g	42%	24g	4g	80mg	225mg	<1g		3	1.5

Cornish Game Hens with Fruit Glaze

(can be made without wheat, gluten, dairy, eggs, or sugar - see page xi about ingredients)

These are especially pretty to serve at company meals. The fruit glaze provides a wonderful complement to the crispy skin and assures a beautifully browned bird.

2 small Cornish game hens, halved	1/4 teaspoon dried tarragon leaves
1/2 teaspoon salt	1 teaspoon olive oil
1/4 teaspoon black pepper	1/4 cup red wine vinegar
1/2 cup fruit-only raspberry jam	1 small garlic clove, minced
1/4 teaspoon dried thyme leaves	Cooking spray

Wash game hens and pat dry. Season with salt and pepper. Arrange game hens skin side up in roasting pan that has been coated with cooking spray. If possible, place hens on roasting rack in pan so they do not sit in fat while roasting.

Combine remaining ingredients in small bowl to make glaze and microwave until jam is melted. Stir mixture thoroughly.

Bake hens, covered, in 400° oven for 45 minutes to 1 hour, brushing frequently with glaze. Serves 4.

								Exchanges		
Calories	Fat	% Fat Cal	Protein	Carb	Chol	Sodium	Fiber	Carb	Meat	Fat
400	25g	57%	29g	12g	170mg	400mg	1g	1	4	2.5

Chicken Earl Grey

(can be made without wheat, gluten, dairy, eggs, or sugar - see page xi about ingredients)

Stacking food! It's all the rage in trendy, upscale restaurants. But it's also quite practical and a very attractive way to display some dishes. Place the cooked chicken on top of the mashed potatoes, drizzle the whole stack with sauce, and you'll have a dish that looks just like those served in upscale restaurants these days. Serve with brightly colored vegetables, such as sautéed green, yellow, and red bell peppers.

And the Earl Grey tea? You'll find that tea is used to flavor many foods these days.

2 tablespoons gf rice wine or gf sherry	3/4 teaspoon black pepper
1/3 cup orange juice or pineapple juice	1/4 teaspoon salt
1/4 cup brewed Earl Grey tea	1 tablespoon olive oil
2 tablespoons gf tamari soy sauce	1 teaspoon cornstarch
1 tablespoon honey or maple syrup	or arrowroot
1 small garlic clove, minced	1 tablespoon water
4 chicken breast halves (1 1/4 pounds)	Garlic Mashed Potatoes (page 186)
1/2 teaspoon ground allspice	or plain mashed potatoes
3/4 teaspoon ground ginger	1 teaspoon paprika for garnish

Combine rice wine (or sherry), orange juice, brewed tea, soy sauce, honey, and minced garlic in glass measuring cup. Set aside.

Wash chicken breasts and pat dry with paper towels. Combine allspice, ginger, black pepper, and salt. Rub onto chicken breasts.

In heavy skillet, brown chicken breasts in olive oil over medium-high heat until golden brown. Transfer chicken to plate and keep warm.

Add rice wine mixture to skillet and bring to boil, scraping up any browned bits. Reduce heat to medium and cook until mixture is reduced by half.

Meanwhile, mix cornstarch with water to form paste. Reduce heat to low-medium and stir paste gently into rice-wine mixture until slightly thickened. Return chicken to skillet and bring to serving temperature. Remove chicken to cutting board or platter and quickly slice each piece diagonally.

To serve, place a mound of Garlic Mashed Potatoes on each plate. Top with the sliced chicken breast. Drizzle remaining sauce over chicken. Garnish with a dusting of paprika. Serve immediately. Serves 4.

See page 186 for nutritional content for Garlic Mashed Potatoes

Calories	Fat	% Fat Cal	Protein	Carb	Chol	Sodium	Fiber	Carb	Meat	Fat
								\multicolumn{3}{c}{Exchanges}		
145	5g	32%	15g	9g	36mg	682mg	.5g		2	1

Chicken Breasts with Mango Chutney

(can be made without wheat, gluten, dairy, eggs, or sugar - see page xi about ingredients)

Mango chutney has been called the "king of chutneys". You'll see it in many gourmet recipes and, of course, there are commercial versions on the shelf. But, you can make your own and have complete control over what goes into it. Prepare the chutney ahead of time and bring to room temperature before serving.

Chicken Breasts
4 chicken breast halves
1 teaspoon salt
1/4 teaspoon black pepper
1 tablespoon cooking oil

Mango Chutney
1/3 cup cider vinegar
3/4 cup sugar or fructose powder
1/2 cup seedless raisins or dried currants
1 small onion, finely chopped
2 teaspoons mustard seed
1 jalapeño or serrano chile pepper, diced
1 large garlic clove, minced
1 tablespoon grated fresh ginger
1 teaspoon ground ginger
1/4 teaspoon salt
1/2 teaspoon ground nutmeg
1/2 teaspoon ground allspice
1/2 teaspoon ground mace
1/8 teaspoon cayenne pepper
1/8 teaspoon ground cloves
1 large mango, peeled and diced

Chutney: Combine all chutney ingredients, except mangoes, in a large kettle. Cook over low heat, uncovered, 45 minutes or until liquid is clear and syrupy. Add mango and continue cooking until fruit is tender, about 20-25 minutes. Stir occasionally to prevent scorching. Remove from heat and cool while chicken is browning.

Chicken: As chutney simmers, wash chicken breasts and pat dry with paper towels. Season with salt and pepper. Brown chicken in olive oil in heavy skillet over medium heat until nicely browned on both sides. Serve with warm chutney. Serves 4.

								Exchanges		
Calories	Fat	% Fat Cal	Protein	Carb	Chol	Sodium	Fiber	Carb	Meat	Fat
370	6g	14%	15g	67g	36mg	768mg	3g	2	2	1

Grilled Chicken with Mango/Black Bean Salsa

(can be made without wheat, gluten, dairy, eggs, or sugar - see page xi about ingredients)

Salsas are very popular in fine restaurants, but you can produce the same results at home. Salsas are very colorful, healthy, and introduce fiber and a variety of interesting flavors into our meals. This one is also great on grilled fish.

Salsa
1 medium ripe mango (peeled, diced)
1/2 cup minced red onion
1/4 cup chopped red bell pepper
1/4 cup cooked black beans
1/4 cup chopped fresh cilantro, packed
1 tablespoon fresh lime or lemon juice
1 tablespoon honey or sugar
1 tablespoon red wine vinegar or
   rice vinegar
1 chipotle pepper*
1 tablespoon olive oil
1/4 teaspoon ground cumin
1/4 teaspoon salt
1/4 teaspoon black pepper

Chicken
4 chicken breast halves
1 teaspoon salt
1/4 teaspoon black pepper
1 tablespoon olive oil

Salsa: Combine ingredients in medium-size bowl. Cover and chill. Leave at room temperature for 15 minutes before serving.

Chicken: Wash chicken and pat dry with paper towels. Season with salt and pepper. Brown in olive oil in heavy skillet over medium heat until nicely browned on both sides. Or, grill on barbecue grill. Serve immediately with salsa. Serves 4.

*Bring 2 tablespoons water to a boil. Remove from heat. Soak 1 dry chipotle pepper in water for 20 minutes. Finely chop the pepper and add it with the water to the salsa. If you have never used chipotle peppers before (they're actually smoked, dried jalapeños), use 1/2 chipotle pepper and 1 tablespoon rather than 2 tablespoons of the chipotle-flavored water. Taste the salsa and add the remaining 1/2 chipotle and tablespoon of water, if desired, for a hotter dish. Or, if you prefer, use one finely chopped fresh jalapeño pepper in place of the chipotle pepper. Wear rubber gloves to protect hands while cutting chiles.

Calories	Fat	% Fat Cal	Protein	Carb	Chol	Sodium	Fiber	Exchanges Carb	Meat	Fat
195	9g	39%	15g	15g	36mg	760mg	3g		2	1.5

Southwestern Chicken with Grilled Peaches

(can be made without wheat, gluten, dairy, eggs, or sugar - see page xi about ingredients)

You've seen fancy restaurant dishes v.ith multiple sauces, decoratively placed on the plate in exotic patterns. The secret? Fill empty, plastic squeeze bottles such as those that contain mustard or ketchup. Store the unused sauces in the refrigerator for up to 1 week. Chipotle peppers (actually dried, smoked jalapeños) are available in the Mexican food section of your grocery store and natural food store. This recipe is a little more work than most, but it is well worth the effort.

<u>Chicken & Peaches</u>
4 chicken breast halves
Fresh cilantro or parsley and cherry
   tomatoes for garnish
2 firm, ripe peaches (unpeeled)
<u>Chipotle Sauce</u>
1 dried chipotle pepper
1/4 cup boiling water
1/2 cup milk (cow, rice, soy)
1 teaspoon grated fresh ginger
1/4 teaspoon salt
1 teaspoon fresh lemon or lime juice
1 teaspoon nut butter (almond
   or cashew)

<u>Southwestern Marinade</u>
3/4 cup fresh lime juice
1/2 cup minced fresh cilantro
2 tablespoons olive oil
2 small garlic cloves, minced
2 teaspoons chili powder
2 teaspoons dried oregano
1/2 teaspoon cayenne pepper
1/2 teaspoon cumin powder
1/2 teaspoon salt
1/2 teaspoon cornstarch
   or arrowroot
2 teaspoons water
<u>Balsamic Syrup</u>
1 cup balsamic vinegar
1 teaspoon sugar or honey
1 teaspoon ground coriander

Chicken: Wash and pat chicken breasts dry with paper towels. Assemble marinade ingredients (except cornstarch and water) in shallow, glass or ceramic dish. Arrange chicken breasts, turn to coat thoroughly, cover, and chill for 2-4 hours. Grill over coals or brown in a ridged skillet until done.
Southwestern Marinade Sauce: While chicken is cooking, bring marinade juices to boil in small, heavy saucepan. Reduce heat and keep warm until ready to serve. Bring sauce to serving temperature before using.
Chipotle Sauce: Bring 1/4 cup water to a boil. Place dried chipotle pepper in water and soak for 5-10 minutes. Finely chop chipotle pepper (wearing rubber gloves to protect hands), and reserve liquid. In food processor, combine chopped chipotle, chipotle soaking liquid, milk, ginger, salt, lemon (or lime) juice, and nut butter. Purée until very, very smooth. Heat mixture in a small, heavy saucepan over medium heat until thick.
Balsamic Syrup: Bring balsamic vinegar, sugar (or honey), and ground coriander to a boil in small, heavy saucepan. Reduce heat to low and simmer until liquid is reduced to about 2/3 cup. The syrup is ready when it coats the back of a spoon. Remove from heat. Bring to serving temperature when ready to serve. (continued on next page)

Grilled Peaches: During the last 5 minutes of grilling time, cut peaches in half and remove pits. Place cut side down on grill. Brush with Balsamic Syrup. Turn to grill other side when grill marks are visible on cut side of peach. Brush Balsamic Syrup on cut side and continue grilling another 2-3 minutes.

Just before serving, stir cornstarch into 2 teaspoons water to form paste. Stir paste into marinade over medium heat until it thickens slightly.

To serve, place 2 tablespoons hot Southwestern Marinade in pool on plate. Place cooked chicken breast in pool.

Spoon Chipotle Sauce over each chicken breast. Using a spoon or a fork or a plastic squeeze bottle, drizzle Balsamic Syrup over chicken breasts in decorative fashion such as zig-zags. Add 1 peach half. Garnish plate with fresh cilantro sprigs and cherry tomatoes. Serve immediately. Serves 4.

| | | | | | | | | Exchanges | | |
Calories	Fat	% Fat Cal	Protein	Carb	Chol	Sodium	Fiber	Carb	Meat	Fat
240	10g	35%	16g	24g	37mg	513mg	2g	1.5	1.5	1.5

SpecialDiet*Celebrations*

Raspberry-Basil Chicken

(can be made without wheat, gluten, dairy, eggs, or sugar - see page xi about ingredients)

Raspberry and basil seem to complement one another and, when they're mixed with other ingredients that enhance this marriage, the result is truly delicious.

6 chicken breast halves
1/3 cup fruit-only raspberry jam
1/4 cup apple, pineapple, or pear juice
3 tablespoons gf tamari soy sauce
1 tablespoon rice or gf balsamic vinegar
1 teaspoon dried basil leaves
1/4 teaspoon salt
1/4 teaspoon black pepper

1/4 teaspoon gf dry mustard
1/4 teaspoon gf garlic powder
    or 1 small garlic clove, minced
1/4 teaspoon chili powder
1/4 teaspoon curry powder
Fresh basil leaf for garnish
Cooking spray

Wash chicken breast halves and pat dry with paper towel. Place in shallow baking dish that has been coated with cooking spray.

Whisk together remaining ingredients and pour half over chicken, reserving the other half. Marinate chicken for 30-45 minutes in refrigerator.

Preheat oven to 350°. Bake chicken, basting occasionally, for 30-45 minutes or until done. Heat remaining sauce and serve over chicken. Garnish with a sprig of fresh basil, if desired. Serves 6.

| | | | | | | | | Exchanges | | |
Calories	Fat	% Fat Cal	Protein	Carb	Chol	Sodium	Fiber	Carb	Meat	Fat
108	2g	14%	14g	89g	37mg	635mg	1g	1	2	

Chicken Cacciatore

(can be made without wheat, gluten, dairy, eggs, or sugar - see page xi about ingredients)

The aroma of this dish will fill your k:tchen, inviting you and your guests to a marvelous dining experience. Serve with hot cooked rice or pasta and a crunchy tossed salad. It is especially wonderful on a cold winter day.

4 chicken breast halves	2 tablespoons fresh lemon juice
1 tablespoon olive oil	2 teaspoons dried basil leaves
3 cups fresh mushrooms, halved	1 teaspoon sugar or honey
1 small green bell pepper, chopped	1 teaspoon dried thyme leaves
1 large onion, sliced	1/4 teaspoon crushed red peppers
1 garlic clove, minced	1/2 teaspoon salt
1/2 cup gf dry red wine	1/4 teaspoon black pepper
1 can (20 oz.) tomatoes, chopped	2 tablespoons tapioca flour
2 tablespoons gf tomato paste	2 tablespoons water

In large, heavy skillet or Dutch oven, brown chicken on all sides in olive oil. Add mushrooms, green bell peppers, onion, and garlic to skillet. Cook until vegetables are tender. Add wine, bring to boiling and simmer, uncovered, until liquid is nearly evaporated. Add undrained canned tomatoes, tomato paste, lemon juice, basil, sugar, thyme, crushed red peppers, salt, and pepper.

Return chicken to pan and simmer, uncovered, for 15 minutes—either on the range or in a 350° oven. If sauce is not thick enough, stir 2 tablespoons tapioca flour with 2 tablespoons water and add to sauce, stirring until thickened. Serves 6.

								Exchanges		
Calories	Fat	% Fat Cal	Protein	Carb	Chol	Sodium	Fiber	Carb	Meat	Fat
148	4g	23%	12g	15g	24mg	233mg	3g	2	1	1

Coq Au Vin

(can be made without wheat, gluten, dairy, eggs, or sugar - see page xi about ingredients)

A popular French dish, this is actually just chicken cooked in wine. It is an elegant blend of flavors and the dish cooks slowly on its own, leaving you free to do other things. It's absolutely delicious and perfect for a fall or winter day.

1 bacon slice, uncooked	1 teaspoon dried rosemary, crushed
1 teaspoon olive oil	1 teaspoon paprika
4 chicken breast halves	1/2 teaspoon gf celery salt
1 package (9 oz.) frozen pearl onions, thawed	1/2 teaspoon black pepper
3 garlic cloves, peeled	1 pound small new potatoes
1/2 pound fresh mushrooms	1 pound baby carrots
1 cup low-sodium chicken broth	1/4 teaspoon salt
1/2 cup gf dry red wine	1 tablespoons cornstarch
1 teaspoon dried thyme	or arrowroot
1 teaspoon sugar or honey	2 tablespoons water
	1/2 cup chopped fresh parsley

In heavy, ovenproof Dutch oven, brown the bacon slice until crisp. Remove bacon from pan and remove pan from heat, leaving bacon drippings in pan.

Wash chicken and pat dry with paper towels. Return Dutch oven to medium heat. Add 1 teaspoon olive oil to bacon fat. Cook chicken pieces until browned on all sides. Remove chicken from pan and set aside.

In same Dutch oven, brown onions and garlic for about 5 minutes. Add the mushrooms and sauté 5 minutes more. Slowly pour in the chicken broth and wine. Add the thyme, sugar, rosemary, paprika, celery salt, and black pepper. Return chicken to the pan and add potatoes and bacon slice.

Bake, covered, for 30 minutes in 400° oven. Reduce heat to 350°, add carrots and continue cooking for another 30 minutes. Check chicken to make sure it's done.

Remove chicken and vegetables from Dutch oven with slotted spoon. Keep warm on serving platter or bowl. If sauce does not need thickening, it may be served at this point by pouring over chicken and vegetables.

If sauce needs thickening, combine cornstarch and water to form paste. With Dutch oven over low-medium heat, stir in cornstarch mixture and boil until sauce thickens. Use more cornstarch for thicker sauce.

Pour sauce over chicken and vegetables. Garnish with parsley. Serves 4.

								Exchanges		
Calories	Fat	% Fat Cal	Protein	Carb	Chol	Sodium	Fiber	Carb	Meat	Fat
318	8g	24%	20g	37g	42mg	688mg	4g	4	2	1

Stir-Fry Lemon Chicken

(can be made without wheat, gluten, dairy, eggs, or sugar - see page xi about ingredients)

One of the secrets to attractive stir-fry dishes is to vary the shapes and colors of the various vegetables. For example, I like to cut the carrots into 1/4-inch ridged diagonals, the red or green bell peppers into long, 1/4-inch thin slices, and the green onions into 1-inch diagonals.

1 pound chicken (1-inch pieces)	1 tablespoon olive oil
1/4 cup gf tamari soy sauce	3 green onions (1-inch diagonals)
1/4 cup fresh lemon juice	2 medium carrots, sliced diagonally
1 tablespoon grated lemon peel	1/2 cup red bell pepper (1/4-inch strips)
1/4 cup water	2 teaspoons cornstarch or arrowroot
1 teaspoon honey	2 cups hot cooked white rice
2 teaspoons crushed red peppers	Additional green onion & lemon
2 medium garlic cloves, minced	peel strips for garnish
1/2 teaspoon ground ginger	

Wash chicken and pat dry with paper towels. Place in shallow, glass dish. Set aside. Combine soy sauce, lemon juice, lemon peel, water, honey, crushed red peppers, garlic, and ginger. Pour half of marinade over chicken in glass dish and reserve the remaining half. Marinate chicken, refrigerated, for 30 minutes.

Meanwhile, prepare vegetables. Set aside. Drain chicken and discard marinade.

In heavy skillet over medium heat, sauté chicken in olive oil until lightly browned. Transfer meat to plate, cover with foil.

In same skillet, sauté onions, carrots, and red bell pepper until crisp-tender. Whisk cornstarch or arrowroot into reserved marinade. Stir into vegetables and stir-fry until thickened. Return chicken to skillet; bring to serving temperature.

Serve immediately over cooked rice. Garnish with additional chopped green onions and lemon strips, if desired. Serves 4.

								Exchanges		
Calories	Fat	% Fat Cal	Protein	Carb	Chol	Sodium	Fiber	Carb	Meat	Fat
415	7g	15%	30g	57g	63mg	999mg	3g	4	3	1

Rice contributes 45mg of the 57g of carbohydrate per serving.

Stir-Fry Orange Chicken

(can be made without wheat, gluten, dairy, eggs, or sugar - see page xi about ingredients)

This is a beautiful dish and one that you can prepare in front of your guests. For some reason, guests love to watch the cook—at least at my house! So, make the food preparation part of the entertainment. You may use shrimp in place of chicken, if you wish.

<u>Sauce</u>
1/2 cup low-sodium chicken broth
1/2 cup fresh orange juice
3 tablespoons gf tamari soy sauce
2 teaspoons rice vinegar
1 teaspoon sesame oil
1 tablespoon cooking oil
1 teaspoon molasses
   (cane or sorghum)
1 teaspoon sugar or honey
3 tablespoons cornstarch
   or arrowroot

<u>Chicken & Vegetables</u>
1 teaspoon cooking oil
4 chicken breast halves
   (sliced diagonally)
3 tablespoons grated orange peel
1 garlic clove, minced
1/4 teaspoon crushed red peppers
1 cup sliced red and/or
   yellow bell pepper
1 cup snow peas, fresh or frozen
1/4 cup diagonally sliced carrots
1/4 cup chopped fresh cilantro, packed
4 cups hot cooked white rice

Sauce: Whisk together sauce ingredients and set aside.
Chicken & Vegetables: In a large skillet or wok, heat oil over medium-high heat. Add the chicken slices and cook until nicely browned. Add the orange peel, garlic, crushed red pepper, bell peppers, snow peas, and carrots. Sauté for 2-3 minutes. Stir in the sauce mixture and simmer for 4-5 minutes until mixture thickens and reduces slightly. Add cilantro. Serve over cooked rice. Serves 4.

								Exchanges		
Calories	Fat	% Fat Cal	Protein	Carb	Chol	Sodium	Fiber	Carb	Meat	Fat
205	6g	29%	17g	64g	37mg	810mg	3g	2	2	1

Rice contributes 44g of the total 64g of carbohydrates per serving.

Baked Ham

(can be made without wheat, gluten, dairy, eggs, or sugar - see page xi about ingredients)

Baked ham is the perfect dish for a Sunday dinner. Leftovers are great, too.

5 pound ham, fully cooked
2 cups gf chicken stock (page 213)
1/2 cup gf dry sherry
1 bay leaf
1/4 cup frozen orange juice concentrate

1/2 teaspoon dried thyme leaves
1/8 teaspoon ground cloves
1 cup raisins
1 tablespoon tapioca flour
2 tablespoons water

Bake ham at 325° for 1 hour, or until heated through. Meanwhile, in heavy medium saucepan combine chicken stock, dry sherry, bay leaf, orange juice concentrate, thyme, and cloves. Bring to boil; remove from heat to cool. Add raisins.

When ready to serve, return sauce to medium heat. Cook for about 10 minutes, or until sauce is slightly reduced. Stir tapioca flour with 2 tablespoons water, then stir into sauce. Continue stirring constantly until mixture thickens slightly. Makes about 2 cups of sauce. Serve sauce over sliced ham. Serves 12.

								Exchanges		
Calories	Fat	% Fat Cal	Protein	Carb	Chol	Sodium	Fiber	Carb	Meat	Fat
460	18g	36%	56g	14g	178mg	230mg	1g	1	8	3

Pork Chops with Anise-Prune Sauce

(can be made without wheat, gluten, dairy, eggs, or sugar - see page xi about ingredients)

Prunes contribute wonderful flavor, interesting texture, and considerable nutrients.

4 medium pork chops
   (1 1/4 pounds)
1 tablespoon olive oil
1 large garlic clove, minced
1 teaspoon grated fresh ginger
2 tablespoons gf tamari soy sauce

2 tablespoons gf red wine vinegar
1/4 cup water
1 tablespoon brown sugar or maple sugar
1/2 teaspoon anise seed or 1 teaspoon
   gf anise extract
1/4 cup prunes, finely chopped

Wash pork chops and pat dry with paper towel. In large, heavy skillet brown pork chops in olive oil over medium heat. Remove meat from skillet.

Add garlic, ginger, soy sauce, vinegar, water, sugar, anise, and prunes. Bring to simmer. Return pork chops to skillet and simmer, covered, for 15 minutes. Remove cover. Let sauce simmer to desired consistency. Serves 4.

								Exchanges		
Calories	Fat	% Fat Cal	Protein	Carb	Chol	Sodium	Fiber	Carb	Meat	Fat
350	13g	34%	45g	11g	130mg	585mg	1g	1	6	2

Barbecued Ribs with 19th Hole Sauce

(can be made without wheat, gluten, dairy, eggs, or sugar - see page xi about ingredients)

This is one of our favorite summertime dishes. By pre-cooking the ribs, they turn out deliciously tender and succulent.

8 pounds pork ribs	1/2 teaspoon black pepper
1 cup gf Tomato Ketchup	2 teaspoons paprika
(page 218)	1 teaspoon chili powder
1/2 cup molasses	1/2 teaspoon salt
(cane or sorghum)	1 bay leaf
2 tablespoons gf onion flakes	1 garlic clove, minced
2 tablespoons brown sugar or	1 teaspoon grated orange peel
maple sugar	1/2 cup fresh orange juice
1 tablespoon mustard seeds	2 tablespoons olive oil
1 teaspoon crushed red peppers	1/4 cup red wine vinegar
1 teaspoon dried oregano leaves	2 tablespoons gf Worcestershire sauce

Wash ribs and pat dry with paper towel. Wrap in aluminum foil and bake in very slow oven (250°) for 3-4 hours. This step can be done the day before. Refrigerate, covered.

To make the sauce, combine remaining ingredients in small saucepan. Bring to boil, reduce heat to low, and simmer sauce for 10-15 minutes. Brush sauce on ribs as they cook on the grill. Serves 12.

								Exchanges		
Calories	Fat	% Fat Cal	Protein	Carb	Chol	Sodium	Fiber	Carb	Meat	Fat
690	45g	62%	42g	20g	170mg	270mg	1g	1	6	6

Grilled Pork with Orange-Rosemary Sauce

(can be made without wheat, gluten, dairy, eggs, or sugar - see page xi about ingredients)

This dish can also be transformed into a last-minute quick dinner—if you skip marinating the pork in the sauce. For a smoother sauce, be sure to grate rather than chop the onion.

4 pork chops (1 1/4 pounds)
2 tablespoons molasses
  (cane or sorghum)
1/2 cup fresh orange juice, strained
1 teaspoon grated orange peel
2 teaspoons Dijonnaise mustard
1 teaspoon olive oil
1 teaspoon gf balsamic vinegar
1/4 teaspoon salt
1/4 teaspoon black pepper

1 teaspoon crushed dried rosemary
  or 1 tablespoon finely snipped
  fresh rosemary
1 small garlic clove, minced
2 tablespoons grated fresh onion or
  1 teaspoon gf onion powder
1 teaspoon cornstarch or arrowroot
1 tablespoon water
Fresh rosemary sprigs for garnish

Wash pork chops and pat dry with paper towel. Place in shallow dish or heavy-duty plastic freezer bag. Combine all sauce ingredients (molasses through onion) and pour over pork. Marinate pork for 6-8 hours. Remove pork and grill until done.

Meanwhile, while pork is cooking, bring marinade to boil in small saucepan over medium heat, reduce to low, and simmer for 5 minutes. Baste chops with the cooked sauce as they grill, if you wish.

Just before serving, mix cornstarch or arrowroot with a tablespoon of water. Whisk into sauce, continuing to stir until mixture thickens. Remove from heat. Serve over pork and garnish with fresh rosemary sprigs, if desired. Serves 4.

								Exchanges		
Calories	Fat	% Fat Cal	Protein	Carb	Chol	Sodium	Fiber	Carb	Meat	Fat
252	8g	29%	31g	13g	90mg	268mg	1	.5	4	1

Pork Chops with Apple-Dijon Sauce

(can be made without wheat, gluten, dairy, eggs, or sugar - see page xi about ingredients)

*The combination of apples and Dijonnaise mustard makes a tantalizing sauce. Serve
with grilled apple rings or applesauce, if desired. You may also use this sauce on
chicken breasts, as well.*

4 pork chops (1 1/4 pounds)	1 tablespoon olive oil
1/2 teaspoon dried thyme leaves	1/2 cup apple juice
1/2 teaspoon dried marjoram leaves	1/4 cup finely chopped green onions
1/2 teaspoon black pepper	2 tablespoons gf Dijonnaise mustard
1/2 teaspoon salt	1 teaspoon cornstarch or arrowroot
1/8 teaspoon ground allspice	1 tablespoon water
1/8 teaspoon cayenne pepper	Fresh apple wedges for garnish

Wash pork chops and pat dry with paper towel. Combine thyme, marjoram,
black pepper, salt, allspice, and cayenne pepper. Rub spice mixture onto both
sides of meat. (You can do this step the night before or morning of the day you
plan to serve this dish. Refrigerate meat until ready to cook.)

In large, heavy skillet over medium heat, brown meat on both sides in olive
oil. Cook about 15 minutes, or until meat is no longer pink.

Transfer to plate and cover with foil. In same skillet, bring apple juice, green
onions, and Dijonnaise to a boil. Mixture will look grainy at first, but becomes
smoother after cooking. Cook over low-medium heat, scraping up browned
bits, for 5 minutes.

Combine cornstarch with 1 tablespoon water to form paste. Whisk into
sauce, stirring constantly, until thickened slightly.

Return meat to pan and bring to serving temperature. Serve with garnishes of
fresh apple wedges. Serves 4.

									Exchanges	
Calories	Fat	% Fat Cal	Protein	Carb	Chol	Sodium	Fiber	Carbo	Meat	Fat
250	11g	39%	31g	6g	90mg	538mg	1g		4	2

Pork Fried Rice

(can be made without wheat, gluten, dairy, eggs, or sugar - see page xi about ingredients)

This is a great way to use up leftover rice. It's quick and easy and the perfect answer when someone says, "Let's order Chinese take-out tonight."

1 tablespoon cooking oil
1/2 pound pork (1/4-inch thick cubes)
1 small onion, finely chopped
2 small garlic cloves, minced
1 large carrot (1/4-inch diagonals)
1/2 cup chopped shitake mushrooms
1 large egg, beaten (optional)
4 cups cooked white rice

2 tablespoons gf tamari soy sauce
3 green onions, cut in 1/4-inch diagonals
1/2 cup snow peas
1/4 pound bean sprouts
1 teaspoon sesame oil
1/2 teaspoon salt
1/4 teaspoon black pepper

In wok or high-edged skillet, sauté pork cubes in oil until lightly browned and cooked through. Remove from pan. Add the onion and stir-fry until onion is translucent. Add the garlic, carrots, and mushrooms and cook for 2 minutes. Add this mixture to the cooked pork. Remove all ingredients from wok and set aside.

In wok, stir-fry egg (if using) and cook until set. Break up the pieces using a spatula. Add the rice and all the cooked ingredients back to the wok. Add the soy sauce, green onions, snow peas, bean sprouts, oil, salt, and pepper. Stir to combine and bring to serving temperature. Serve immediately. Serves 4.

								Exchanges		
Calories	Fat	% Fat Cal	Protein	Carb	Chol	Sodium	Fiber	Carb	Meat	Fat
330	15	40%	17g	35g	86mg	890mg	3g	3	2	2

Pork Medallions with Cherry Sauce

(can be made without wheat, gluten, dairy, eggs, or sugar - see page xi about ingredients)

2 pounds pork tenderloin
1 teaspoon black pepper
1 cup dried tart cherries
1 cup gf port wine or red grape juice

1 teaspoon unsalted butter
   or cooking oil
1/4 cup gf balsamic vinegar
1/2 teaspoon dried marjoram leaves

Wash pork tenderloins; pat dry with paper towels. Season with pepper. Roast in 325° oven until thermometer registers 160°. (About 25 minutes per pound.)

In a small saucepan over medium heat, combine cherries with 1/3 cup port wine (or grape juice). Bring to a simmer; turn off heat. Let cherries soak in liquid for 15 minutes. Return mixture plus remaining port wine to medium heat. Add remaining ingredients and boil one minute over high heat to thicken. Spoon over sliced pork tenderloins. Serves 6.

| | | | | | | | | Exchanges | | |
Calories	Fat	% Fat Cal	Protein	Carb	Chol	Sodium	Fiber	Carb	Meat	Fat
360	8g	20%	43g	21g	122mg	91mg	1g	1	6	2

Thai Pork Noodle Bowl

(can be made without wheat, gluten, dairy, eggs, or sugar - see page xi about ingredients)

1/2 pound pork (1/2-inch cubes)
1/4 cup chopped green onions
1 garlic clove, minced
1 tablespoon cooking oil
1/2 cup chopped red bell pepper
1/4 cup rice vinegar
3 tablespoons gf tamari soy sauce
6 tablespoons brown sugar or
   maple sugar

4 teaspoons paprika
1 teaspoon Reese's anchovy paste or
   gf fish sauce (optional)
3/4 teaspoon cayenne pepper
1/4 cup chopped fresh cilantro, packed
2 cups mung bean sprouts
12 ounces rice noodles, cooked
1/4 cup cashews (optional)

In large, heavy skillet over medium heat, sauté pork, green onions, and garlic in oil until pork is cooked through. Add red bell peppers; cook 1 minute.

In a small bowl, combine vinegar, soy sauce, sugar, paprika, anchovy paste or fish sauce, and cayenne pepper. Add mixture to skillet and toss, along with cilantro, until hot.

Place bean sprouts and cooked noodles in individual serving bowls and top with meat mixture. Garnish with chopped cashews. Serves 6.

| | | | | | | | | Exchanges | | |
Calories	Fat	% Fat Cal	Protein	Carb	Chol	Sodium	Fiber	Carb	Meat	Fat
262	7g	25%	25g	27g	67mg	487mg	1g	2	3	1

Pork Tenderloin with Ginger Sauce

(can be made without wheat, gluten, dairy, eggs, or sugar - see page xi about ingredients)

Fruit and ginger complement pork, so this sauce greatly enhances the pork tenderloin.

1 pound pork tenderloin	1/4 teaspoon gf curry powder
1/2 teaspoon salt	1 tablespoon honey or sugar
1/2 teaspoon black pepper	1 1/4 cups apple juice or pineapple juice
1 tablespoon olive oil	1/3 cup dried tart cherries or apricots
1 clove garlic, minced	1/4 teaspoon salt
1/4 cup fresh grated onion or	1/4 teaspoon black pepper
1 teaspoon gf onion powder	1 teaspoon cornstarch or arrowroot
1 inch fresh ginger, grated or	2 tablespoons water
1 teaspoon ground ginger	

Cut pork tenderloin into medallions and sprinkle with salt and pepper. Brown medallions in olive oil in large skillet over medium heat. Transfer to plate and keep warm while preparing sauce.

In same skillet, add garlic, onion, ginger, and curry powder and sauté for one minute. Add honey, apple juice, cherries, and 1/4 teaspoon salt and pepper—scraping up browned bits. Bring to boil, then reduce to low and simmer, un-covered, until mixture is reduced by half (about 5 minutes).

Stir arrowroot (or cornstarch) into 2 tablespoons water until smooth and gradually stir into mixture. Increase heat to medium and stir until mixture thickens slightly. Serve sauce over pork tenderloins. Serves 4.

								Exchanges		
Calories	Fat	% Fat Cal	Protein	Carb	Chol	Sodium	Fiber	Carb	Meat	Fat
262	7g	25%	25g	26g	67mg	487mg	1g	2	3.5	1

Bayou Red Beans & Rice

(can be made without wheat, gluten, dairy, eggs, or sugar - see page xi about ingredients)

A crock pot is an ideal way to cook the beans. Assemble the ingredients in the morning and cook all day. You'll be greeted with a wonderful aroma when you arrive home from work.

1 celery stalk, chopped
1 small yellow onion, chopped
3 garlic cloves, minced
1 teaspoon olive oil
1 pound dried red beans (not kidney)
1 teaspoon dried basil leaves
1 teaspoon crushed dried rosemary
1/2 teaspoon dried oregano leaves
1/2 teaspoon dried thyme leaves
2 teaspoons salt

1 teaspoon black pepper
2 tablespoons brown sugar or maple
    sugar, packed
1/8 teaspoon cayenne pepper
2 bay leaves
1/4 pound Canadian bacon, chopped
Water to cover beans
4 cups hot cooked white rice
1 tablespoon parsley (optional)

In large, heavy saucepan over medium heat, sauté celery, onion, and garlic in olive oil until translucent.

Rinse and pick over beans to remove stones or debris. Add to saucepan along with basil, rosemary, oregano, thyme, salt, black pepper, sugar, cayenne pepper, bay leaves, and Canadian bacon.

Add enough water to cover beans and simmer over medium heat for 2 hours —or until beans are done. Serve over cooked rice. Garnish with parsley, if desired. Serves 8.

								Exchanges		
Calories	Fat	% Fat Cal	Protein	Carb	Chol	Sodium	Fiber	Carb	Meat	Fat
220	2g	9%	9g	40g	7mg	910mg	6g	2	1	

Rice contributes 22 of the total 40g of carbohydrates per serving.

Sweet-and-Sour Pork

(can be made without wheat, gluten, dairy, eggs, or sugar - see page xi about ingredients)

This is an old standby, but a real favorite. It makes a great answer to "Let's eat Chinese tonight." For the prettiest effect, be sure to vary the shapes of the vegetables. Cut the carrots into 1/4-inch ridge diagonals, the bell peppers into 1/4-inch long slices, and the onions into quarters.

Marinade & Pork
1 tablespoon gf tamari soy sauce
1 teaspoon ground ginger
1 tablespoon cornstarch
  or arrowroot
1 garlic clove, minced
1 tablespoon pineapple juice
1 pound pork, cubed

Vegetables & Sauce
1 small onion, coarsely chopped
1 medium carrot, in 1/4-inch thick slices
1/2 cup chopped red bell pepper
1 small green bell pepper, chopped
1 tablespoon cooking oil
8 ounces pineapple chunks in juice
2 tablespoons brown or maple sugar
3 tablespoons cider vinegar
1 tablespoon grated fresh ginger
2 tablespoons gf tamari soy sauce
1/8 teaspoon white pepper
1 tablespoon tapioca flour
1 tablespoon water
4 cups hot cooked white rice

Marinade & Pork: Combine first 5 ingredients in bowl. Rinse pork cubes and pat dry with paper towel. Add pork cubes to bowl and marinate while chopping the vegetables.

Vegetables & Sauce: In a heavy skillet over medium heat, brown onion, carrots, and pork cubes in oil until lightly browned, stirring frequently. Remove from skillet. Sauté red and green bell peppers for 3 minutes, stirring frequently. Remove from skillet. Set aside.

To skillet, add pineapple chunks (including juice and water to equal 2/3 cup liquid), sugar, vinegar, ginger, soy sauce, and pepper over medium heat. Stir tapioca flour with 1 tablespoon water until paste forms. Stir slowly into skillet, continuing to stir until mixture thickens slightly.

Return pork, onions, and carrots to skillet. Cover and simmer gently for 10 minutes. Add red and green bell peppers and bring to serving temperature. Serve over hot cooked rice. Serves 6.

| | | | | | | | | Exchanges | | |
Calories	Fat	% Fat Cal	Protein	Carb	Chol	Sodium	Fiber	Carb	Meat	Fat
390	14g	33%	18g	47g	52mg	553mg	2g	3	2	2

Rice contributes 25g of the total 47g of carbohydrates per serving.

Coconut Shrimp with Orange Marmalade

(can be made without wheat, gluten, dairy, or sugar - see page xi about ingredients)

If eggs are inappropriate, dip shrimp in flour mixture only.

1 pound jumbo shrimp
1/4 cup soy flour or Jowar flour
1/4 cup arrowroot powder
1/2 cup unsweetened shredded coconut
1/2 teaspoon gf garlic powder
1/2 teaspoon gf onion powder

1/2 teaspoon baking powder
1/2 teaspoon salt
1/4 teaspoon cayenne pepper
1 large egg, beaten to a foam
Oil for frying
Orange Marmalade (see below)

Peel and clean the shrimp, removing the intestinal vein. To butterfly the shrimp, use a paring knife to open the shrimp down the back without cutting all the way through. Press each shrimp flat. Set aside.

In a large bowl, whisk together the flour, arrowroot powder, shredded coconut, garlic powder, onion powder, baking powder, salt, and cayenne pepper.

In large bowl, whisk egg until it has a foamy texture. Set aside. Heat enough cooking oil to cover shrimp in a deep fryer or deep, heavy pot. Dip each shrimp in the egg mixture, then in coconut-flour mixture. Fry shrimp in small batches, turning twice to ensure even browning. Transfer to plate lined with paper towels for draining. Continue with remaining shrimp. Serve with Orange Marmalade as dip. Serves 4.

| | | | | | | | | | Exchanges | |
Calories	Fat	% Fat Cal	Protein	Carb	Chol	Sodium	Fiber	Carb	Meat	Fat
287	7g	20%	19g	40g	188mg	525mg	2g	2	2.5	1

Orange Marmalade

(can be made without wheat, gluten, dairy, eggs, or sugar - see page xi about ingredients)

1 large thin-skinned orange, seeded   1/2 cup granulated sugar or fructose

Chop orange (peel and pulp) coarsely. Pulverize pieces in food processor or blender. Measure mixture in glass measuring bowl and add equal amount of sugar or fructose.

Place bowl in microwave oven. Microwave on high, covered, for 2 minutes. Stir. Microwave again for 2 minutes. Stir again. Continue to microwave for 1 minute periods, stirring at each interval, until mixture thickens. Cool. Refrigerate in glass jar, covered, for up to 1 week. Serves 16 (1 tablespoon each).

| | | | | | | | | | Exchanges | |
Calories	Fat	% Fat Cal	Protein	Carb	Chol	Sodium	Fiber	Carb	Meat	Fat
28	0g	0	1g	7g	0mg	0mg	.2g	.5		

Salmon in Parchment

(can be made without wheat, gluten, dairy, eggs, or sugar - see page xi about ingredients)

The recipes on this page make great company dishes because they can be prepared ahead of time and look very elegant. To julienne means to cut into matchstick shapes.

4 salmon fillets (1 1/4 pounds)
1 teaspoon dried dill weed
1 teaspoon dried thyme
1/2 teaspoon salt
1/4 teaspoon black pepper
1 small carrot, julienne
1 small red bell pepper, julienne

1 small zucchini, julienne
1 tablespoon grated fresh onion
2 teaspoons grated lemon peel
1 tablespoon olive oil
Parchment paper or aluminum foil
Cooking spray

Preheat oven to 425°. Cut parchment paper (or foil) into four 13-inch squares. Lay each piece flat on counter top and lay a salmon fillet on each.

Combine remaining ingredients and distribute evenly on each salmon fillet. Fold parchment paper together. Crimp or fold edges attractively. Twist ends tightly to seal. Spray with cooking spray. Don't spray aluminum foil.

Bake for 15-20 minutes or until packages puff and are lightly browned. Place on individual serving plates. Open carefully to avoid steam burns. Serves 4.

| | | | | | | | | Exchanges | | |
Calories	Fat	% Fat Cal	Protein	Carb	Chol	Sodium	Fiber	Carb	Meat	Fat
211	.5	37%	29g	4g	74mg	393mg	1g		4	1

Red Snapper in Parchment

(can be made without wheat, gluten, dairy, eggs, or sugar - see page xi about ingredients)

4 red snapper fillets (1 1/4 pounds)
1/4 cup chopped sun-dried tomatoes
2 tablespoons fresh lemon juice
2 teaspoon grated lemon peel
2 teaspoons crushed dried rosemary

1 small garlic clove, minced
1/2 teaspoon salt
1/4 cup black pepper
Parchment paper or aluminum foil
Cooking spray

Preheat oven to 425°. Cut parchment paper (or foil) into four 13-inch squares. Set aside.

Combine all ingredients in small bowl, except red snapper. Arrange parchment squares on counter top. Place one red snapper fillet on center of each square. Top with tomato mixture. Fold parchment paper together. Crimp or fold edges attractively. Twist ends tightly to seal. Spray with cooking spray (parchment paper only).

Bake for about 15-20 minutes or until packages puff up and are lightly browned. Cut open carefully to avoid steam burns. Serves 4.

| | | | | | | | | Exchanges | | |
Calories	Fat	% Fat Cal	Protein	Carb	Chol	Sodium	Fiber	Carb	Meat	Fat
110	2	12%	20g	3g	35mg	405mg	1g	.5	3	

Shrimp Creole

(can be made without wheat, gluten, dairy, eggs, or sugar - see page xi about ingredients)

This dish makes an excellent buffet dish since the sauce can be served in a crock pot or chafing dish. The rice and vegetables can be arranged in a molded pan for a very pretty presentation.

1 tablespoon olive oil	1/2 teaspoon gf celery salt
1/2 cup chopped onion	3/4 teaspoon gf chili powder
1 garlic clove, minced	1/8 teaspoon cayenne pepper
1/2 cup chopped celery	2 teaspoons cornstarch or arrowroot
1 can (16 oz.) peeled tomatoes	1 tablespoon cold water
1 can (8 oz) gf tomato sauce	1 pound shrimp (peeled, de-veined)
1 tablespoon gf Worcestershire sauce	1/2 cup chopped green bell pepper
1 teaspoon salt	4 cups hot cooked white rice
1 teaspoon sugar or honey	1/4 cup fresh chopped parsley

In large, heavy Dutch oven, sauté onion, garlic, and celery in olive oil until tender, but not brown. Add tomatoes, tomato sauce, Worcestershire sauce, salt, sugar, chili powder, and cayenne pepper. Simmer, uncovered, for 30 minutes.

Mix cornstarch (or arrowroot) with cold water until smooth. Stir into sauce. Cook, stirring until bubbly. Add shrimp and green bell pepper. Cover and simmer another 5 minutes.

To mold cooked rice, spray Bundt pan or other decoratively shaped pan with cooking spray. Pack hot, cooked rice in pan. It works better to fill a pan all the way to the top, rather than using a larger pan that you only fill halfway. Turn out on serving place. For an even more decorative presentation, serve a vegetable such as hot cooked green peas in the center hole (if using Bundt pan). Serve immediately. Serves 4.

								Exchanges		
Calories	Fat	% Fat Cal	Protein	Carb	Chol	Sodium	Fiber	Carb	Meat	Fat
430	7g	14%	30g	62g	170mg	13mg	4g	6	3	1

Paella

(can be made without wheat, gluten, dairy, eggs, or sugar - see page xi about ingredients)

All you need with this dish is a tossed salad and bread. Serve it in a large, attractive dish—perhaps the one you cook it in. I cook mine in a large, flat copper pan that goes from oven to tabletop. It makes a great centerpiece.

3 pounds chicken drumsticks
2 tablespoons olive oil
1/4 pound gf Sausage (page 47)
1/2 cup chopped onions
1/2 pound medium tomatoes, chopped
1/2 pound shrimp (peeled, de-veined)
1 package (9 oz.) frozen artichoke hearts
   or 1 can (16 oz.) artichoke hearts
1 clove garlic or 1/4 teaspoon gf garlic
   powder
1/4 cup chopped parsley or
1 tablespoon dried parsley

1 teaspoon paprika
1 teaspoon Beau Monde or
   gf seasoning salt
1/2 teaspoon crushed saffron
1 teaspoon salt
1/4 teaspoon black pepper
3 cups low-sodium chicken stock
1 1/2 cups uncooked white rice
3 ounces pimientos (optional)
1 dozen mussels or clams
1/2 pound fish fillets (cod, perch)
1 cup green peas

In large skillet, brown chicken on all sides in olive oil. Remove. Add sausage, onions, and tomatoes and cook until onion is lightly browned.

Return chicken to pan, add shrimp and remaining ingredients, except green peas. Cover and simmer 30 minutes. (If using an ovenproof skillet, you may also place skillet in oven to cook). Uncover, add green peas and cook for another 5 minutes. Serves 6.

| | | | | | | | | Exchanges | | |
Calories	Fat	% Fat Cal	Protein	Carb	Chol	Sodium	Fiber	Carb	Meat	Fat
676	23g	32%	59g	55g	195mg	999mg	6g	3	7	2

Poached Salmon

(can be made without wheat, gluten, dairy, eggs, or sugar - see page xi about ingredients)

Serve this atop a bed of mixed greens or mesclun. Arrange several spears of cooked, chilled asparagus alongside the salmon and drizzle your favorite salad dressing over the whole dish. Very refreshing on a hot summer day!

4 salmon steaks (1 1/4 pounds)
4 cups vegetable stock (page 213)
1 teaspoon salt
2 tablespoons rice vinegar or
   fresh lemon juice
10 whole black peppercorns
6 whole dill seeds
2 whole cloves
1 bay leaf

1 small garlic clove
1 tablespoon chopped fresh parsley or
   1 teaspoon dried parsley
1 tablespoon fresh thyme or 1 teaspoon
   dried thyme leaves
1 tablespoon fresh tarragon or 1
   teaspoon dried tarragon leaves
Fresh herb sprigs for garnish
Vinegar-Free Herb Dressing (page 165)

Wash salmon and set aside.

In large, deep pan or skillet place remaining ingredients and bring to a boil. Reduce heat and bring liquid to a simmer. Add as many salmon steaks as will comfortably fit in a single layer. Cover, and simmer for 5-10 minutes or until thoroughly cooked—depending on thickness of steak. Check to make sure salmon is thoroughly cooked before removing from poaching liquid.

Remove from liquid with large spatula or slotted spoon. Chill before serving. Serve garnished with fresh herbs and a dollop of Vinegar-Free Herb Dressing. Serves 4.

| | | | | | | | | Exchanges | | |
Calories	Fat	% Fat Cal	Protein	Carb	Chol	Sodium	Fiber	Carb	Meat	Fat
200	5g	27%	35g	2g	74mg	685mg	.5g		4	.5

Spicy Shrimp & Pasta

(can be made without wheat, gluten, dairy, eggs, or sugar - see page xi about ingredients)

This beautiful dish is especially appropriate for guests. It is very attractive and colorful, with the contrast of the snow peas and red bell peppers against the pasta. If you like extra-spicy foods, increase the cayenne pepper a bit. Also, if you prefer not to use wine, you may use the same amount of chicken broth instead.

1 tablespoon cooking oil
8 ounces snow peas, fresh or frozen
1 red bell pepper (1/4-inch strips)
1 medium garlic clove, minced
1 tablespoon tapioca flour
1 cup low-sodium chicken broth
1/2 cup dry gf white wine
1/2 teaspoon dried basil
1/2 teaspoon paprika
1/2 teaspoon dried thyme leaves
1/4 teaspoon cayenne pepper

1/4 teaspoon black pepper
1/4 teaspoon crushed red peppers
1 pound medium-size shrimp
2 cups cooked gf fettuccini or
 spaghetti, uncooked
6 quarts water
1/2 cup Parmesan cheese (cow, rice,
 soy) for garnish
1 tablespoon chopped fresh parsley,
 divided
1 teaspoon grated lemon peel, divided

Place oil in large, heavy skillet. Over low-medium heat, sauté peas, red bell pepper, and minced garlic until vegetables are crisp-tender—about 3 minutes. Remove vegetables and set aside.

In same skillet, combine tapioca flour with two tablespoons of the chicken broth to form a smooth paste. Then add paste, along with wine and remaining chicken broth. Stir in basil, paprika, thyme, cayenne pepper, black pepper, and crushed red peppers. Bring mixture to boil until it thickens slightly.

Add shrimp. Reduce heat and cook five minutes or until shrimp are pink and curled. Return vegetables to skillet and cook one minute longer. Keep warm.

Cook pasta in 6 quarts boiling, salted water until al dente. Drain, leaving two tablespoons hot water in pot. Return pasta to pot and set aside.

To serve, divide pasta among four serving plates. Garnish with fresh parsley and a sprinkle of grated Parmesan cheese. Just before serving, toss shrimp mixture with remaining lemon peel and chopped parsley. Serve over hot noodles. Sprinkle with more Parmesan cheese, if desired. Serves 4.

Exchanges

Calories	Fat	% Fat Cal	Protein	Carb	Chol	Sodium	Fiber	Carb	Meat	Fat
427	10g	20%	33g	47g	171mg	790mg	5g	3	2.5	1

Tuna Burgers with Grilled Pineapple Slices

(can be made without wheat, gluten, dairy, eggs, or sugar - see page xi about ingredients)

These burgers are an interesting change from hamburgers. The sauce can be prepared ahead of time (maybe the night before while you're preparing dinner) and refrigerated until dinner the next evening. Grilled pineapple slices add flavor, color, variety, and nutrients to any meal. If you're not using the outdoor barbecue grill, try using a ridged skillet on top of the range.

Oriental Sauce
1 cup pineapple or apple juice
1/2 cup rice vinegar
1 teaspoon ground ginger
1/4 cup gf tamari soy sauce
1/4 cup brown sugar or maple sugar
1/4 cup fresh lemon juice
1 teaspoon white pepper
1/8 teaspoon ground allspice
1/2 teaspoon cornstarch
   or arrowroot
1 tablespoon cold water

Tuna Burgers
1 pound fresh tuna steaks or
   3 cans (6 oz. each) gf canned tuna
1/2 cup gf bread crumbs
1 large egg or 1/4 cup flax mix
   (page 211)
1 teaspoon gf dry mustard
1/2 teaspoon dried thyme leaves
1/2 teaspoon salt
1 tablespoon gf tamari soy sauce
1/2 teaspoon black pepper
Paprika for garnish

Grilled Pineapple Slices
8 pineapple slices (16 oz. can)
1 teaspoon cooking oil

Oriental Sauce: Combine all ingredients in small saucepan. Bring to boil over medium heat, reduce to low and simmer until liquid is reduced by half. Just before serving, stir 1/2 teaspoon cornstarch with 1 tablespoon water until smooth. Add to sauce, stirring until mixture thickens slightly. Set aside.

Tuna Burgers: While sauce cooks, grind tuna in food processor (if not already ground.) (You can also use 3 cans—6 oz. each—of tuna in spring water, drained.) Combine with burger ingredients and shape into 4 patties. In a large cast-iron skillet, a nonstick skillet, or a barbecue grill, cook tuna burgers on both sides. Serve burgers with sauce and pineapple slices. Garnish with dash of paprika.

Grilled Pineapple Slices: Coat pineapple slices with oil. Then grill for 3-5 minutes, turning when grill marks are visible on underside. Handle carefully so slices don't slip through grate or use metal basket specially designed for grilling. Serves 4.

Tuna Burgers & Pineapple Slices   Exchanges

Calories	Fat	% Fat Cal	Protein	Carb	Chol	Sodium	Fiber	Carb	Meat	Fat
390	9g	21%	33g	44g	96mg	999mg	2g	2.5	3.5	1

Pineapple Slices only   Exchanges

Calories	Fat	% Fat Cal	Protein	Carb	Chol	Sodium	Fiber	Carb	Meat	Fat
251	3g	11%	2	59g	51mg	51mg	3g	4		1

Walnut Shrimp Salad

(can be made without wheat, gluten, eggs, or sugar - see page xi about ingredients)

This fabulous dish is best eaten immediately after it's prepared. Unfortunately, the dish loses a lot of flavor without the sour cream, so . . . it is not dairy-free.

2 pounds medium shrimp
(peeled, cooked)
1 tablespoon gf tamari soy sauce
1 cup walnut halves
1 cup diagonally sliced celery
1/2 cup green onions, sliced diagonally
1 can (8 oz.) water chestnuts, sliced

1 cup mandarin oranges, drained
6 red-leaf lettuce leaves
1 cup gf sour cream
2 tablespoons apple cider vinegar
1/2 teaspoon salt
paprika for garnish

Toss shrimp with soy sauce. Add walnuts, celery, onions, oranges, and water chestnuts and mix well. Arrange on 6 serving plates lined with lettuce leaves.

To make dressing, combine sour cream, vinegar, and salt. Drizzle over each salad plate. Garnish with paprika. Serves 6.

Calories	Fat	% Fat Cal	Protein	Carb	Chol	Sodium	Fiber	Exchanges		
								Carb	Meat	Fat
361	22g	53%	28g	15g	232mg	653mg	3g		3.5	3.5

Lamb Chops with Rosemary Marinade

(can be made without wheat, gluten, dairy, eggs, or sugar - see page xi about ingredients)

3 pounds lamb chops (1/2-inch thick)
3/4 cup fresh orange or pineapple juice
2 tablespoons olive oil
3 tablespoons gf tamari soy sauce
2 teaspoons crushed dried rosemary or
2 tablespoons minced fresh rosemary

1/4 teaspoon cayenne pepper
1/4 teaspoon salt
1/8 teaspoon black pepper
1 teaspoon cornstarch or arrowroot
2 teaspoons water

Arrange chops in single layer in shallow glass dish. Combine remaining ingredients (except cornstarch and water) and pour over chops. Cover and refrigerate 4 hours.

Grill lamb chops over grill or on a ridged skillet until desired doneness.

Meanwhile, in a small saucepan over medium heat, bring the remaining marinade to a boil. Reduce heat to medium. Stir cornstarch into water to form paste. Stir mixture into heated marinade, whisking until mixture thickens. Serve lamb chops with thickened marinade. Serves 4.

Calories	Fat	% Fat Cal	Protein	Carb	Chol	Sodium	Fiber	Exchanges		
								Carb	Meat	Fat
563	30g	50%	60g	8g	200mg	880mg	.5	.5	8.5	1

Chorizo

(can be made without wheat, gluten, dairy, eggs, or sugar - see page xi about ingredients)

Boldly flavored, chorizo is the Mexican version of sausage.

1 **pound ground round**
2 **pounds ground pork**
1 **tablespoon paprika**
1/3 **cup apple cider vinegar**
1 **teaspoon salt**
1 **teaspoon crushed red peppers**

2 **teaspoons dried oregano leaves**
3 **garlic cloves, minced**
1 **teaspoon ground coriander**
1 **teaspoon ground cumin**
1/2 **teaspoon ground cloves**
Cooking spray

In large bowl, mix ground meats together. Add remaining ingredients. Mix thoroughly, using spatula or your hands. Shape into large ball or log and chill.
Shape meat mixture into patties, 1/2-inch thick and two inches in diameter. (For link sausage, shape into links about 3 inches long and 3/4-inch wide.
In non-stick pan coated with cooking spray, fry patties until nicely browned on both sides. Freeze for up to 2 weeks. Makes 12 patties, depending on size.

| | | | | | | | | Exchanges | | |
Calories	Fat	% Fat Cal	Protein	Carb	Chol	Sodium	Fiber	Carb	Meat	Fat
230	15g	59%	22g	1g	64mg	260mg	<1g		3	1

Sausage

(can be made without wheat, gluten, dairy, eggs, or sugar - see page xi about ingredients)

Shape this sausage into meatballs, bake, and freeze. For crumbled sausage, simply brown loose meat in skillet.

1 **pound ground round**
1 **pound ground pork**
1 **pound ground turkey**
4 **garlic cloves, minced**
6 **green onions or 1/2 cup finely chopped yellow onion**
1/2 **cup finely minced green bell pepper**
1/2 **cup finely minced red bell pepper**

2 **teaspoons chopped fresh cilantro**
2 **teaspoons ground cumin**
2 **teaspoons dried thyme leaves**
2 **teaspoons fennel seed**
1/4 **teaspoon ground nutmeg**
1/2 **teaspoon crushed red peppers**
1 **teaspoon salt**
Cooking spray

In large bowl, mix together all ingredients with your hands or large spatula. Shape meat into large ball or log. Refrigerate for 4 hours. Shape mixture in patties or meatballs. Brown on baking sheet in 350° oven for 20-25 minutes. Serves 12.

| | | | | | | | | Exchanges | | |
Calories	Fat	% Fat Cal	Protein	Carb	Chol	Sodium	Fiber	Carb	Meat	Fat
215	13g	54%	22g	2g	66mg	270mg	.5g		3	1

Corned Beef & Cabbage

(can be made without wheat, gluten, dairy, eggs, or sugar - see page xi about ingredients)

On a recent trip to Ireland, I couldn't find this dish on Irish menus. The reason? It's like our turkey dinners at Thanksgiving—reserved for special occasions only. But, it sure makes a great St. Patrick's Day dinner. Serve this with Colcannon (page 184) and Irish Griddle Cakes (page 68).

1 **lean corned beef brisket (4 pounds)**	2 **garlic cloves, peeled**
2 **medium onions, peeled**	16 **small new red potatoes, scrubbed**
6 **whole cloves**	1 **small head cabbage, quartered**
4 **whole allspice berries**	1 **3-inch strip orange peel**
6 **whole black peppercorns**	1/2 **cup chopped fresh parsley**
1/2 **teaspoon whole mustard seeds**	**Salt and pepper to taste**
Water to cover beef	**Cooking spray**
1 **pound carrots (peeled, 2-inch pieces)**	**Additional fresh parsley for garnish**

Wash and pat beef dry. Place in large ovenproof casserole dish that has been sprayed with cooking spray. Add onions, cloves, allspice, peppercorns, and mustard seeds. Cover with water and bake, covered, in 325° oven for about 3 hours, or until meat is tender. Remove beef and keep warm.

Strain the liquid and discard the solids. Return beef and liquid to casserole dish along with remaining ingredients. Cover and bake for another 30-45 minutes, or until vegetables are fork-tender.

Place beef on serving platter, surrounded by cooked vegetables. Garnish with additional fresh parsley. Strain liquid, ladle some over platter, and serve remainder in a gravy boat. Serve with your favorite sauces or condiments. Serves 8.

| | | | | | | | | Exchanges | | |
Calories	Fat	% Fat Cal	Protein	Carb	Chol	Sodium	Fiber	Carb	Meat	Fat
563	34g	55%	37g	25g	122mg	362mg	7g	.5	5	4

Orange Beef Stir Fry

(can be made without wheat, gluten, dairy, eggs, or sugar - see page xi about ingredients)

Looking for a change of pace for your next dinner? This dish is different, easy to prepare, and looks great on your plate. Your family and your guests will love it.

1 cup fresh orange juice	1 tablespoon cooking oil
1/4 cup grated orange peel	1 large garlic clove, minced
1 tablespoon molasses (cane or sorghum)	1 tablespoon grated fresh ginger
1/4 cup gf tamari soy sauce	1/2 teaspoon crushed red peppers
1 tablespoon rice vinegar	1/2 pound broccoli florets, sliced
2 tablespoons cornstarch or arrowroot	1 small red bell pepper, chopped
1 pound lean beef (cut in 1/4-inch diagonal slices)	1/2 cup sliced green onions
	4 cups hot cooked white rice

Combine orange juice, orange peel, molasses, soy sauce, rice vinegar, and cornstarch and set aside.

Slice beef diagonally into 1/4-inch thick slices. (For easier slicing, freeze meat for 30 minutes before slicing). In large, heavy skillet or wok, brown meat in oil until lightly seared and no longer pink. Remove from pan and keep warm.

In same pan, add garlic, ginger, crushed red peppers, broccoli florets, and red bell pepper and stir over medium heat for 1 minute. Cover and cook for 1 more minute. Remove cover and add orange juice mixture to pan, stirring until mixture thickens. Return beef to pan, add chopped green onions, and bring to serving temperature. Serve over rice. Serves 4.

Exchanges

Calories	Fat	% Fat Cal	Protein	Carb	Chol	Sodium	Fiber	Carb	Meat	Fat
500	10g	18%	35g	67g	77mg	999mg	4g	.5	3.5	1.5

Rice contributes 44g of total 67g of carbohydrates per serving.

Spaghetti Sauce & Meatballs

(can be made without wheat, gluten, dairy, eggs, or refined sugar - see page xi about ingredients)

I've been making this low-fat sauce for nearly 25 years and, even though we've tried several others, it remains our favorite. A crock pot works best.

1 can (48 oz.) tomato juice	1 teaspoon black pepper
3 cans (6 oz. each) gf tomato paste	3 tablespoons sugar or
3 tablespoons dried parsley	1 1/2 tablespoons honey
2 tablespoons dried basil leaves	2 teaspoons salt
1 tablespoon dried rosemary leaves	1/4 cup Romano or Parmesan
2 bay leaves	cheese (optional)
2 teaspoons dried oregano leaves	1/2 pound Sausage meatballs (page 47)

In large crock pot, combine all ingredients. Mix well. Cook all day on low-medium heat. Or, cook in large pot on stovetop all day. Stir occasionally. Makes about 8 cups of sauce. Serve with meatballs and your favorite pasta. Serves 12 (3/4 cup each).

								Exchanges		
Calories	Fat	% Fat Cal	Protein	Carb	Chol	Sodium	Fiber	Carb	Meat	Fat
118	5g	31%	5g	17g	9mg	553mg	3g	.5	.5	1

Fresh Tomato Basil Sauce with Pasta

(can be made without wheat, gluten, dairy, eggs, or sugar - see page xi about ingredients)

Choose the most flavorful tomatoes you can find for this easy, fresh-tasting sauce.

4 cups plum tomatoes	1/2 cup chopped fresh basil, packed
2 large garlic cloves, minced	or 2 tablespoons dried basil
1/4 cup extra virgin olive oil, divided	4 cups hot cooked pasta
1/2 teaspoon salt	1/4 cup Parmesan cheese for garnish
1/4 teaspoon black pepper	

Dip tomatoes in boiling water, then peel. Quarter and seed each tomato.

In large bowl, crush tomatoes with potato masher. Drain again and reserve juice for another use.

In medium-sized, non-reactive pan sauté garlic in 1 tablespoon oil for 2 minutes. Add tomatoes, salt, pepper, basil, and remaining oil. Simmer gently for 15 minutes, uncovered. Serve with pasta and Parmesan cheese. Serves 4.

								Exchanges		
Calories	Fat	% Fat Cal	Protein	Carb	Chol	Sodium	Fiber	Carb	Meat	Fat
190	16g	72%	4g	9g	5mg	423mg	2g	2	.5	3

Pad Thai

(can be made without wheat, gluten, dairy, eggs, or sugar - see page xi about ingredients)

This dish sounds difficult, but it's actually quite easy. Egg-sensitive people can simply omit the eggs. To julienne means to cut into thin, matchstick shapes.

8 ounces rice noodles, uncooked
2 quarts water
2 teaspoons salt
1/4 cup fresh lemon or lime juice
1 tablespoon gf fish sauce (optional)
1/4 cup gf tamari soy sauce
1 tablespoon brown sugar
   or maple sugar
1/4 teaspoon crushed red peppers
1 tablespoon sesame oil or olive oil

1 pound shrimp (peeled, de-veined)
1 cup snow peas
1/4 cup red bell pepper, julienne
1/2 cup green onions
2 large garlic cloves, minced
2 large eggs, lightly beaten
   (optional)
2 cups bean sprouts
1/4 cup cashews
1/2 cup fresh cilantro, divided

This dish cooks quickly, so have all ingredients assembled beforehand. Cook rice noodles in boiling water with 2 teaspoons salt. Drain thoroughly.

Meanwhile, while noodles are cooking combine lemon juice, fish sauce, soy sauce, sugar, and crushed red peppers. Set aside.

Heat oil in wok or heavy skillet. Sauté shrimp, snow peas, red bell pepper, green onions, and garlic cloves for 2-4 minutes over medium heat until shrimp turn pink. Add eggs, if using, and continue stirring until eggs are cooked. Add cooked noodles and lemon juice mixture and heat, stirring constantly, for another 2-3 minutes.

Just before serving, stir in bean sprouts, cashews, and half of the cilantro. Garnish with additional nuts and remaining cilantro, if desired. Serves 4.

Exchanges

Calories	Fat	% Fat Cal	Protein	Carb	Chol	Sodium	Fiber	Carb	Meat	Fat
294	10g	31%	26g	26g	240mg	999mg	3g	2	3	2

Veal (Pork) Scaloppini

(can be made without wheat, gluten, dairy, eggs, or sugar - see page xi about ingredients)

For a dairy-free version, omit butter and use 1/2 teaspoon arrowroot mixed in 2 teaspoons water to form paste. Stir into reduced liquid until mixture thickens slightly.

4 veal or pork cutlets (1 1/4 pound)
Salt and pepper to taste
2 tablespoons olive oil
2 tablespoons fresh lemon juice
1/2 cup chicken broth
  or gf white wine

2 tablespoons unsalted butter or oleo
2 tablespoons gf capers (packed in salt
  or salt brine, not vinegar)
1 tablespoon dried parsley or 1/4 cup
  chopped fresh parsley
1/8 teaspoon ground nutmeg

Season veal (or pork) with salt and pepper. (If using pork cutlets, pound to 1/4-inch thickness.) In large, heavy skillet brown meat in batches in the oil—about 2 minutes on each side. Remove meat from skillet, but keep warm.

Increase heat to high and add lemon juice and broth to skillet. Continue cooking until reduced by half. Add chilled butter and whisk until thoroughly melted. Or, use arrowroot mixture (see note above.) Add capers, parsley, and nutmeg and serve over meat. Serves 4.

| | | | | | | | | Exchanges | | |
Calories	Fat	% Fat Cal	Protein	Carb	Chol	Sodium	Fiber	Carb	Meat	Fat
238	18g	69%	17g	1g	64mg	234mg	.5		2.5	3

Pasta Salad

(can be made without wheat, gluten, dairy, eggs, or sugar - see page xi about ingredients)

For a heartier dish suitable for an entrée, simply add your favorite meat such as cooked shrimp or diced, cooked chicken. I prefer using fusilli style pasta by Pastariso.

2 cups pasta of choice, uncooked
1/4 cup red wine vinegar
2 tablespoons fresh lemon juice
1 teaspoon Dijonnaise mustard
1 tablespoon dried basil leaves
1 small garlic clove, minced
1/4 teaspoon each salt and white pepper

1/4 cup olive oil
1 cup snow peas, blanched
1 cup broccoli flowerets, blanched
1 small red bell pepper
1/4 cup black olives, halved
1/4 cup toasted pine nuts
1/4 cup Parmesan cheese (optional)

Cook pasta in boiling, salted water until desired degree of doneness. Drain; chill. Meanwhile, whisk together vinegar, lemon juice, mustard, basil, garlic, salt, pepper, and olive oil. Combine remaining ingredients in large bowl. Add cooked pasta. Toss with dressing to taste. Chill. Serves 4.

| | | | | | | | | Exchanges | | |
Calories	Fat	% Fat Cal	Protein	Carb	Chol	Sodium	Fiber	Carb	Meat	Fat
494	22g	40%	10g	65g	5mg	402mg	2.5g	3	1	4

Pizza Crust & Pizza Sauce

(can be made without wheat, gluten, dairy, eggs, or sugar - see page xi about ingredients)

This is one of the most often requested recipes from my cookbooks. It has received national acclaim, appeared in several national magazines, and is the recipe most people mention when they refer to my books. I've changed it a little from the previous books by omitting the dry milk powder. The crust is now totally dairy-free.

Pizza Crust
1 tablespoon gf active dry yeast
2/3 cup brown rice flour or
    garbfava flour
1/2 cup + 2 tablespoons tapioca flour
2 teaspoons xanthan gum
1/2 teaspoon salt
1 teaspoon unflavored gelatin powder
1 teaspoon Italian seasoning
2/3 cup warm milk (105°)
    (cow, rice, soy)
1/2 teaspoon sugar or honey
1 teaspoon olive oil
1 teaspoon cider vinegar
Cooking spray
Extra rice flour for sprinkling

Pizza Sauce
8 ounces gf tomato sauce or use
    recipe on page 216
1/2 teaspoon dried oregano leaves
1/2 teaspoon dried basil leaves
1/2 teaspoon crushed dried
    rosemary leaves
1/2 teaspoon fennel seeds
1/4 teaspoon gf garlic powder
2 teaspoons sugar or 1 teaspoon
    honey
1/2 teaspoon salt
Toppings of your choice

Sauce: Combine all ingredients in small saucepan and bring to boil over medium heat. Reduce heat to low and simmer for 15 minutes, while Pizza Crust is being assembled. Makes about 1 cup.

Crust: Preheat oven to 425°. In medium mixer bowl using regular beaters (not dough hooks), blend the yeast, flours, xanthan gum, salt, gelatin powder, and Italian seasoning on low speed. Add warm milk, sugar, oil, and vinegar.

Beat on high speed for 3 minutes. (If the mixer bounces around the bowl, the dough is too stiff. Add water if necessary, one tablespoon at a time, until dough does not resist beaters.) The dough will resemble soft bread dough. (You may also mix in bread machine on dough setting.)

Put mixture on 12-inch pizza pan or baking sheet (for thin, crispy crust), 11 x 7-inch pan (for deep-dish version) that has been coated with cooking spray. Liberally sprinkle rice flour onto dough, then press dough into pan, continuing to sprinkle dough with flour to prevent sticking to your hands. Make edges thicker to hold the toppings.

Bake pizza crust for 10 minutes. Remove from oven. Top Pizza Crust with sauce and your preferred toppings. Bake for another 20-25 minutes or until top is nicely browned. Serves 6 (1 slice per serving).

| | | | | | | | | Exchanges | | |
Calories	Fat	% Fat Cal	Protein	Carb	Chol	Sodium	Fiber	Carb	Meat	Fat
153	1.5g	9%	4g	33g	1mg	635mg	3g	1.5		

Spice Rub for Meat

(can be made without wheat, gluten, dairy, eggs, or sugar - see page xi about ingredients)

Spice rubs are one of the hottest food trends of the 90's. This is a great one to keep on hand. When I'm not sure about what to fix for dinner, I simply sprinkle this on the meat we're having and presto— we have flavor!

1 tablespoon paprika	3/4 teaspoon gf onion powder
1 teaspoon gf garlic powder	1/2 teaspoon dried oregano leaves
1 teaspoon salt	1/2 teaspoon dried thyme leaves
3/4 teaspoon black pepper	1/8 teaspoon ground allspice
1/4 teaspoon cayenne pepper	

Combine in glass, airtight container. Use about 2 tablespoons per pound of meat. Store in dark, dry place for up to 1 month. Makes less than 1/4 cup.

Spicy Fettuccini with Basil

(can be made without wheat, gluten, dairy, eggs, or sugar - see page xi about ingredients)

So very simple to make and so impressive and tasty. The perfect entrée for a meatless meal. If you absolutely must have meat, try adding shrimp or cubed chicken.

1/2 cup extra virgin olive oil	1/3 cup gf Italian bread crumbs
2 large garlic cloves, minced	(toasted)
1/2 teaspoon crushed red peppers	1/2 cup grated Parmesan cheese
3 cups gf fettuccini, uncooked	(cow, rice, soy)
6 quarts boiling, salted water	4 plum tomatoes, finely chopped
1/2 cup chopped fresh basil, firmly	1 lemon cut into 4 wedges
packed or 2 teaspoons dried basil	1/4 cup chopped fresh parsley

Heat 1 tablespoon of oil in medium skillet over low heat. Sauté garlic and crushed red peppers for 2-3 minutes, stirring frequently. Set aside.

Cook pasta in 6 quarts boiling, salted water until al dente—about 2-3 minutes. Drain, leaving 1/3 cup hot water in pot. Return pasta to pot; remove pot from heat. Add garlic-pepper mixture, remaining oil, basil, bread crumbs, and Parmesan cheese and toss gently. Garnish with chopped tomatoes, parsley, and a squeeze of fresh lemon juice. Serve immediately. Serves 4.

								Exchanges		
Calories	Fat	% Fat Cal	Protein	Carb	Chol	Sodium	Fiber	Carb	Meat	Fat
500	32g	56%	8g	47g	10mg	333mg	3g	3.5	1	6

Asparagus Soup

(can be made without wheat, gluten, dairy, eggs, or sugar - see page xi about ingredients)

Spring-time green, smooth, and creamy—a wonderful choice for a spring luncheon.

1 1/2 pounds fresh asparagus spears
1 small onion, finely chopped
1 large garlic clove or 1/2 teaspoon
  gf garlic powder
1 large peeled carrot (1-inch pieces)
6 large basil leaves or 1/2 teaspoon
  dried basil leaves
1 tablespoon chopped fresh tarragon
  or 1 teaspoon dried tarragon leaves
1 tablespoon chopped fresh parsley or
  1 teaspoon dried parsley

1 teaspoon chopped fresh thyme
  or 1/2 teaspoon dried thyme
1/2 teaspoon salt
1/4 teaspoon black pepper
1/8 teaspoon cayenne pepper
3 cups low-sodium chicken broth
1/2 cup sour cream or puréed
  soft silken tofu
1/4 teaspoon paprika for garnish

Wash and trim woody ends from asparagus. Cut the stalks into 1-inch pieces. Reserve the tips, which will be added later.

Place all ingredients (except sour cream, if using, asparagus tips, and paprika) in heavy, large saucepan and cook, covered tightly, for 30-40 minutes or until vegetables are done. Remove soup from heat and cool.

Place mixture in food processor and process until very smooth. Strain soup through a medium-size sieve to remove woody fibers.

Return soup to saucepan and add asparagus tips. Simmer until tips are done, about 10 minutes. Just before serving, stir in all but 2 tablespoons of sour cream (if using) and heat to serving to serving temperature.

To serve, ladle soup into serving bowls. Top with a dollop of the remaining sour cream or tofu and a sprinkle of paprika. Serves 4.

								Exchanges		
Calories	Fat	% Fat Cal	Protein	Carb	Chol	Sodium	Fiber	Carb	Meat	Fat
100	3g	24%	8g	13g	0mg	999mg	4g	2.5		

Sour cream adds additional 45 calories, 12mg cholesterol, and 5g fat.

Chinese Hot-Sour Soup

(can be made without wheat, gluten, dairy, eggs, or sugar - see page xi about ingredients)

If you don't use the egg, the soup might not be quite as thick. But it will still be delicious. To julienne means to cut into thin matchsticks.

4 cups low sodium beef broth	1/2 cup tofu, cut in 1/4-inch cubes
2 green onions, thinly sliced	1 cup turkey dark meat, diced
1 small carrot, julienne	1/8 teaspoon cayenne pepper
1 tablespoon grated fresh ginger	1 teaspoon fish sauce (optional)
1/2 teaspoon white pepper	1 tablespoon cornstarch or arrowroot
1 teaspoon cooking oil	2 tablespoons rice vinegar
1 cup fresh, sliced shitaki mushrooms	1 egg white, well-beaten (optional)

In large saucepan, combine beef broth, green onions (reserve 2 tablespoons for garnish), carrot, ginger, and white pepper. Bring to boil over high heat, simmering for 15 minutes.

In a medium skillet, sauté mushrooms in cooking oil over high heat for about 1 minute. To beef stock, add mushrooms plus tofu, turkey meat, cayenne, and fish sauce (if using).

In small bowl, dissolve cornstarch in vinegar. Add to the soup and stir until thickened, about 1 minute.

Remove soup from heat and, stirring constantly, slowly pour in the beaten egg white (if using). Cook until egg is done. Taste and adjust seasonings, adding more vinegar or white pepper. Ladle soup into four serving bowls. Garnish with sliced green onions. Serves 4.

Exchanges

Calories	Fat	% Fat Cal	Protein	Carb	Chol	Sodium	Fiber	Carb	Meat	Fat
154	5g	27%	17g	12g	30mg	999mg	2g	3	.5	1

Colorado Chili

(can be made without wheat, gluten, dairy, eggs, or sugar - see page xi about ingredients)

Cook in a crock pot and let guests help themselves as they wish. If the chili thickens too much as it cooks, add a bit of water.

1 pound ground round
1 cup finely chopped onions
1 can (15 oz.) pinto or kidney beans, undrained
1 can (15 oz) canned tomatoes, undrained
2 teaspoons chili powder

1/2 teaspoon ground allspice
1/2 teaspoon ground cumin
1/2 teaspoon ground coriander
1/4 teaspoon ground cloves
1/4 teaspoon ground cinnamon
1 teaspoon salt

In large Dutch oven or skillet, combine ground round and chopped onion. Brown over medium heat. Add remaining ingredients, cover, and simmer on low for 2 hours. Or, cook in crock pot 4-6 hours. Serve with crackers and various garnishes—green onions, shredded cheese, chopped cilantro. Serves 6.

								Exchanges		
Calories	Fat	% Fat Cal	Protein	Carb	Chol	Sodium	Fiber	Carb	Meat	Fat
210	7g	31g	20%	16g	28mg	466mg	5g	1	2	.5

Green Chile Stew

(can be made without wheat, gluten, dairy, eggs, or sugar - see page xi about ingredients)

This is one of the most common dishes we find on menus when we visit Santa Fe—one of our favorite cities. For easy entertaining, cook and serve this in a crock pot.

1 pound lean pork (1-inch pieces)
1/2 cup chopped onion
2 carrots, cut in 1/2-inch pieces
1 tablespoon olive oil
1 can (4 oz.) diced green chiles or 1/3 cup diced fresh green chiles
3 cups low-sodium beef broth
2 medium white potatoes, diced

4 plum tomatoes, diced
1 large garlic clove, minced
1/2 teaspoon ground cumin
1/2 teaspoon ground coriander
1/2 teaspoon dried oregano leaves
1/2 teaspoon salt
1/4 teaspoon black pepper
1/2 cup chopped fresh cilantro, packed

In heavy Dutch oven, brown pork, onion, and carrots in olive oil over medium heat until lightly browned. Add remaining ingredients (except cilantro) and simmer, covered, for one hour. Alternatively, transfer mixture to a slow cooker (crock pot) and simmer all day on low. Add cilantro just before serving. Serves 4.

								Exchanges		
Calories	Fat	% Fat Cal	Protein	Carb	Chol	Sodium	Fiber	Carb	Meat	Fat
340	16g	41%	26g	25g	72mg	480mg	4g	2.5	4	2.5

Notes

Breads

Hearty, flavorful breads complement any meal. They add wonderful flavor, help "fill you up", and provide a very important tactile element (they're fun to chew). Think of breads as the "rising stars" at any meal.

Many of you have asked for gluten-free breads that also contain no dairy or eggs. So . . . I'm happy to introduce a new set of bread recipes in this section. Some are yeast-leavened; others are quick breads that use baking soda or baking powder (or a combination of cream of tartar and baking soda).

You'll notice that the egg-free, dairy-free yeast breads are considerably heavier, more dense, and won't rise as high as those containing eggs. In fact, these breads are remarkably similar to the heavy breads I ate in Germany before my wheat-free days. They're still wonderful, just heavier and chewier. I think you'll like them.

Easy directions for each gluten-free recipe show you how to make the bread with or without eggs and milk—so you leave out only the ingredients you don't want. Enjoy!

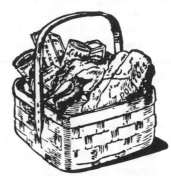

For additional breads without wheat, gluten, or dairy see ***Wheat-Free Recipes & Menus: Delicious Dining Without Wheat or Gluten, 1997***. For additional wheat and gluten-free bread recipes that can also be made without eggs, sugar, or yeast see ***Special Diet Solutions: Healthy Cooking Without Wheat, Gluten, Dairy, Eggs, Yeast, or Refined Sugar, 1998***. Both books are published by Savory Palate, Inc.

"Cracked Wheat" Bread

(can be made without wheat, gluten, dairy, eggs, or sugar - see page xi about ingredients)

Cracked Wehani rice (by Lundberg) or brown rice imitate the texture of whole wheat bread. Place rice in a blender or coffee grinder and whirl until kernels are 1/4 to 1/3 their original size. If you use tofu in place of eggs, bread will be heavy and dense—much like some European breads. Jowar flour and soy milk are best (see Mail-Order Sources).

Ingredients	1 lb.	1 1/2 to 2 lb.
	Serves 10	Serves 16
Gf active dry yeast (hand)	1 1/2 tablespoons	2 1/4 tablespoons
(machine)	1 1/2 teaspoons	2 1/4 teaspoons
Jowar flour or brown rice flour	1 3/4 cups	2 1/4 cups
Potato starch	1/2 cup	3/4 cup
Tapioca flour	1/4 cup	1/3 cup
Wehani or brown rice, cracked	1/4 cup	1/3 cup
Xanthan gum	1 teaspoon	1 1/2 teaspoons
Salt	1 teaspoon	1 1/2 teaspoons
Brown sugar or maple sugar	1 tablespoon	2 tablespoons
Ener-G® egg replacer	1 teaspoon	1 1/2 teaspoons
Eggs	2 large eggs or 1/2 cup soft silken tofu	3 large eggs or 3/4 cup soft silken tofu
Butter (melted) or cooking oil	3 tablespoons	1/3 cup
Apple cider vinegar	1 teaspoon	2 teaspoons
Milk (cow, rice, soy)	1 cup	1 1/2 cups
	Bake in three 5x3-inch pans or one 9x5-inch pan	Bake in five 5x3-inch pans or two 8x4-inch pans

Hand: Combine yeast, 2 teaspoons of the sugar, and the warmed milk (105°) and set aside to let yeast foam for 5 minutes.

In large mixer bowl using electric beaters (not dough hooks), combine flours, cracked rice, xanthan gum, salt, remainder of sugar, and egg replacer. In separate bowl, cream together eggs (or tofu), butter (or oil), and vinegar until very smooth.

With mixer on low speed, add egg mixture to dry ingredients and blend. Add yeast-milk mixture, increase speed to high and beat for full 2 minutes.

Coat pans with cooking spray. Divide dough among pans. Rise in warm place—small pans 35-40 minutes; large pans 45-60 minutes—or until doubled.

Preheat oven to 350°. Bake small loaves for 25-30 minutes; large loaves for 40-50 minutes—or until tops are nicely browned. Cool 5 minutes in pan. Remove from pan; cool on wire rack.

Machine: Spray pan with cooking spray. Have ingredients at room temperature. Add ingredients in order listed by manufacturer. Set controls and bake.

								Exchanges		
Calories	Fat	% Fat Cal	Protein	Carb	Chol	Sodium	Fiber	Carb	Meat	Fat
200	4g	18%	4g	38g	1mg	290mg	2g	1.5	0	.5

Eggs and butter add additional 52mg cholesterol per serving.

Focaccia

(can be made without wheat, gluten, dairy, eggs, or sugar - see page xi about ingredients)

This is a great bread because it is a success—no matter how it turns out.

Bread
3/4 cup warm water (105°)
1 teaspoon sugar or honey
2 large eggs*
2 tablespoons olive oil
1/2 teaspoon cider vinegar
1 1/2 teaspoons gf active dry yeast
1 cup brown rice flour or garbfava flour
1/2 cup tapioca flour
1 teaspoon unflavored gelatin powder

1 1/2 teaspoons xanthan gum
1 teaspoon dried rosemary leaves
1/2 teaspoon gf onion powder
3/4 teaspoon salt
Topping
1 1/4 teaspoons Italian Seasoning
1/4 teaspoon salt
1 tablespoon olive oil
Cooking spray
Parmesan cheese (cow, rice, soy)

Bread: Combine warm water, sugar (or honey), eggs (or tofu—see Focaccia without Eggs below), oil, and vinegar in medium mixer bowl. Beat dough with mixer (using regular beaters, not dough hooks) until very, very smooth. Add yeast, flours, gelatin powder, xanthan gum, rosemary, onion powder, and salt. Beat for 2 minutes. The dough will be soft and sticky—like thick cake batter.

Transfer dough to 11 x 7-inch nonstick pan, 8-inch round nonstick pan, or 15 x 10-inch nonstick pan sprayed with cooking spray. Cover with aluminum foil and let rise in warm place for 30 minutes or until desired height.

Topping: Preheat oven to 400°. Sprinkle Focaccia with Italian seasoning, salt, and oil (or to taste). Bake for 15 minutes or until golden brown. You may drizzle additional olive oil on baked Focaccia. (A sprinkle of Parmesan cheese is optional.) Makes 8-inch or 11 x 7-inch or 15 x 10-inch loaf. Serves 6.

Focaccia without Eggs: Omit eggs. Use 1/2 cup soft silken tofu.

| | | | | | | | | Exchanges | | |
Calories	Fat	% Fat Cal	Protein	Carb	Chol	Sodium	Fiber	Carb	Meat	Fat
215	8g	33%	4g	32g	20mg	396mg	3g	1.5	.5	1.5

Eggs add additional 42mg cholesterol per serving.

Additional Toppings

Herb Focaccia: Combine 1/2 teaspoon dried rosemary, 1/2 teaspoon dried sage, 1/2 teaspoon dried thyme, 1/4 teaspoon black pepper, and 2 tablespoons Parmesan cheese (cow, rice, soy).

Sun-Dried Tomato & Olive Focaccia: Sauté 1/4 cup chopped sun-dried tomatoes, 1/4 cup sliced black olives, and 1/4 cup chopped onion in 1 teaspoon oil.

Pesto Focaccia: Purée the following in food processor just until smooth, leaving a bit of texture: 1 cup fresh basil leaves, 1 garlic clove, 1/2 cup pine nuts. With motor running, slowly add 1/4 cup olive oil through feed tube. Add 1/4 cup Parmesan cheese (cow, rice, soy) and dash of freshly ground black pepper.

French Bread

(can be made without wheat, gluten, dairy, eggs, or sugar - see page xi about ingredients)

French bread is a typical accompaniment to a pasta meal. This one is so easy—and it can be ready in a little over an hour. Double the recipe to make two loaves.

1 1/2 teaspoons gf active dry yeast
1 teaspoon sugar or honey
1 cup warm (105°) milk (cow, rice, soy)
1 teaspoon cornmeal for pan (optional)
1/4 cup soft silken tofu
2 tablespoons melted butter or cooking oil
1 teaspoon apple cider vinegar

1 3/4 cups brown or
   white rice flour
1/2 cup potato starch
1/3 cup tapioca flour
1 teaspoon xanthan gum
1/4 teaspoon soy lecithin
1 teaspoon salt
Cooking spray

Dissolve the yeast and sugar (or honey) in the warm milk. Set aside to foam for 5 minutes.

Coat baking pan or cookie sheet or French-loaf shaped pan with cooking spray. Lightly dust with cornmeal, if desired.

In bowl of food processor, purée the yeast mixture along with the tofu, butter (or oil), and vinegar until very, very smooth. Add flours, xanthan gum, soy lecithin, and salt. Blend until thoroughly mixed. Mixture will be stiff.

Spoon onto prepared pan, smoothing the top of the dough with a spatula. Cover and let rise in a warm place until doubled in bulk, about 30-40 minutes. Spray with oil (or brush with milk) for a glossier shine. (An egg wash made of beaten egg white makes the glossiest sheen, but only use this method if eggs are approved for your diet.)

Place bread in oven, turn heat to 425°. Bake for approximately 30 minutes, or until bread is nicely browned. Remove bread from pans and cool on wire rack. Cool thoroughly before slicing. Makes 1 loaf. Serves 12.

								Exchanges		
Calories	Fat	% Fat Cal	Protein	Carb	Chol	Sodium	Fiber	Carb	Meat	Fat
140	2g	13%	3g	28g	.5mg	229mg	1g	1		.5

Garlic French Bread: Spread slices of French Bread with a mixture of 1/2 cup softened butter, oleo, or canola oil spread and 1 garlic clove, minced. A tablespoon of butter adds 100 calories.

Italian Breadsticks

(can be made without wheat, gluten, dairy, eggs, or sugar - see page xi about ingredients)

Breadsticks are one of the easiest ways to serve bread at any meal. For an attractive presentation, stand the sticks on end in a decorative pitcher or container.

1 tablespoon gf active dry yeast
2/3 cup warm milk (105°)
  (cow, rice, soy)
1/2 teaspoon sugar or honey
1/2 cup brown rice flour
1/2 cup + 1 tablespoon tapioca flour
2 teaspoons xanthan gum
1/2 cup grated Parmesan cheese
  (cow, rice, soy)

1/2 teaspoon salt
1 teaspoon gf onion powder
1 teaspoon unflavored gelatin powder
1 tablespoon olive oil
1 teaspoon cider vinegar
1 large egg white, beaten to a foam*
1 teaspoon Italian Seasoning
Cooking spray

Combine yeast, warm milk, and sugar in a small bowl. Set aside for 5 minutes or until yeast is foamy.

Preheat oven to 400° for 5 minutes, then turn off.

In medium-size mixer bowl while oven is preheating, blend yeast-milk mixture, flours, xanthan gum, Parmesan cheese, salt, onion powder, gelatin, oil, and vinegar on low speed of electric mixer. Beat on high for 3 minutes. Dough will be soft and sticky.

Place dough in large, heavy-duty plastic freezer bag that has 1/2-inch opening cut diagonally on one corner. (This makes a 1-inch circle.) Coat a large baking sheet with cooking spray. Squeeze dough out of plastic bag onto sheet in 10 strips, each 1-inch wide by 6 inches long. For best results, hold bag of dough upright as you squeeze, rather than at an angle. Also, hold bag with corners perpendicular, rather than horizontal, to baking sheet for a more authentic-looking breadstick. Brush with beaten egg white for crispier, shinier breadstick. Then sprinkle with Italian Seasoning.

Place in warmed oven to rise for 20-30 minutes. Leaving breadsticks in oven, turn oven to 400° and bake until golden brown, about 15-20 minutes. Rotate cookie sheet halfway through baking to assure even browning. Cool on wire rack. Serves 10.

*Egg Alternative: Omit egg wash and spray with cooking spray of choice.

| | | | | | | | | Exchanges | | |
Calories	Fat	% Fat Cal	Protein	Carb	Chol	Sodium	Fiber	Carb	Meat	Fat
100	3g	27%	4g	15g	4mg	231mg	1.5g	.5	.5	.5

Pumpernickel Bread

(can be made without wheat, gluten, dairy, eggs, or sugar - see page xi about ingredients)

The tofu makes this bread fairly heavy and dense—similar to some European breads.

Ingredients	1 lb.	1 1/2 to 2 lb.
	Serves 10	Serves 16
Gf active dry yeast (hand)	1 1/2 tablespoons	2 1/4 tablespoons
(machine)	1 1/2 teaspoons	2 1/4 teaspoons
Jowar flour or brown rice flour	1 3/4 cups	2 cups
Potato starch	1/2 cup	3/4 cup
Tapioca flour	1/4 cup	1/3 cup
Xanthan gum	1 teaspoon	1 1/2 teaspoons
Salt	1 teaspoon	1 1/2 teaspoons
Brown sugar or maple sugar	1 tablespoons	1 1/2 tablespoons
Ener-G egg replacer	1 teaspoon	1 1/2 teaspoons
Caraway seeds	1 tablespoon	1 1/2 tablespoons
Unsweetened cocoa powder	1 tablespoon	1 1/2 tablespoons
Instant coffee powder	1 teaspoon	1 1/2 teaspoons
Gf onion powder	1/2 teaspoon	3/4 teaspoon
Eggs	2 large eggs or 1/2 cup soft silken tofu	3 large eggs or 3/4 cup soft silken tofu
Butter (melted) or cooking oil	2 tablespoons	3 tablespoons
Molasses (cane or sorghum)	2 tablespoons	3 tablespoons
Apple cider vinegar	1 teaspoon	1 1/2 teaspoons
Milk (cow, rice, soy)	1 cup	1 1/2 cups
	Bake in three 5x3-inch pans or one 9x5-inch pan	Bake in five 5x3-inch pans or two 8x4-inch pans

Hand: Combine yeast, warm milk 105°, and 2 teaspoons sugar in small bowl. Set aside to foam—about 5-10 minutes.

In large mixer bowl, combine remaining dry ingredients (including remaining brown sugar) and blend on low speed. With mixer on low, add eggs (or tofu), oil, molasses, and vinegar to dry mixture. Add yeast/milk mixture. Once liquid is incorporated, increase mixer speed to high and beat for full 2 minutes.

Coat pans with cooking spray. Divide dough among pans. Rise in warm place—small pans 35-40 minutes; large pans 45-60 minutes—or until doubled.

Preheat oven to 350°. Bake small loaves for 25-30 minutes; large loaves for 40-50 minutes.

Machine: Spray pan with cooking spray and have ingredients at room temperature. Add ingredients in order listed by manufacturer. Set controls and bake.

Exchanges

Calories	Fat	% Fat Cal	Protein	Carb	Chol	Sodium	Fiber	Carb	Meat	Fat
160	4g	24%	4g	27g	0mg	260mg	2g	1		1

Eggs and butter add additional 56mg cholesterol per serving.

Sandwich Bread

(can be made without wheat, gluten, dairy, eggs, or sugar - see page xi about ingredients)

This dairy-free, egg-free bread will remind you of heavy, European breads. This is typical of egg-free gluten-free breads since egg actually provides some additional leavening (and lightness). Jowar flour and soy milk produce the best results.

Ingredients	1 lb.	1 1/2 to 2 lb.
	Serves 10	Serves 16
Gf active dry yeast (hand) (machine)	1 1/2 tablespoons 1 1/2 teaspoons	2 1/4 tablespoons 2 1/4 teaspoons
Jowar flour or brown rice flour	1 3/4 cups	2 cups
Potato starch	1/2 cup	3/4 cup
Tapioca flour	1/4 cup	1/3 cup
Xanthan gum	1 teaspoon	1 1/2 teaspoons
Salt	1 teaspoon	1 1/2 teaspoons
Brown sugar or maple sugar	1 tablespoon	2 tablespoons
Ener-G® egg replacer	1 teaspoon	1 1/2 teaspoons
Eggs	2 large eggs or 1/2 cup soft silken tofu	3 large eggs or 3/4 cup soft silken tofu
Butter (melted) or cooking oil	3 tablespoons	1/4 cup
Apple cider vinegar	1 teaspoons	2 teaspoons
Milk (cow, rice, soy)	1 cup	1 1/2 cups
	Bake in three 5x3-inch pans or one 9x5-inch pan	Bake in five 5x3-inch pans or two 8x4-inch pans

Hand: Have all ingredients at room temperature. Combine yeast, 2 teaspoons of the sugar (or all of the honey), and milk (105°). Set aside for 5 minutes.

In large mixer bowl using regular beaters (not dough hooks), combine flours, xanthan gum, salt, remainder of sugar, and egg replacer. Add eggs (or tofu), melted butter (or oil), vinegar, and yeast mixture.

Mix ingredients together on low speed until liquid is incorporated, then increase mixer speed to high and beat for 2 minutes—or until mixture is very smooth. Occasionally, scrape sides of bowl with spatula.

Coat pans with cooking spray. Divide dough among pans. Rise in warm place—small pans 35-40 minutes; large pans 45-60 minutes—or until doubled.

Preheat oven to 350°. Bake small loaves for 25-30 minutes; large loaves for 40-50 minutes—or until tops are nicely browned. Cool 5 minutes in pan. Remove from pan; cool on wire rack.

Machine: Spray pan with cooking spray. Have all ingredients at room temperature. Add ingredients in order listed by manufacturer. Set controls and bake.

								Exchanges		
Calories	Fat	% Fat Cal	Protein	Carb	Chol	Sodium	Fiber	Carb	Meat	Fat
180	3.5g	17%	3.5g	35g	1mg	290mg	1g	1.5		.5

Eggs and butter add additional 56mg cholesterol per serving.

Bacon Onion Muffins

(can be made without wheat, gluten, dairy, eggs, or sugar - see page xi about ingredients)

I often brown a pound of bacon at a time and freeze the strips. They defrost quickly in the microwave. Then you have bacon ready to be used at a moment's notice. These muffins are best eaten right after they come out of the oven.

1/2 cup bacon or gf bacon bits
1/2 cup finely chopped onion or 1 tablespoon gf dried minced onions
1 1/2 cups brown rice flour or garbfava flour
3/4 cup potato starch
3/4 cup tapioca flour
1 1/2 teaspoons unflavored gelatin powder
1 1/2 teaspoons xanthan gum

1 tablespoon baking powder
1 tablespoon sugar or honey
1 teaspoon salt
1 teaspoon dried thyme leaves
1 cup milk (cow, rice, soy)
1/3 cup cooking oil
3 large eggs, lightly beaten*
Cooking spray

Brown bacon and onion until bacon is crisp and onion is golden brown—the darker the bacon, the fuller the flavor. Preheat oven to 400°. Coat standard 12-muffin tin with cooking spray or oil. Set aside.

In medium mixer bowl, combine all dry ingredients. In separate small bowl, whisk together milk, oil, and eggs (or tofu—see below) until very, very smooth. Add bacon and onion to milk mixture.

Make well in center of dry ingredients. Add milk mixture all at once, stirring just until moistened. Divide evenly in standard 12-muffin tin, filling each tin to just below the top.

Bake for 20-25 minutes or until tops are golden brown and crusty. Serve immediately. Makes 12.

								Exchanges		
Calories	Fat	% Fat Cal	Protein	Carb	Chol	Sodium	Fiber	Carb	Meat	Fat
200	6g	28%	4g	32g	4mg	430mg	1.5g	1	.5	1

Eggs add additional 70mg cholesterol per serving.

*Egg Alternative: 3/4 cup soft silken tofu in place of 3 large eggs. Muffins will be heavier and somewhat dense.

Corn Bread with Green Chiles

(can be made without wheat, gluten, dairy, eggs, or sugar - see page xi about ingredients)

Some cornbread experts insist on baking cornbread in a pre-heated 9-inch cast-iron skillet. That method works fine with this recipe, producing a slightly crispy crust. If you are not accustomed to eating green chiles, you might reduce the amount to 2 tablespoons the first time you make this corn bread.

1 can (4 oz.) diced green chiles or
   1/4 cup chopped fresh green chiles
2 tablespoons chopped fresh cilantro
1/4 cup garbfava flour or
   brown rice flour
3 tablespoons tapioca flour
3 tablespoons potato starch
1/2 teaspoon xanthan gum
1/2 cup yellow cornmeal
2 tablespoons sugar or honey

1 teaspoon baking powder
1/2 teaspoon baking soda
1/2 teaspoon salt
1 large egg*
2/3 cup buttermilk or 1 tablespoon
   cider vinegar and enough non-
   dairy milk to equal 2/3 cup
2 tablespoons cooking oil
Cooking spray

Preheat oven to 375°. Coat 8 x 8-inch pan (or 9-inch cast-iron skillet) with cooking spray. Set aside.

If using canned green chiles, drain thoroughly. If using fresh chiles, wear rubber gloves while finely chopping them. Set aside. Finely chop fresh cilantro and set aside.

In medium bowl, combine flours, xanthan gum, cornmeal, sugar (or honey), baking powder, baking soda, and salt. Make a well in center. Set aside.

In another bowl, beat egg, buttermilk, and oil until well blended. Add egg mixture all at once to dry mixture, stirring just until moistened. Gently stir in chiles and cilantro.

Bake for 20-25 minutes or until top is firm and edges are lightly browned. Serve warm. Serves 6.

*Corn Bread without Eggs: Omit egg, add 2 teaspoons Ener-G® egg replacer and increase buttermilk to 1 cup. Bake for 20-25 minutes or until top is firm and lightly browned.

| | | | | | | | | Exchanges | | |
Calories	Fat	% Fat Cal	Protein	Carb	Chol	Sodium	Fiber	Carb	Meat	Fat
150	4g	23%	4g	25g	37mg	485mg	2g	1		.5

Eggs add additional 36mg cholesterol per serving.

Irish Griddle Cakes

(can be made without wheat, gluten, dairy, eggs, or sugar - see page xi about ingredients)

This is a great way to use up left over mashed potatoes and it provides a great way to have crispy, chewy bread in relatively little time.

1 cup mashed potatoes	1/2 teaspoon crushed dried rosemary
1/4 cup brown rice flour	1/2 teaspoon gf onion powder
1/4 cup potato starch	1/2 teaspoon baking powder
1/4 cup tapioca flour	1 tablespoon cooking oil
1/2 teaspoon xanthan gum	1 tablespoon milk (cow, rice, soy)
1/2 teaspoon salt	1 tablespoon cooking oil for frying

Combine all ingredients together (except oil for frying) in food processor until thoroughly mixed. Roll out between sheets of waxed paper into 1/4-inch thick circle. Dust with additional rice flour to prevent sticking.

With a sharp knife, cut circle in half, then cut each half into three wedges.

Heat griddle or cast-iron skillet until medium-hot. Add oil and fry cakes for 5-7 minutes on each side or until golden brown, turning once. Serve hot. Serves 6.

								Exchanges		
Calories	Fat	% Fat Cal	Protein	Carb	Chol	Sodium	Fiber	Carb	Meat	Fat
115	3g	25%	1g	21g	1mg	390mg	1g	1		.5

Irish Soda Bread with Dried Cherries

(can be made without wheat, gluten, dairy, eggs, or sugar - see page xi about ingredients)

Serve this bread with your favorite Irish meal. It is also great just on its own. The dried tart cherries are not traditional, but provide a contemporary touch.

1 cup garbfava flour or brown rice flour
2/3 cup potato starch
1/3 cup tapioca flour
2 teaspoons sugar or honey
1 teaspoon xanthan gum
3/4 teaspoon salt
1/2 teaspoon unflavored gelatin powder
1/2 teaspoon cream of tartar

1/2 teaspoon baking soda
1 large egg*
1 1/3 cups low-fat yogurt**
2 tablespoons cooking oil
1 tablespoon caraway seed
1/2 cup finely chopped dried cherries
Cooking spray

Coat two 5 x 3-inch nonstick pans (or 8 x 8-inch nonstick pan) with cooking spray. Preheat oven to 350°.

Combine dry ingredients in large mixing bowl and mix well. With electric mixer on low, add egg, yogurt (or milk) oil, and caraway seeds. Blend on medium speed for 2 minutes. Stir in dried cherries.

Spoon into prepared pans, smooth tops with wet spatula (if necessary), and bake small pans for 45-50 minutes, large pan for 50-55 minutes or until top is deeply browned and loaf sounds hollow when tapped. Cool on wire rack. Slice with serrated knife or electric knife when bread reaches room temperature. Serves 8.

*Irish Soda Bread without Eggs: Omit egg. Add 1 tablespoon Ener-G® egg replacer and 1/4 cup water. Bake as directed. Bread will be heavy and dense.

**Dairy Alternative: 1 cup milk (rice, soy) in place of 1 1/3 cups yogurt

| | | | | | | | | Exchanges | | |
Calories	Fat	% Fat Cal	Protein	Carb	Chol	Sodium	Fiber	Carb	Meat	Fat
200	4g	16%	4g	40g	2mg	365mg	2g	1		.5

Egg adds additional 27mg cholesterol per serving.

Notes

BREAKFAST & BRUNCH

S pecial occasions take on a different atmosphere when they're celebrated in the morning, at breakfast, or mid-day—such as a brunch. I especially love to use brunch as an occasion to celebrate with friends or family. In the wintertime, we make sure to have the fireplace roaring. In summer, you'll likely find us on our sun-drenched patio, enjoying the late morning rays.

In fact, brunch is probably my favorite way to entertain. When guests enter my home, I want them to be greeted with the aroma of freshly-brewed coffee, fresh-baked muffins or scones—piping hot from the oven, pleasant music, and table decorations to complete the ambience. Nothing terribly fancy—but I like to use lots of color to set the mood. It's just a great way to begin the day!

Bread, Doughnuts, Muffins, Rolls, & Scones

Blueberry Muffins with Lemon Curd 72-73
Cappuccino Chocolate Chip Muffins 74
Bran Muffins 75
Pumpkin Doughnuts 76
Pumpkin Muffins 77
Sally Lunn (Soleit et Lune) Bread 78
Scones with Citrus Butter 79
Scones 79-81
Scones with Ham 80
Scones with Sun-Dried Tomatoes & Olives 80

Main Dishes & Miscellaneous

Breakfast Sausage 90
Breakfast Trifle 90
Citrus Butter 79
Lemon Curd 72
Orange Marmalade 39

Pancakes & Waffles

Banana-Pecan Waffles
with Maple Raisin Syrup 86
Pancakes 87
Sweet Potato Waffles 88
Waffle 89

Grains & Cereals

Bircher-Muesli 91
Gourmet Granola 92

Bars & Cakes

Blueberry Apricot Coffee Cake 82
Breakfast Fruit Pizza 83
Caffe Borgia Coffee Cake 84
Granola Bars 93
Lemon Poppy Seed Raspberry Cake 85

For a wide variety of additional wheat/gluten/dairy-free breakfast dishes, see ***Wheat-Free Recipes & Menus: Delicious Dining Without Wheat or Gluten*** or ***Special Diet Solutions: Healthy Cooking Without Wheat, Gluten, Dairy, Eggs, Yeast, or Refined Sugar***. Both are published by Savory Palate, Inc.

Blueberry Muffins with Lemon Curd

(can be made without wheat, gluten, dairy, or sugar - see page xi about ingredients)

These delightful muffins are perfect for everyday—or special breakfasts or brunches. Use the tangy lemon curd as you would use butter—it adds a delightful twist. See egg-free version on next page.

Muffins
1 cup brown rice flour or garbfava flour
2/3 cup potato starch
2/3 cup tapioca flour
1 teaspoon xanthan gum
1 teaspoon unflavored gelatin powder
2 1/2 teaspoons baking powder
1/2 cup sugar*
1 teaspoon salt
1 cup milk (cow, rice, soy)
1/4 cup cooking oil
2 large eggs
1 teaspoon gf vanilla extract

1 tablespoon grated lemon peel or
  2 teaspoons gf lemon extract
1 cup blueberries (fresh or frozen)
Cooking spray or paper liners
Lemon Curd
1 cup thawed pure white grape
  juice frozen concentrate
3/4 cup fresh orange juice
1/4 cup fresh lemon juice
1/4 cup cornstarch or arrowroot
1/4 teaspoon salt
1 tablespoon grated lemon peel
1 teaspoon gf vanilla extract

Muffins: Preheat oven to 400°. Coat 6-cup or standard 12-cup, nonstick muffin tin with cooking spray or use paper liners.

Stir together flours, xanthan gum, gelatin, baking powder, sugar, and salt in large bowl. Make well in center.

In another bowl, combine milk, oil, eggs, vanilla extract, and lemon peel (or extract). Pour into well of flour mixture. Stir just until ingredients are moistened. Add blueberries and gently stir in. (If the blueberries are frozen, add 5 minutes baking time.)

Divide dough among 6 (or 12) muffin tins that are coated with cooking spray or lined with paper liners. Bake larger muffin tins (6-muffin size) for approximately 25 minutes; 12-muffin tins for 20-25 minutes—or until tops of muffins are lightly browned. Remove from oven. Cool.

Lemon Curd: Combine all ingredients in a blender and process until very, very smooth. Place in small, heavy saucepan and cook over medium heat, stirring constantly, until mixture thickens—about 3-5 minutes. Chill, covered, in glass container.

*Sugar Alternative: Use 1/3 cup honey or agave nectar in place of 1/2 cup sugar. Reduce milk to 3/4 cup.

Per muffin   Exchanges

Calories	Fat	% Fat Cal	Protein	Carb	Chol	Sodium	Fiber	Carb	Meat	Fat
182	4g	20%	3g	34g	36mg	367mg	1g	1		.5

Per 2 1/2 tablespoons Lemon Curd   Exchanges

Calories	Fat	% Fat Cal	Protein	Carb	Chol	Sodium	Fiber	Carb	Meat	Fat
64	<1g	1%	<1g	16g	0mg	50mg	0g	1		

Blueberry Muffins without Eggs

(can be made without wheat, gluten, dairy, eggs, or sugar - see page xi about ingredients)

If you love Blueberry Muffins but can't eat eggs—this is the recipe for you. These muffins will be somewhat heavier than the muffins on the previous page, but they'll taste fabulous! They're best warm from the oven. If any are left over, store in airtight container. For a luscious Lemon Curd, see previous page.

<u>Muffins</u>
1 1/4 cups garbfava or brown rice flour
3/4 cup potato starch
1/2 cup tapioca flour
1 teaspoon unflavored gelatin powder
1 teaspoon xanthan gum
1 1/4 teaspoons baking powder
1 1/4 teaspoons baking soda
1 teaspoon salt
1/2 cup sugar*
1 1/4 cups milk (cow, rice, soy, or nut)
1/4 cup cooking oil
1 teaspoon gf vanilla extract

1 tablespoon grated lemon peel
1 cup blueberries (fresh or frozen)
Cooking spray or paper liners

<u>Streusel Topping</u>
2 tablespoons garbfava flour or
   brown rice flour
1/4 cup brown sugar or
   maple sugar
1/2 teaspoon ground cinnamon
1/4 cup chopped pecans
1 tablespoon cooking oil

Muffins: Preheat oven to 375°. Coat standard 12-cup muffin pan with cooking spray or use paper liners. In large mixing bowl, combine flours, gelatin, xanthan gum, baking powder, baking soda, salt, and sugar. Make well in center. Set aside.

   In medium bowl, whisk together milk, oil, vanilla, and lemon peel. Stir liquid mixture into dry ingredients. Gently fold blueberries into batter, which will be the consistency of thick cake batter. Distribute batter evenly in pan.
Streusel Topping: Combine ingredients thoroughly. Sprinkle topping evenly on muffins. Bake for 20-25 minutes or until toothpick inserted in center comes out clean. Remove from oven. Serves 12.

*Sugar Alternative: 1/3 cup honey instead of 1/2 cup sugar. Reduce milk to 1 cup.

								Per Muffin	Exchanges	
Calories	Fat	% Fat Cal	Protein	Carb	Chol	Sodium	Fiber	Carb	Meat	Fat
233	7g	26%	5g	39g	1mg	452mg	2g	.5		1

Cappuccino Chocolate Chip Muffins

(can be made without wheat, gluten, dairy, eggs, or sugar - see page xi about ingredients)

These delicious muffins combine two favorite flavors—coffee and chocolate. These muffins travel well and are sure to delight your chocoholic friends and family.

1 cup cocoa powder (not Dutch)
1 cup brown rice flour or
  garbfava flour
1/2 cup potato starch
1/2 cup tapioca flour
1 teaspoon unflavored gelatin powder
1 teaspoon xanthan gum
1 1/4 teaspoons baking soda
1/3 cup brown sugar or maple sugar
1 teaspoon gf instant coffee granules
  or espresso powder

1 teaspoon ground cinnamon
3/4 teaspoon salt
1/2 cup milk (cow, rice, soy)
1/2 cup warm (105°) brewed coffee
1/4 cup cooking oil
2 large eggs*
1 teaspoon gf vanilla extract
1/2 cup gf/df chocolate chips
1/2 cup chopped nuts
Cooking spray or paper liners

Preheat oven to 375°. Coat 6-cup or 12-cup standard muffin tin with cooking spray. Stir together cocoa, flours, gelatin, xanthan gum, baking soda, sugar, coffee, cinnamon, and salt in large bowl. Make well in center.

In another bowl, whisk together milk, brewed coffee, oil, eggs (or tofu—see below), and vanilla extract until very, very smooth. Pour into well of flour mixture. Stir just until ingredients are moistened. Gently stir in chocolate chips and nuts.

Divide dough among muffin pans. Bake 6-muffin pans for approximately 25-30 minutes; 12-muffin pans for 20-25 minutes—or until tops of muffins are very firm. Remove from oven. Serve slightly warm so chocolate chips are soft.

*Egg Alternative: Use 1/2 cup soft silken tofu in place of 2 eggs. Muffins will be heavier and denser. For best results, use garbfava flour.

| | | | | | | | | Exchanges | | |
Calories	Fat	% Fat Cal	Protein	Carb	Chol	Sodium	Fiber	Carb	Meat	Fat
226	9g	34%	5g	36g	1mg	336mg	4g	1.5	.5	1.5

Egg adds additional 35mg cholesterol per muffin.

Bran Muffins

(can be made without wheat, gluten, dairy, eggs, or sugar - see page xi about ingredients)

If you prefer a hearty muffin for breakfast, but one that isn't too sweet—this muffin is for you. If you like to bake only a few muffins at a time, this batter keeps in the refrigerator for up to 2 days.

1 cup brown rice flour or
   garbfava flour
2/3 cup potato starch
1/3 cup tapioca flour
3 tablespoons rice bran or rice polish
1 1/2 teaspoons baking powder
3/4 teaspoon baking soda
1 1/4 teaspoons xanthan gum
1/2 teaspoon soy lecithin
1/4 teaspoon ground nutmeg
1 1/4 teaspoons ground cinnamon
1/2 teaspoon ground ginger

1/2 teaspoon ground allspice
3/4 teaspoon salt
1 cup milk (cow, rice, soy)
3 tablespoons cider vinegar
1 large egg*
3 tablespoons cooking oil
1/2 cup molasses (cane or sorghum)
1 teaspoon gf vanilla extract
2/3 cup raisins
1/3 cup chopped walnuts
1 tablespoon grated orange peel
Cooking spray or paper liners

Preheat oven to 375°. Spray 6-cup or standard 12-cup muffin pan with cooking spray or use paper liners.

In large bowl, mix together flours with other dry ingredients. In separate bowl, use electric mixer to combine milk, vinegar, egg (or tofu—see below), oil, molasses, and vanilla until very, very smooth. Stir into dry ingredients until moistened. Gently stir in raisins, nuts, and orange peel.

Distribute evenly into muffin pan. Bake 12-muffin pans for 25-30 minutes or until tops are firm; six-cup muffin tins for 30-40 minutes.

*Egg Alternative: 1/4 cup soft silken tofu in place of 1 egg. Increase baking soda to 1 teaspoon. Muffins will be heavier and denser. For best results, use garbfava flour.

								Exchanges		
Calories	Fat	% Fat Cal	Protein	Carb	Chol	Sodium	Fiber	Carb	Meat	Fat
210	6g	22%	3g	40g	1mg	344mg	2g	1		1

Egg adds additional 17mg cholesterol per muffin.

Pumpkin Doughnuts

(can be made without wheat, gluten, dairy, eggs, or sugar - see page xi about ingredients)

Although the idea of pumpkin seems appropriate for fall and winter, you can make these doughnuts any time you like.

3 tablespoons sugar or fructose powder
1 cup brown rice flour or
   garbfava flour
1/2 cup potato starch
1/4 cup tapioca flour
1 teaspoon xanthan gum
2 1/4 teaspoons ground cinnamon
1/2 teaspoon ground nutmeg
1 1/2 teaspoons baking powder
1 1/2 teaspoons baking soda

1/2 teaspoon salt
1 large egg*
1 cup buttermilk or 2 tablespoons
   cider vinegar with enough
   non-dairy milk to equal 1 cup
3/4 cup brown sugar**
1/2 cup canned pumpkin
3 tablespoons cooking oil
1 teaspoon grated lemon peel
Cooking spray

Preheat oven to 400°. Spray 6-cup mini-Bundt pan with cooking spray or lightly coat with oil. Sprinkle molds with 3 tablespoons sugar, tapping out excess.

In large bowl, combine flours, xanthan gum, cinnamon, nutmeg, baking powder, baking soda, and salt. Set aside.

In another bowl, whisk together the egg (or tofu—see below), buttermilk, brown sugar, pumpkin, oil, and lemon peel until very, very smooth. Add dry ingredients and stir just until combined. Spoon 1/4 cup batter into prepared molds.

Bake 15-18 minutes or until doughnuts brown around edges. Cool 2 minutes. Then loosen edges and invert doughnuts onto wire rack to cool. Repeat with remaining half of batter. Makes 12 doughnuts.

Egg Alternative: Use 1/4 cup soft silken tofu in place of 1 large egg
****Sugar Alternative:** Use 3/4 cup maple sugar in place of 3/4 cup brown
  sugar. Add 1/8 teaspoon baking soda.

Calories	Fat	% Fat Cal	Protein	Carb	Chol	Sodium	Fiber	Exchanges Carb	Meat	Fat
175	3g	16%	2g	36g	1mg	385mg	1.5g	1.5		.5

Egg adds 18mg cholesterol per doughnut.

Pumpkin Muffins

(can be made without wheat, gluten, dairy, eggs, or sugar - see page xi about ingredients)

These muffins are perfect for a crisp, fall morning. The heavenly aroma makes your kitchen a very appealing place! You can make the batter, refrigerate (covered), and bake the next morning.

3/4 cup canned pumpkin	1 teaspoon xanthan gum
1/2 cup pure maple syrup or honey	1/2 teaspoon salt
2 tablespoons molasses (cane or sorghum)	1 1/2 teaspoons baking powder
1/3 cup cooking oil	1 1/2 teaspoons baking soda
2 large eggs*	2 teaspoons pumpkin pie spice
1 teaspoon cider vinegar	1/2 teaspoon ground allspice
3/4 cup garbfava flour or brown rice flour	1/2 cup chopped nuts (optional)
1/2 cup potato starch	1/2 cup raisins
1/3 cup tapioca flour	Cooking spray or paper liners

Preheat oven to 350°. Spray standard 12-muffin pan with cooking spray or use paper liners. Combine pumpkin, maple syrup, molasses, oil, egg (or tofu—see below), and vinegar in large mixing bowl. Beat on low until very, very smooth—about 1 minute.

Combine remaining ingredients (except nuts and raisins) and add to pumpkin mixture. Blend at low speed until moistened. Stir in nuts and raisins. Transfer batter to prepared pan (use spring-action ice cream scoop for uniformly-sized muffins) and bake for 25-30 minutes or until firm. Cool in pan on wire rack for 10 minutes. Remove from pan and cool on wire rack. Serves 12.

*Egg Alternative: Omit eggs. Use 1/2 cup soft silken tofu. For best results, use garbfava flour.

								Exchanges		
Calories	Fat	% Fat Cal	Protein	Carb	Chol	Sodium	Fiber	Carb	Meat	Fat
230	10g	38%	3g	34g	0mg	330mg	2g	1.5		2

Eggs add 35mg cholesterol per muffin.

Sally Lunn (Soleil et Lune) Bread

(can be made without wheat, gluten, dairy, or sugar - see page xi about ingredients)

Serve this bread with a dusting of powdered sugar or with Orange Marmalade (page 39). If you wish, assemble the dough the night before and let rise, covered, in refrigerator all night. Next morning, remove from refrigerator and bake for an extra 10 minutes—or until done. Because eggs provide part of the leavening, this is not an egg-free bread.

<u>Cake</u>
1 tablespoon gf active dry yeast
1/4 cup sugar or fructose powder, divided
1/2 cup warm water (105°)
2 cups white or brown rice flour
1 cup potato starch
1/2 cup tapioca flour
2 teaspoons xanthan gum
1 teaspoon unflavored gelatin powder
1 1/4 teaspoons salt
3/4 teaspoon ground mace
1 1/2 tablespoons grated orange peel

1 cup hot fresh orange juice (115°)
6 tablespoons butter or oleo or Spectrum™ canola oil spread or or 1/4 cup cooking oil
3 large eggs (room temperature)
3 teaspoons gf vanilla extract
Cooking spray

<u>Glaze</u>
3 tablespoons fresh orange juice
3 tablespoons powdered sugar or fructose powder
2 tablespoons grated orange peel

Dissolve yeast and 1 teaspoon sugar in 1/2 cup warm water. Set aside until foamy.

Combine flours, remaining sugar, xanthan gum, gelatin, salt, and mace in large mixing bowl with electric mixer. Add orange peel, orange juice, butter (or oleo), eggs, vanilla, and yeast mixture. Beat with regular beaters (not dough hooks) for 3 minutes. Batter will be very soft and sticky.

Transfer dough to 10-inch Bundt pan (coated with cooking spray). Cover loosely with oiled plastic wrap and let rise at room temperature until doubled in volume, 45 minutes to 1 hour.

Ten minutes before baking, preheat oven to 350°. Remove plastic wrap and bake bread for 30-35 minutes, or until cake tester inserted into center comes out clean. (If refrigerated, bake 10 minutes longer.) Turn bread out of pan on to wire rack to cool.

In small saucepan (or in microwave oven), heat orange juice and sugar until sugar melts. Brush warm bread with glaze. Serves 12.

								Exchanges		
Calories	Fat	% Fat Cal	Protein	Carb	Chol	Sodium	Fiber	Carb	Meat	Fat
235	5g	17%	4g	45g	53mg	260	0g	1.5		1

Butter adds additional 30 calories, 3g fat, and 15mg cholesterol per serving.

Scones with Citrus Butter

(can be made without wheat, gluten, dairy, eggs, or sugar - see page xi about ingredients)

Scones are fool proof because any way you make them they're a success. See egg-free version (page 81).

1/4 cup butter or oleo or Spectrum™
    canola oil spread
2/3 cup plain yogurt*
1 large egg, lightly beaten
1 1/4 cups brown rice flour
    or garbfava flour
1/2 cup tapioca flour
1 1/2 teaspoons cream of tartar
3/4 teaspoon baking soda

1 teaspoon xanthan gum
1/4 teaspoon soy lecithin (optional)
1/2 teaspoon salt
2 tablespoons sugar or
    fructose powder
1/2 cup currants
Cooking spray
Citrus Butter (see below)

Preheat oven to 425°. Coat baking sheet with cooking spray. Set aside.

In food processor, blend butter (or oleo), yogurt (or milk), and egg until well mixed. Add flours, cream of tartar, baking soda, xanthan gum, lecithin, salt, and sugar. Blend just until mixed. Add currants and pulse a few times to incorporate. Dough will be soft.

Transfer dough to baking sheet; pat into 8-inch circle, 3/4-inch thick. Bake for 15-20 minutes or until deeply browned. For crispier, wedge-shaped pieces, cut into 8 wedges and return to oven for final 5 minutes of baking. Serves 8.

*Dairy Alternative: 1/2 cup milk (rice, soy) in place of 2/3 cup yogurt

								Exchanges		
Calories	Fat	% Fat Cal	Protein	Carb	Chol	Sodium	Fiber	Carb	Meat	Fat
230	7g	28%	4g	38mg	43mg	290mg	2g	1		1

Citrus Butter

(can be made without wheat, gluten, dairy, eggs, or sugar - see page xi about ingredients)

1 tablespoon grated orange peel
1 teaspoon grated lemon peel
1 teaspoon grated lime peel
1 tablespoon fresh orange juice

1 stick butter or oleo or 1/2 cup
    Spectrum™ canola oil spread
1/8 teaspoon salt

Bring butter to room temperature. Using a spatula, combine all ingredients thoroughly until well blended. Chill until ready to serve. Serve at room temperature. Makes about 2/3 cup. Serves 8 (1 tablespoon each).

								Exchanges		
Calories	Fat	% Fat Cal	Protein	Carb	Chol	Sodium	Fiber	Carb	Meat	Fat
100	11g	98%	<1g	.5g	31mg	37mg	<1g			2

Scones with Ham

(can be made without wheat, gluten, dairy, eggs, or sugar - see page xi about ingredients)

Hearty scones are almost a meal by themselves. For an egg-free version, see page 81.

1/4 cup butter or oleo or
   Spectrum™ canola oil spread
2/3 cup plain yogurt*
1 large egg, lightly beaten
1 1/4 cups brown rice flour or
   garbfava flour
1/2 cup tapioca flour
1 1/2 teaspoons cream of tartar

3/4 teaspoon baking soda
1 teaspoon xanthan gum
1/2 teaspoon salt
2 tablespoons sugar or fructose powder
1 1/2 teaspoon dried sage leaves
1/2 cup finely chopped ham
Cooking spray

Preheat oven to 425°. Coat nonstick baking sheet with cooking spray. Set aside.

In food processor, blend butter(or oleo or canola oil spread), yogurt (or milk), and egg together until well mixed. Add flours, cream of tartar, baking soda, xanthan gum, salt, sugar, and sage. Blend just until mixed. Remove bowl from stand and gently stir in chopped ham. Work quickly so the leavening doesn't lose its power. Dough will be soft.

Transfer dough to baking sheet, patting with spatula into 8-inch circle, 3/4-inch thick. Bake for 15-20 minutes or until deeply browned. For crispier, wedge-shaped pieces, cut into 8 wedges and return to oven for final 5 minutes of baking. Serves 8.

*Dairy Alternative: 1/2 cup milk (rice, soy) in place of 2/3 cup yogurt

| | | | | | | | | Exchanges | | |
Calories	Fat	% Fat Cal	Protein	Carb	Chol	Sodium	Fiber	Carb	Meat	Fat
210	8g	32%	5g	31g	46mg	390mg	2g	1	.5	1

Scones with Sun-Dried Tomatoes & Olives: Omit sage and chopped ham. Add 1 teaspoon crushed rosemary leaves, 1/2 cup sun-dried tomatoes (see page 214 for Oven-Dried Tomatoes) and 1/2 cup sliced black olives. Bake as directed as above.

| | | | | | | | | Exchanges | | |
Calories	Fat	% Fat Cal	Protein	Carb	Chol	Sodium	Fiber	Carb	Meat	Fat
220	8g	33%	4g	33g	42mg	407mg	2g	1		1

Scones without Eggs

(can be made without wheat, gluten, dairy, eggs, or sugar - see page xi about ingredients)

If at all possible, make these scones with the garbfava four. You'll be pleased with the results because the scones will rise higher and have a smoother crust. If you want this to be a sweeter scone, increase the sugar to 1/4 cup. Use this recipe to make egg-free versions of the other scones in this chapter.

1/4 cup butter, oleo, or Spectrum™ canola oil spread
3/4 cup milk (cow, rice, soy)
1 1/4 cups garbfava flour or brown rice flour
1/2 cup tapioca flour
1 1/2 teaspoons cream of tartar
3/4 teaspoon baking soda

1 teaspoon xanthan gum
1/4 teaspoon soy lecithin
1/2 teaspoon salt
2 tablespoons sugar or
  1 tablespoon honey
1/2 cup currants
Cooking spray

Preheat oven to 425°. Coat nonstick baking sheet with cooking spray. Set aside.

In food processor, blend butter, milk, flours, cream of tartar, baking soda, xanthan gum, lecithin, salt, and sugar. Blend just until mixed. Add currants and pulse a few times to incorporate. Work quickly so the leavening doesn't lose its power. Dough will be soft.

Transfer dough to baking sheet, patting with spatula into 8-inch circle, 3/4-inch thick. Bake for 15-20 minutes or until deeply browned. For crispier, wedge-shaped pieces, cut into 8 wedges and return to oven for final 5 minutes of baking. Serves 8.

								Exchanges		
Calories	Fat	% Fat Cal	Protein	Carb	Chol	Sodium	Fiber	Carb	Meat	Fat
220	8g	30%	7g	33g	16mg	300mg	3g	.5		1

Blueberry Apricot Coffee Cake

(can be made without wheat, gluten, dairy, eggs, or sugar - see page xi about ingredients)

Cake

1/3 cup butter or oleo Spectrum™
  canola oil spread or
  1/4 cup cooking oil
3/4 cup sugar*
2 large eggs**
1 tablespoon grated orange peel
1 cup brown rice flour or garbava flour
6 tablespoons potato starch
2 tablespoons tapioca flour
1 teaspoon xanthan gum
1/2 teaspoon baking powder

1/2 teaspoon baking soda
1/2 teaspoon salt
2 tablespoons cider vinegar
1/2 cup + 2 tablespoons milk
  (cow, rice, soy)
1 teaspoon gf vanilla extract
1/2 cup dried blueberries,
  chopped
1/2 cup dried apricots,
  finely chopped
Cooking spray

Topping

1/4 cup brown sugar or maple sugar
1/2 teaspoon ground cinnamon
1/4 teaspoon ground nutmeg
2 tablespoons cooking oil

2 tablespoons brown rice flour
  or garbfava flour
1/4 cup chopped nuts of choice
1/4 cup rolled rice flakes

Preheat oven to 350°. Coat 11 x 7-inch nonstick pan with cooking spray. Set aside.

Using an electric mixer and large mixer bowl, cream together oil, sugar, and eggs (or tofu—see below) on medium speed about 2 minutes—or until very, very, smooth. Add grated orange peel.

In a medium bowl, combine flours, xanthan gum, baking powder, baking soda, and salt. In another medium bowl, combine vinegar, milk, and vanilla.

On low speed, beat dry ingredients into egg (tofu) mixture, alternating with milk mixture, beginning and ending with dry ingredients. Mix just until combined. Stir in blueberries and apricots.

Spoon batter into pan. Mix together topping ingredients and sprinkle on top. Bake 35 minutes or until top is golden brown and cake tester comes out clean. Serves 10.

*Sugar Alternative #1: 3/4 cup fructose powder in place of 3/4 cup sugar
*Sugar Alternative #2: 1/2 cup honey in place of 3/4 cup sugar. Decrease
  milk to 1/2 cup.
**Egg Alternative: Omit eggs. Use 1/2 cup soft silken tofu. Increase baking
  powder and baking soda by 1/4 teaspoon each. For best results, use garbfava
  flour. Cake will be heavier and more dense.

| | | | | | | | | Exchanges | | |
Calories	Fat	% Fat Cal	Protein	Carb	Chol	Sodium	Fiber	Carb	Meat	Fat
340	12g	30%	5g	27g	60mg	264mg	3g	1	.5	2

Breakfast Fruit Pizza

(can be made without wheat, gluten, dairy, eggs, or sugar - see page xi about ingredients)

Surprise your children with this unique pizza. You can do anything you want with the toppings, so feel free to experiment. It also makes a great dish to serve your weekend guests. Cut the pizza into wedges and pick it up and eat it—just like real pizza!

<u>Pizza</u>
1 tablespoon gf active dry yeast
2/3 cup brown rice flour or
   garbfava flour
1/2 cup + 2 tablespoons tapioca flour
2 teaspoons xanthan gum
1/2 teaspoon salt
1 teaspoon unflavored gelatin powder
1 teaspoon cinnamon
1/4 teaspoon ground mace (optional)
2/3 cup warm milk (105°)
   (cow, rice, soy)
1 tablespoon sugar or fructose powder
1 teaspoon cooking oil
1 teaspoon cider vinegar
2 teaspoons grated lemon peel
Cooking spray

<u>Topping</u>
1/2 cup fresh orange juice
2 tablespoons sugar or honey
1 tablespoon cornstarch
   or arrowroot
1/4 teaspoon ground cinnamon
1/4 teaspoon salt
2 cups finely chopped fruit:
   apples, peaches, plums,
   blueberries,
   or use dried fruit:
   cherries, cranberries, apricots
1 cup chopped nuts (optional)

Pizza: Preheat oven to 425°. Coat 12-inch nonstick pizza (thin, crispy crust) or 11 x 7-inch pan (deep-dish) with cooking spray or grease with oil. Set aside.

In medium mixer bowl using regular beaters (not dough hooks), blend yeast, flours, xanthan gum, salt, cinnamon, and gelatin powder on low speed. Add warm milk, sugar, oil, vinegar, and lemon peel.

Beat on high speed for 3 minutes. (If mixer bounces around bowl, the dough is too stiff. Add water if necessary, one tablespoon at a time, until dough does not resist beaters.) The dough will resemble soft bread dough.

Put mixture onto prepared pan. Liberally sprinkle rice flour onto dough, then press dough into pan, continuing to sprinkle dough with flour to prevent sticking to your hands. Make edges thicker to hold toppings. Bake pizza crust for 10 minutes. Remove from oven.

Filling: Combine orange juice, sugar, cornstarch, and cinnamon in small pan and cook over low-medium heat, continuing to stir until mixture thickens. Stir in fruit. Spread filling on baked pizza crust.

Return pizza to oven and bake another 10-15 minutes or until golden brown. Add nuts during last 5 minutes of baking. Cool for 5 minutes before serving. Serves 6 (1 slice each).

| | | | | | | | | Exchanges | | |
Calories	Fat	% Fat Cal	Protein	Carb	Chol	Sodium	Fiber	Carb	Meat	Fat
320	14g	36%	7g	47g	<1mg	320mg	5g	1.5	.5	2

Caffee Borgia Coffee Cake

(can be made without wheat, gluten, dairy, or sugar - see page xi about ingredients)

Borrowed from the chocolate-infused coffee drink that is also flavored with orange, this cake is perfect for brunch. If you're a coffee lover, be sure to try this one.

Cake

3/4 cup brown sugar*
1/4 cup cooking oil
2 large eggs**
2 tablespoons grated orange peel
2 teaspoons gf vanilla extract
1/2 cup brewed coffee
2/3 cup garbfava flour or
  brown rice flour
1/2 cup potato starch

1/4 cup tapioca flour
1 tablespoon cocoa powder (not Dutch)
1 tablespoon espresso powder or 2
  tablespoons gf instant coffee powder
2 1/4 teaspoons baking powder
1/2 teaspoon xanthan gum
1/2 teaspoon salt
1 teaspoon ground cinnamon
Cooking spray

Topping

1 teaspoon cocoa powder
1 teaspoon ground cinnamon
1 tablespoon cooking oil

1/4 cup brown sugar or maple sugar
2 tablespoons brown rice flour
  or garbfava flour

Cake: Preheat oven to 350°. Coat 8 x 8-inch nonstick pan with cooking spray. Set aside.

Using an electric mixer and a large mixer bowl, cream together sugar, oil, eggs (or tofu—see below), orange peel, vanilla extract, and coffee on medium speed until very, very smooth—about 1 minute.

Add remaining cake ingredients and mix just until combined. Pour batter into pan.

Topping: Combine ingredients thoroughly with pastry blender or fork. Sprinkle topping on batter. Bake 25-30 minutes or until tester comes out clean. Serves 10.

*Sugar Alternative #1: 3/4 cup dried cane juice in place of 3/4 cup brown sugar. Add 1/8 teaspoon baking soda.
*Sugar Alternative #2: 1/2 cup honey or maple syrup in place of 3/4 cup brown sugar. Decrease coffee to 1/3 cup.
**Egg Alternative: 1/2 cup soft silken tofu in place of 2 eggs. For best results, use garbfava flour.

| | | | | | | | | | Exchanges | | |
Calories	Fat	% Fat Cal	Protein	Carb	Chol	Sodium	Fiber	Carb	Meat	Fat
230	8g	30%	3.5g	38g	0mgq	220mg	2g	1		1

Eggs add additional 44mg of cholesterol per serving.

Lemon Poppy Seed Raspberry Coffee Cake

(can be made without wheat, gluten, dairy, or sugar - see page xi about ingredients)

Old-fashioned poppy seed cake is updated to include lemon and raspberry flavors. Serve this at your next brunch.

Cake

1/4 cup cooking oil
3/4 cup granulated sugar*
2 large eggs**
3 tablespoons grated lemon peel
1 cup brown rice flour or garbfava flour
6 tablespoons potato starch
2 tablespoons tapioca flour
1 teaspoon xanthan gum
1/2 teaspoon baking powder

1/2 teaspoon baking soda
1/2 teaspoon salt
2 tablespoons cider vinegar
2/3 cup milk (cow, rice, soy)
1 teaspoon gf vanilla extract
1/3 cup poppy seeds
1 cup fresh raspberries
Cooking spray

Topping

1/4 cup brown sugar or maple sugar
1/2 teaspoon ground cinnamon
2 teaspoons poppy seeds

1 tablespoon cooking oil
2 tablespoons brown rice flour
   or garbfava flour

Cake: Preheat oven to 350°. Coat 11 x 7-inch nonstick pan with cooking spray.
   Using an electric mixer and large mixer bowl, cream together oil, sugar, and eggs (or tofu—see below) on medium speed until very, very smooth—about 1 minute. Add grated lemon peel.
   In a medium bowl, combine flours, xanthan gum, baking powder, baking soda, and salt. In another medium bowl, combine vinegar, milk, and vanilla.
   On low speed, beat dry ingredients into egg mixture, alternating with milk mixture, beginning and ending with dry ingredients. Mix just until combined. Spoon 2/3 of batter into pan. Arrange fresh raspberries in single layer on top of batter, then pour remaining batter over raspberries.
Topping: Combine ingredients thoroughly with pastry blender or fork. Sprinkle on batter. Bake 35 minutes or until top is golden brown and cake tester comes out clean. Serves 10.

*Sugar Alternative #1: 3/4 cup fructose powder in place of 3/4 cup granulated sugar
*Sugar Alternative #2: 1/2 cup honey in place of 3/4 cup granulated sugar. Decrease milk to 1/2 cup.
**Egg Alternative: Omit eggs. Use 1/2 cup soft silken tofu. For best results, use garbfava flour.

| | | | | | | | | Exchanges | | |
Calories	Fat	% Fat Cal	Protein	Carb	Chol	Sodium	Fiber	Carb	Meat	Fat
250	7g	25%	4g	44g	1mg	288mg	3g	2	.5	1

Eggs add additional 42mg cholesterol per serving.

Banana-Pecan Waffles with Maple Raisin Syrup

(can be made without wheat, gluten, dairy, eggs, or sugar - see page xi about ingredients)

Save those extra-ripe bananas and surprise your family or impress your guests with this special breakfast dish. For best results, use garbfava flour.

Waffles
1 cup garbfava flour or brown rice flour
1/2 cup potato starch
1/4 cup tapioca flour
2 teaspoons baking powder
1/2 teaspoon salt
1 tablespoon sugar or honey
2 large ripe bananas, mashed
2 tablespoons cooking oil
1 tablespoon cider vinegar
1 cup milk (cow, rice, soy)

1 teaspoon gf vanilla extract
1 teaspoon gf rum extract
1/3 cup finely chopped pecans

Maple Raisin Syrup
1 cup pure maple syrup
1/3 cup dark raisins
1 tablespoon gf rum or
   1 teaspoon gf rum extract
Cooking spray

Waffles: Heat waffle iron. Spray with cooking spray. Combine all waffle ingredients in medium bowl and whisk thoroughly until very smooth.

Pour 1/4 of batter onto heated waffle iron. Close and bake according to manufacturer's instructions or until steaming stops, about 4-6 minutes. Repeat with remaining batter.

Maple Raisin Syrup: While waffles are baking, heat maple syrup, raisins, and rum in a small saucepan over low heat. Simmer until ready to serve with waffles. Makes 4 waffles, each 9 inches.

| | | | | | | | | Exchanges | | |
Calories	Fat	% Fat Cal	Protein	Carb	Chol	Sodium	Fiber	Carb	Meat	Fat
690	16g	29%	16g	125g	108ng	720mg	5g	4.5	.5	2

Pancakes

(can be made without wheat, gluten, dairy, or sugar - see page xi about ingredients)

These pancakes are light, yet filling. See egg-free version below.

1 large egg
1/2 cup nonfat plain yogurt*
1/4 cup brown rice flour or garbfava flour
2 tablespoons potato starch
2 tablespoons tapioca flour
1 teaspoon baking powder

1/2 teaspoon baking soda
1 teaspoon sugar or honey
1/2 teaspoon salt
1 teaspoon gf vanilla extract
1 tablespoon cooking oil
Additional oil for frying

Blend egg and yogurt (or milk) in blender or whisk vigorously in bowl. Add remaining ingredients and blend, just until mixed.

Over medium heat, place large, nonstick skillet lightly coated with oil. Pour batter into skillet and cook until tops are bubbly (3-5 minutes). Turn and cook until golden brown (2-3 minutes). Makes eight 4-inch pancakes. Serves 4 (2 pancakes each).

Dairy Alternative: 1/3 cup milk (cow, rice, soy) in place of 1/2 cup yogurt

Per 2 pancakes:

Exchanges

Calories	Fat	% Fat Cal	Protein	Carb	Chol	Sodium	Fiber	Carb	Meat	Fat
260	4g	15%	4g	52g	55mg	646mg	.5g	.5		.5

Pancakes without Eggs

(can be made without wheat, gluten, dairy, eggs, or sugar - see page xi about ingredients)

2/3 cup milk (cow, rice, soy)
2 teaspoons Ener-G® Egg Replacer powder
1/4 cup brown rice flour or garfava flour
1/4 cup potato starch
1 tablespoon tapioca flour
1 1/4 teaspoons baking powder

3/4 teaspoon baking soda
1 teaspoon sugar or honey
1/2 teaspoon salt
1 teaspoon gf vanilla extract
1 tablespoon cooking oil
Additional oil for frying

Blend milk and egg replacer powder in blender until frothy, about 1 minute. Add remaining ingredients and blend, just until mixed.

Over medium heat, place large, nonstick skillet that's been lightly coated with oil. Pour batter into skillet and cook until tops are bubbly (2-3 minutes). Turn; cook until golden brown (1-2 minutes). Makes eight 4-inch pancakes. Serves 4 (2 each).

Per 2 pancakes:

Exchanges

Calories	Fat	% Fat Cal	Protein	Carb	Chol	Sodium	Fiber	Carb	Meat	Fat
110	3g	21%	2g	20g	1mg	736mg	.5g	.5		.5

Sweet Potato Waffles

(can be made without wheat, gluten, dairy, eggs, or sugar - see page xi about ingredients)

You're probably thinking "Sweet potatoes in waffles?" Remember—sweet potatoes are extremely nutritious and provide an excellent source of beta carotene, they're low-calorie and high in fiber, and they are one of the least allergenic foods on earth. They bind the ingredients in this recipe (no need for eggs) and are absolutely delicious. Try them!

1 cup garbfava flour or brown rice flour
1/2 cup potato starch
1/4 cup tapioca flour
2 teaspoons baking powder
1/2 teaspoon salt
1 teaspoon ground cinnamon
1 tablespoon sugar or fructose powder

1/2 teaspoon xanthan gum
2 tablespoons cooking oil
1 medium cooked sweet potato,
    mashed to yield 1/2 to 3/4 cup
1 1/4 cups milk (cow, rice, soy)
1 teaspoon gf vanilla extract

Combine dry ingredients (flour through xanthan gum) in medium bowl. In separate bowl, whisk together oil, sweet potato, milk, and vanilla extract. Whisk liquid mixture into flour mixture just until combined.

Cook on waffle iron, according to manufacturer directions. Makes 4 waffles, depending on size of waffle iron.

								Exchanges		
Calories	Fat	% Fat Cal	Protein	Carb	Chol	Sodium	Fiber	Carb	Meat	Fat
340	7g	18%	12g	58g	2g	684mg	5g			1

Waffles

(can be made without wheat, gluten, dairy, or sugar - see page xi about ingredients)

This waffle recipe is so easy and dependable. See egg-free version below.

1 cup garbfava flour or brown rice flour
1/2 cup potato starch
1/4 cup tapioca flour
2 teaspoons baking powder
1/2 teaspoon salt
1 tablespoon sugar or honey

2 large eggs
2 tablespoons cooking oil
2 tablespoons cider vinegar
1 1/3 cups milk (cow, rice, soy)
1 teaspoon gf vanilla extract

Combine dry ingredients (flour through sugar) in medium bowl. In separate bowl, whisk together eggs, oil, vinegar, milk, and vanilla. Whisk liquid mixture (including honey, if using) into flour mixture just until combined.

Cook on waffle iron, according to manufacturer instructions. Makes 4 waffles, depending on size of waffle iron.

								Exchanges		
Calories	Fat	% Fat Cal	Protein	Carb	Chol	Sodium	Fiber	Carb	Meat	Fat
350	10g	29%	15g	51g	108mg	644mg	3g	.5	.5	1.5

Waffles without Eggs

(can be made without wheat, gluten, dairy, eggs, or sugar - see page xi about ingredients)

Even without eggs, these waffles are crisp and delicious.

1 cup brown rice flour or
  garbfava flour
1/2 cup potato starch
1/4 cup tapioca flour
1 teaspoon baking soda
1/2 teaspoon salt
1/2 teaspoon xanthan gum

1 tablespoon sugar or honey
2 tablespoons cooking oil
1 1/4 cups buttermilk or 1 tablespoon
  cider vinegar with enough milk (cow,
  rice, soy) to equal 1 1/4 cups
1 teaspoon gf vanilla extract

In a small bowl, mix together flours, baking soda, salt, xanthan gum, and sugar. (If using honey, add to liquid ingredients.) Whisk in oil, buttermilk, and vanilla.

Heat waffle iron. Pour 1/4 of batter onto heated waffle iron. Follow manufacturer's directions for your particular waffle iron. Close and bake until steaming stops, about 4-6 minutes. Repeat with remaining batter. Makes 4 waffles, depending on size of waffle iron.

Per waffle:

								Exchanges		
Calories	Fat	% Fat Cal	Protein	Carb	Chol	Sodium	Fiber	Carb	Meat	Fat
325	9g	24%	6g	58g	3mg	690mg	2g	2		1

Breakfast Sausage

(can be made without wheat, gluten, dairy, eggs, or sugar - see page xi about ingredients)

If you love sausage in the "wurst" way, this recipe makes it easy to include this flavorful meat on your breakfast plate. If you want an even lower fat content, try using half ground turkey and half ground pork. You can either shape the meat into patties or links— or brown the meat in a crumbled fashion. You can sprinkle the crumbles onto your scrambled eggs or your favorite pizza. Yum!!!

1 pound ground pork or turkey or beef	1/2 teaspoon black pepper
1 teaspoon rubbed sage	1/2 teaspoon fennel seed
1/2 teaspoon salt	1/4 teaspoon ground nutmeg
1/2 teaspoon dried thyme leaves	1/8 teaspoon ground cloves
1/2 teaspoon ground cumin	1/8 teaspoon cayenne pepper
1/2 teaspoon dried savory	Cooking spray

Blend all ingredients together in a large bowl using your hands or a large spatula. Form into patties or links (spray your hands with cooking spray first) and fry over medium heat until cooked through. Or, simply brown mixture in skillet in a crumbled fashion. Serves 12.

								Exchanges		
Calories	Fat	% Fat Cal	Protein	Carb	Chol	Sodium	Fiber	Carb	Meat	Fat
110	8g	64%	10g	<1g	36mg	125mg	<1g		1.5	1

Breakfast Trifle

(can be made without wheat, gluten, dairy, eggs, or sugar - see page xi about ingredients)

This dish looks pretty in individual, clear glass goblets or in a straight sided, glass serving dish. This allows the layers of ingredients to be visible from the side. Use whatever fruit you have available—blueberries, raspberries, sliced peaches,etc.

1/2 Basic Cake (pages 98-99) cut in 1-inch cubes	2 small bananas, diced
	2 cups sliced strawberries
4 small containers (8 oz. each) flavored yogurt or use 4 cups pudding of choice	Fresh mint for garnish

Layer the ingredients in serving dish, starting and ending with yogurt. Garnish with a few pieces of whole fruit and mint. Serve chilled. Serves 6.

								Exchanges		
Calories	Fat	% Fat Cal	Protein	Carb	Chol	Sodium	Fiber	Carb	Meat	Fat
450	10g	20%	13g	80g	56mg	500mg	3g	5		1.5

Bircher-Muesli

(can be made without wheat, gluten, dairy, eggs, or sugar - see page xi about ingredients)

I've always loved this cereal and now I have it frequently at home knowing it contains no wheat or gluten. You can assemble the rolled rice flakes, nuts, and spices the night before. Then add the fresh fruit and yogurt (or milk) just before serving. You can double this recipe for big groups. I've enjoyed this wonderful breakfast dish both cold and warm and I prefer the warm version.

2 **cups rolled rice flakes**
2 **teaspoons grated lemon peel**
1 **tablespoon grated orange peel**
1 **cup fresh orange juice**
1/2 **teaspoon ground cinnamon**
1/4 **cup dried tart cherries**
1/4 **cup golden raisins**
1/4 **cup dried apricots**

1/4 **cup dried blueberries**
1/2 **cup nuts of your choice**
1 **apple, finely chopped**
1 **pear, finely chopped**
1 **banana, finely chopped**
1 **cup yogurt or 3/4 cup milk**
    (cow, rice, soy)

Combine all ingredients in large serving bowl. Heat to desired temperature or serve chilled. Makes about 8 cups. Serves 8 (about 1 cup each). (If mixture is too thick, add additional yogurt or milk to achieve desired consistency.)

| | | | | | | | | Exchanges | | |
Calories	Fat	% Fat Cal	Protein	Carb	Chol	Sodium	Fiber	Carb	Meat	Fat
210	6g	22%	4g	40g	0mg	75mg	3g	2.5		1

Gourmet Granola

(can be made without wheat, gluten, dairy, eggs, or sugar - see page xi about ingredients)

This makes a small recipe, but one that fits nicely in a fairly thin layer on a 15 x 10-inch jelly roll pan. If you have a very large oven and/or very large baking pans you can double the recipe. The sweetener you use will affect the flavor somewhat. You can vary the dried fruit as you wish in this morning treat. In fact, dried blueberries or dried peaches will also work nicely.

2 cups rolled rice flakes	2 teaspoons cooking oil or spray
1/2 teaspoon ground cinnamon	1/4 teaspoon salt
1/4 cup sesame seeds	1/4 cup honey or pure maple syrup
1/4 cup sunflower or pumpkin seeds	or agave nectar
1/4 cup almond slivers	1/4 cup golden raisins
1/4 cup unsweetened coconut flakes	1/4 cup dried cherries or cranberries
1 teaspoon gf vanilla extract	1/4 cup finely chopped dried apricots

Combine all ingredients, except dried fruit (raisins, cherries, apricots). Shake all ingredients together in a very large plastic container with a tight fitting lid or in a very large plastic bag. For a lower-fat version, omit cooking oil and spray mix with cooking spray each time you stir it during browning process described below.

Spread granola on baking sheet coated with cooking spray. Bake for 30-40 minutes at 300°, or until lightly browned. Stir every 10 minutes to assure even browning. Remove from oven and cool for 15 minutes. Add dried fruit. Cool completely. Store in airtight container in dark, dry place. Makes about 4 cups. Serves 8 (1/2 cup each).

Exchanges

Calories	Fat	% Fat Cal	Protein	Carb	Chol	Sodium	Fiber	Carb	Meat	Fat
210	9g	37%	4g	31g	<1mg	128mg	3g	1	.5	2

Granola Bars

(can be made without wheat, gluten, dairy, eggs, or sugar - see page xi about ingredients)

You can vary the fruits in this easy, but highly nutritious granola bar. For example, dates or dried blueberries or cranberries also work great. The potato flour (not potato starch) gives the bars a nice, chewy texture that more closely resembles granola bars made with oatmeal. This recipe makes a thin granola bar.

1/4 cup applesauce or
    other fruit purée
1/4 cup honey or pure maple syrup
1/4 cup golden raisins
1/4 cup dried tart cherries
1/4 cup chopped dried apricots
1 tablespoon grated orange peel
1 teaspoon gf vanilla extract
2 teaspoons cooking oil
1/4 cup potato flour
2 cups rolled rice flakes

1 teaspoon xanthan gum
1 teaspoon ground cinnamon
1 teaspoon baking powder
1/4 cup sesame seeds
1/4 cup sunflower or pumpkin seeds
1/4 cup almond slivers
1/4 cup unsweetened coconut flakes
1/2 teaspoon salt
Cooking spray

Preheat oven to 325°. Coat 13 x 9-inch pan with cooking spray or grease thoroughly. Line pan with waxed paper or parchment paper if you plan to invert the pan. Spray again. Set aside.

Combine all ingredients in a food processor. Pulse until mixture is thoroughly combined. Using a food processor is especially good for this recipe because it chops the ingredients evenly, making for a more consistent granola bar.

Spread batter evenly in prepared pan. Bake for 30-35 minutes or until mixture begins to brown around edges. Remove from oven and cool for 10 minutes. If inverting pan onto a cutting surface, do so now. Otherwise, let bars cool to room temperature before cutting. Makes 18 bars.

								Exchanges		
Calories	Fat	% Fat Cal	Protein	Carb	Chol	Sodium	Fiber	Carb	Meat	Fat
100	4g	35%	2g	15g	<1mg	117mg	2g	.5		

Notes

DESSERTS

I like to think of dessert as the "grand finale" to a spectacular meal—similar to the surprise ending to a wonderful play. Dessert should be memorable, like the way you remember the encore performance of a talented entertainer.

Desserts also create an opportunity to establish rituals—such as baking that favorite birthday cake every year . . .or making an apple dish with the first hint of fall . . .or making homemade ice cream on July 4th.

Each time I write a cookbook, the dessert chapter turns out to be the largest. It's also the one I start working on first. That probably tells you where my heart is. But this chapter of desserts is perhaps my favorite because it contains many chocolate desserts. At our house, dessert IS chocolate! If you are not passionate about chocolate, you'll find other tempting desserts in this chapter. So, go ahead and indulge. Just do so in moderation.

More desserts on next page

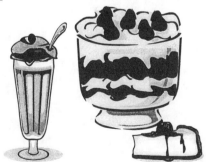

DESSERTS (continued)

Pies, Puddings, & Other Desserts
Baked Alaska 141
Cantaloupe with Cinnamon 142
Cappuccino Pudding 142
Cherry Cobbler 143
Chocolate Covered Strawberries 144
Chocolate Dipped, Filled Strawberries 144
Chocolate Pots De Crème 140
Chocolate Mocha Fudge Trifle 145
Flower Pot Treats 146
Frozen Tiramisu 147
Panna Cotta 148
Peach Melba Ice Cream Pie 149

Wedding Cakes
Chocolate Raspberry Groom's Cake 113
Coconut Wedding Cake 114
Lemon Wedding Cake 115
Spice Wedding Cake 116-117
White Wedding Cake with Fruit Filling 118
Yellow Tiered Wedding Cake 119

Ice Cream, Sherbet, & Sorbet
Chocolate Cappuccino Ice Cream 158
Chocolate Sorbet 158
Lemon Sorbet 159
Peach Ice Cream 160
Raspberry Sherbet 160
Strawberry Sherbet 160
Vanilla Frozen Yogurt without Eggs 161
Vanilla Ice Cream with Eggs 161

Frostings, Toppings, Etc.
Apricot Filling 133
Caramel Sauce 134
Cherry Pie Filling 133
Chocolate Cinnamon Cream 135
Chocolate Ganache 135
Chocolate Syrup 136
Chocolate Frostings 136-137
Espresso Ganache 135
Raspberry Filling 138
Un-chocolate Frosting 138
Whipped Topping (Nut-based) 139
Whipped Topping (Soy-based) 139
White 7-Minute Frosting 140

Applesauce Spice Cake

(can be made without wheat, gluten, dairy, eggs, or sugar - see page xi about ingredients)

Think of a crisp, fall day with the aroma of this cake filling your kitchen. Wonderful!
This recipe makes a small cake, perfect for the smaller (6 cup) Bundt pan.

1/2 cup garbfava flour or
   brown rice flour
1/4 cup potato starch
1/4 cup tapioca flour
1/2 teaspoon xanthan gum
1 teaspoon unflavored gelatin powder
1/2 teaspoon salt
1 1/2 teaspoons baking soda
1 1/2 teaspoons baking powder
1 teaspoon ground cinnamon
1/2 teaspoon ground cloves
1/4 teaspoon ground nutmeg

1/4 teaspoon ground allspice
1/2 cup chopped walnuts
1/2 cup currants or dark raisins
1/3 cup butter or oleo or
   Spectrum™ canola oil spread
   or 1/4 cup cooking oil
2/3 cup brown sugar*
2 large eggs**
1/2 cup applesauce
1 tablespoon apple cider vinegar
Cooking spray

Preheat oven to 350°. Spray 6-cup nonstick Bundt cake pan or 8 x 8-inch nonstick cake pan with cooking spray or grease thoroughly. Set aside.

Sift dry ingredients together (flour through allspice). Toss walnuts and currants with 2 tablespoons of the flour mixture. Set aside.

In large mixing bowl, cream butter, sugar, egg (or tofu—see below), applesauce, and vinegar until thoroughly blended and very, very smooth. Slowly add dry ingredients, mixing just until combined. Fold in nuts and currants.

Transfer to prepared pan and bake for 25-30 minutes. Cool in pan for 5-10 minutes. Remove cake to wire rack to cool completely. Serves 8.

| | | | | | | | | Exchanges | | |
Calories	Fat	% Fat Cal	Protein	Carb	Chol	Sodium	Fiber	Carb	Meat	Fat
300	13g	37%	5g	43g	0mg	500mg	2g	1		2

Eggs and butter add additional 75mg cholesterol per serving.

*Sugar Alternative: 2/3 cup maple sugar in place of 2/3 cup brown sugar. Add 1/8 teaspoon baking soda.

**Egg Alternative: 1/2 cup soft silken tofu in place of 2 eggs. For best results, use garbfava flour. Cake will be heavy and dense.

Basic Cake

(can be made without wheat, gluten, dairy, or sugar - see page xi about ingredients)

This is an all-purpose basic cake that you can use for many occasions. For a white cake, use 3 egg whites rather than 2 whole eggs. For an egg-free version, see next page.

1/3 cup butter or oleo or Spectrum™
   canola oil spread or cooking oil
1 cup sugar*
2 large eggs (or 3 egg whites)
1 tablespoon grated lemon peel
1 cup white rice flour or brown rice flour
1/3 cup potato starch
3 tablespoons tapioca flour
1 teaspoon xanthan gum

1/2 teaspoon baking powder
1/2 teaspoon baking soda
1/4 teaspoon salt
1/2 cup buttermilk or 2 teaspoons
   cider vinegar and enough
   non-dairy milk to equal 1/2 cup
1 teaspoon gf vanilla extract
Cooking spray

Preheat oven to 325°. Coat two 8-inch round pans with cooking spray and line with parchment paper or waxed paper. Or, spray two 5 x 3-inch small cake pans with cooking spray. Set aside.

Using an electric mixer and large mixer bowl, cream together butter (or oleo) and sugar (or fructose) on medium speed until thoroughly blended. Mix in eggs and grated lemon peel on low speed until blended.

In a medium bowl, sift together flours, xanthan gum, baking powder, baking soda, and salt. In another medium bowl, combine buttermilk and vanilla extract.

On low speed, beat dry ingredients into butter mixture, alternating with buttermilk, beginning and ending with dry ingredients. Mix just until combined. Spoon batter into prepared pans and smooth tops.

Bake 8-inch cakes for about 30-35 minutes or small loaf pans for 30-40 minutes —or until tops are golden brown and a cake tester inserted in the center comes out clean. Let cakes cool in pans for 5 minutes, then remove from pan, remove paper, and cool on rack. Serves 12.

| | | | | | | | | Exchanges | | |
Calories	Fat	% Fat Cal	Protein	Carb	Chol	Sodium	Fiber	Carb	Meat	Fat
195	6g	29%	2g	33g	35mg	144mg	1g	1.5		1

Butter adds additional 15mg cholesterol per serving.

*Sugar Alternative #1: 1 cup fructose powder in place of 1 cup sugar
*Sugar Alternative #2: 2/3 cup pure fruit juice concentrate (thawed but not reconstituted) instead of 1 cup sugar. Reduce milk to 1/2 cup. For a sweeter, stronger fruit flavor, simmer 1 cup concentrate on low heat until reduced to 2/3 cup. Cool. You may also use 2/3 cup honey—reduce milk to 1/2 cup.

Basic Cake without Eggs

(can be made without wheat, gluten, dairy, eggs, or sugar - see page xi about ingredients)

This cake was designed for people who don't want to eat eggs. It can be baked as cupcakes, a layer cake, or used for any dessert requiring a basic cake.

1 cup garbfava flour or
  brown rice flour
1/2 cup potato starch
1/4 cup tapioca flour
1/2 teaspoon xanthan gum
2 1/4 teaspoons baking powder
1/4 teaspoon salt
3/4 cup granulated sugar*

1/2 cup butter or oleo or Spectrum™
  canola oil spread or 1/3 cup
  cooking oil
2 teaspoons gf vanilla extract
1/2 cup soft silken tofu
Grated lemon peel of 1 lemon
1/2 cup boiling water
Cooking spray

Preheat oven to 350° and lightly coat 11 x 7-inch nonstick pan (or two 5 x 3-inch pans—or other pan sizes, see below) with cooking spray. (Cake rises better in smaller pans.) Sift together flours, xanthan gum, baking powder, and salt. Set aside.

In food processor, cream together sugar, butter (at room temperature), vanilla, tofu, and lemon peel. Process on high until completely smooth and glossy. Add boiling water and process on high until completely mixed. Add flour mixture and process until smooth. Scrape down sides of bowl with spatula, if necessary.

Spoon batter into prepared pan(s) and bake 11 x 7-inch pan for 25-30 minutes; small loaf pans for 30-40 minutes or until tops are firm. Cake will not brown very much. Remove from oven and cool for 10 minutes before removing from pan(s). Cool completely before cutting. Serves 12.

								Exchanges		
Calories	Fat	% Fat Cal	Protein	Carb	Chol	Sodium	Fiber	Carb	Meat	Fat
200	9g	39 %	4g	28g	0mg	154mg	<1 g	1		1.5

Butter adds additional 20mg cholesterol per serving.

*Sugar Alternative: 2/3 cup honey or pure maple syrup in place of 3/4 cup granulated sugar. Reduce boiling water to 1/3 cup. Reduce oven to 325°.

Cupcakes: Bake 12 standard-size cupcakes for 20-25 minutes or until tops are firm.
Layer Cake: Line 8 or 9-inch round nonstick pan with waxed paper or parchment paper and spray with cooking spray. Spread batter in pan and bake at 350° for 35-40 minutes or until top is firm. Or, bake in two 8-inch round, nonstick pans for 25-30 minutes or until tops are firm. Cool cake for 10 minutes before removing from pan. Cool on wire rack.

Basic Chocolate Cake

(can be made without wheat, gluten, dairy, or sugar - see page xi about ingredients)

This basic chocolate cake is extremely versatile and it will become one of your favorites. Though it makes a somewhat small cake, it is virtually fail-proof. If you prefer a larger cake, double the recipe. For an egg-free version, see next page.

1/2 cup brown rice flour	1 cup brown sugar*
or garbfava flour	2 teaspoons gf vanilla extract
1/2 cup potato starch	1/2 cup milk (cow, rice, soy)
1/4 cup tapioca flour	1/2 cup butter or oleo or
1/2 cup cocoa powder (not Dutch)	Spectrum™ canola oil spread
1 teaspoon xanthan gum	1 large egg
1 1/4 teaspoons baking soda	3/4 cup warm (105°) coffee or water
3/4 teaspoon salt	Cooking spray

Preheat oven to 350°. Coat 9 x 9-inch round or square nonstick pan or 11 x 7-inch nonstick pan with cooking spray. Set aside.

Place all ingredients, except hot water or coffee, in large bowl and blend with electric mixer. Add hot water or coffee and mix until thoroughly blended. Pour into prepared pan and bake for 30-35 minutes or until toothpick placed in center of cake comes out clean. Serves 12.

Cupcakes: Bake 12 cupcakes for 20-25 minutes or until toothpick comes out clean.
Layer Cake: Double the recipe and bake in a 9-inch round nonstick pan for 35-40 minutes, or two 8-inch round nonstick pans for 25-30 minutes or until toothpick inserted in center comes out clean. Be sure to line pan(s) with waxed paper or parchment paper and spray with cooking spray for easier cake removal.

								Exchanges		
Calories	Fat	% Fat Cal	Protein	Carb	Chol	Sodium	Fiber	Carb	Meat	Fat
210	9g	36%	2g	33g	18mg	300mg	2g	1		1.5

Egg adds additional 20mg cholesterol per serving.

*Sugar Alternative #1: 1 cup maple sugar or dried cane juice in place of 1 cup brown sugar. Add 1/4 teaspoon baking soda.
*Sugar Alternative #2: 2/3 cup maple syrup in place of 1 cup brown sugar. Add 1/4 teaspoon baking soda. Decrease coffee or water to 1/2 cup.

Mexican Chocolate Cake: Add 1 1/2 tablespoons gf almond extract and 1 tablespoon ground cinnamon. Bake as directed.

Basic Chocolate Cake without Eggs

(can be made without wheat, gluten, dairy, eggs, or sugar - see page xi about ingredients)

*This version can be used just like the Chocolate Cake recipe on the previous page.
If you prefer a larger cake, double the recipe. For best results, use garbfava flour.*

1/2 cup garbfava flour or brown rice
   flour
1/2 cup potato starch
1/4 cup tapioca flour
1/2 cup cocoa powder (not Dutch)
1/2 teaspoon xanthan gum
2 1/4 teaspoons baking powder
1/2 teaspoon salt

3/4 cup brown sugar*
1/4 cup butter or oleo or Spectrum™
   canola oil spread or cooking oil
1/2 cup soft silken tofu
2 teaspoons gf vanilla extract
2/3 cup boiling hot coffee or water
Cooking spray

Preheat oven to 350°. Lightly coat 9-inch round or square nonstick pan (may use 8-inch springform pan) with cooking spray. Combine flours, cocoa, xanthan gum, baking powder, and salt. Set aside.

In food processor, cream together sugar, butter (at room temperature), tofu, and vanilla extract until very, very smooth. Add boiling coffee (or water) and blend until completely mixed. Add flour mixture and mix at low speed until smooth.

Spoon batter into prepared pan. Bake for 25-30 minutes or until top is firm and toothpick inserted in center comes out clean. Remove from oven. Cool 5 minutes before removing from pan (if using springform pan). Serves 12.

Cupcakes: Bake 12 cupcakes for 20-25 minutes or until toothpick comes out clean.

Layer Cake: Double the recipe and bake in 9-inch round nonstick pan for 30-35 minutes or two 8-inch round nonstick pans for 25-30 minutes or until toothpick inserted in center comes out clean. Be sure to line pan(s) with waxed paper or parchment paper and spray with cooking spray for easier cake removal.

								Exchanges		
Calories	Fat	% Fat Cal	Protein	Carb	Chol	Sodium	Fiber	Carb	Meat	Fat
150	5 g	28 %	3g	10g	10mg	200 mg	2 g	1		1

Butter adds additional 10mg cholesterol per serving.

*Sugar Alternative #1: 3/4 cup dried cane juice or maple sugar instead of 3/4 cup brown sugar. Add 1/4 teaspoon baking soda.

*Sugar Alternative #2: 2/3 cup honey or pure maple syrup in place of brown sugar. Reduce coffee or water to 1/3 cup. Add 1/4 teaspoon baking soda. Reduce oven to 325°.

Black Forest Brownie Torte

(can be made without wheat, gluten, dairy, eggs, or sugar - see page xi about ingredients)

If you love chocolate and cherry, you'll love this dessert. Commercial cherry pie filling may contain corn syrup and red food coloring (plus thickeners of unknown origin), so consider making your own using the recipe on page 133.

1/2 cup brown rice flour or garbfava flour	1/2 cup sugar*
1/2 cup potato starch	1/2 cup brown sugar*
1/4 cup tapioca flour	1 large egg**
1/2 cup cocoa (not Dutch)	2 teaspoons gf vanilla extract
1 teaspoon baking powder	1/4 cup hot (115°) water or brewed coffee
1/2 teaspoon salt	1 can (22 oz.) gf cherry pie filling (page 133)
1/4 teaspoon xanthan gum	1 cup Chocolate Syrup (page 136)
1/4 cup butter or oleo or cooking oil	Cooking spray

Preheat oven to 350°. Grease two 8-inch round, nonstick pans. Line bottom of pans with parchment paper or waxed paper. Spray again and set aside.

Stir together the flours, cocoa, baking powder, salt, and xanthan gum. In large mixing bowl, beat butter and sugar with electric mixer on medium speed until well combined.

Add egg and vanilla; beat until well combined. With mixer on low speed, add dry ingredients and hot water or coffee. Mix until just blended; a few lumps may remain.

Divide batter between greased pans and bake for 20-25 minutes or until a toothpick inserted in center comes out almost clean. Cool brownies for 10 minutes. Run knife around edges of pan to loosen brownies. Turn out onto cooling rack.

To assemble, place one brownie layer on serving plate. Top with 2/3 of the cherry pie filling. Place second brownie layer on top of cherry pie filling. Top with remaining cherry pie filling. Serve with Whipped Topping (page 139). Serves 10.

								Exchanges		
Calories	Fat	% Fat Cal	Protein	Carb	Chol	Sodium	Fiber	Carb	Meat	Fat
310	6g	18%	3g	64g	12mg	200mg	3g	1		1

Butter and egg add additional 22mg cholesterol per serving.

*Sugar Alternative: 1 cup dried cane juice or maple sugar in place of the 1/2 cup brown and 1/2 cup granulated sugar. Add 1/4 teaspoon baking soda.

**Black Forest Brownie Torte without Eggs: Omit egg and 1 tablespoon Ener-G® egg replacer powder. Increase hot water or coffee to 1/2 cup. Bake as directed.

Caramelized Pear Torte

(can be made without wheat, gluten, dairy, eggs, or sugar - see page xi about ingredients)

The perfect fall finale—when pears are at their best. This beautiful, delicious dessert is best made in a cast-iron skillet so you don't have to pour the caramel into another dish. Remember, this torte is turned upside-down before serving so arrange the pears as attractively as possible.

3/4 cup brown sugar or maple sugar
2 tablespoons water
3 firm ripe pears
1/3 cup butter or oleo or Spectrum™ canola oil spread or cooking oil
1 cup sugar or fructose powder
2 large eggs*
1 tablespoon grated lemon peel
1 cup white or brown rice flour
1/3 cup potato starch

3 tablespoons tapioca flour
1 teaspoon xanthan gum
1/2 teaspoon baking powder
1/2 teaspoon baking soda
1/4 teaspoon salt
1/2 cup buttermilk or 2 teaspoons cider vinegar and enough non-dairy milk to equal 1/2 cup
1 teaspoon gf vanilla extract
Cooking spray

Preheat oven to 350°. In 10-inch cast iron skillet sprayed with cooking spray, combine sugar and water. Bring to simmer over low heat, swirling pan occasionally, until sugar dissolves. Cook for another minute, gently swirling pan if sugar is coloring unevenly. Remove from heat. Let cool for 10 minutes. Mixture will firm slightly as it cools.

Wash and peel pears. Cut in half, lengthwise; then cut in quarters. Remove core from each piece. Cut each quarter into 3 uniformly-sized wedges. Arrange pears in pin-wheel design, as close together as possible, in caramel. Set aside.

Using electric mixer and large mixer bowl, cream together butter (or oleo) and sugar (or fructose) on medium speed until thoroughly blended. Mix in eggs and grated lemon peel on low speed until mixture is very, very smooth.

In a medium bowl, sift together flours, xanthan gum, baking powder, baking soda, and salt. In another medium bowl, combine buttermilk and vanilla.

On low speed, beat dry ingredients into butter mixture, alternating with buttermilk, beginning and ending with dry ingredients. Mix just until combined. Spoon batter gently over the pears.

Bake for about 30-35 minutes or until cake tester inserted in center comes out clean. Let cool for 5 minutes. Loosen edges with a knife. To invert torte onto a serving plate, place plate top down over skillet. Wearing oven mitts on both hands, hold plate and skillet together and flip so plate is on bottom; skillet on top. Remove skillet. Cool to room temperature. Serves 12.

| | | | | | | | | Exchanges | | |
Calories	Fat	% Fat Cal	Protein	Carb	Chol	Sodium	Fiber	Carb	Meat	Fat
295	7.5g	22%	2.5g	57g	36mg	150mg	2g	3		1.5

Butter adds additional 14mg cholesterol per serving.

*Caramelized Pear Torte without Eggs: Use Basic Cake without Eggs on page 99.

Chocolate Cake
with Espresso Sauce & Orange Coulis

(can be made without wheat, gluten, dairy, eggs, or sugar - see page xi about ingredients)

This is absolutely, wonderfully decadent— combining the wonderful flavors of chocolate, orange, and coffee. As an alternative to the espresso beans, dissolve 3 tablespoons espresso powder in milk or cream.

Cake
1/2 cup brown rice flour
   or garbfava flour
1/2 cup potato starch
1/4 cup tapioca flour
1/2 cup cocoa powder (not Dutch)
1 teaspoon xanthan gum
1 1/4 teaspoons baking soda
3/4 teaspoon salt
1 cup brown sugar*
2 teaspoons gf vanilla extract
1/2 cup milk (cow, rice, soy)
1/3 cup cooking oil
1 teaspoon flaxseed meal
1 tablespoon grated orange peel
1 tablespoon espresso powder
3/4 cup warm (105°) strongly brewed
   coffee
Cooking spray

Orange Coulis
3/4 cup fresh orange juice
1/3 cup sugar or fructose powder
1 tablespoon grated orange peel
1 teaspoon cornstarch or arrowroot

Espresso Sauce
1/4 cup espresso beans or 3
   tablespoons espresso powder
1 cup heavy cream or 3/4 cup milk
   (cow, soy, rice)
1/3 cup brown sugar or maple sugar,
   packed
1 small package (6 oz.) gf/df
   chocolate chips
2 tablespoons unsalted butter or oleo
   or 1 tablespoon cooking oil
1 teaspoon gf vanilla extract
Grated orange peel for garnish

Espresso Sauce: Roast espresso beans in 325° oven for 5-10 minutes, or until you can smell their aroma. Remove beans and cool. Place in a coffee grinder and grind coarsely. (Or, use 2 tablespoons espresso powder dissolved in milk.)

Place beans in a small saucepan with heavy cream (or non-dairy beverage) and bring to a boil. Remove from heat and let sit 30 minutes. Proceed to baking the cake.

Cake: Preheat oven to 350°. Coat 9-inch nonstick springform pan with cooking spray. Set aside.

Place all ingredients, except hot water or coffee, in large bowl and blend with electric mixer. Add warm water or coffee and mix until thoroughly blended. Pour into prepared pan and bake for 35-40 minutes or until toothpick placed in center of cake comes out clean. Cool on wire rack.

After cake is in oven, return to espresso sauce. Strain espresso bean mixture through a fine mesh strainer into a bowl. Return mixture to saucepan, add sugar, and bring to a boil. Remove from heat and add chocolate, butter (or oil), and vanilla extract. Stir until completely smooth. Or, make ahead of time and bring to room temperature at serving time. (continued on next page)

Orange Coulis: While cake is baking, prepare orange coulis. Combine orange juice, sugar, and orange peel over low heat. Stir constantly until mixture is thick and syrupy and reduced by half—about 5-10 minutes. If mixture is not thick enough, mix 1/2 teaspoon cornstarch into tablespoon of water and stir into orange coulis until thickened. Set aside to cool.

When ready to serve, place a small pool of orange coulis on each plate. Place espresso sauce in a measuring cup with a spout or a squeeze bottle (e.g., an empty ketchup bottle) and drizzle the sauce in concentric circles over the orange coulis, beginning in the center and ending at the edge of the orange coulis pool.

Holding a kitchen knife perpendicular to the plate, draw it through sauce beginning at the center and ending at the edge of the orange coulis. Repeat at even intervals around the entire plate. This gives a radiating "star" design to the sauce.

Cut the cake into wedges and very carefully place a wedge of cake in the center of the sauce. Top with a dollop of remaining espresso sauce and additional grated orange peel, if desired. Serves 12.

| | | | | | | | | Exchanges | | |
Calories	Fat	% Fat Cal	Protein	Carb	Chol	Sodium	Fiber	Carb	Meat	Fat
340	13g	33%	3g	57g	6mg	300mg	3g	2.5		2

*Sugar Alternative: 1 cup maple sugar in place of 1 cup brown sugar. Add 1/4 teaspoon baking soda.

Chocolate Cherry Cake

(can be made without wheat, gluten, dairy, eggs, or sugar - see page xi about ingredients)

If you like the combination of chocolate and cherries, then try this recipe. For variety, try the sweeter Bing cherries. This produces a heavy, dense cake—especially if you use the tofu.

1/2 cup brown rice flour or garbfava flour
1/2 cup potato starch
1/4 cup tapioca flour
1/2 cup cocoa (not Dutch)
1 teaspoon xanthan gum
1 1/4 teaspoons baking soda
3/4 teaspoon salt
3/4 cup brown sugar*
2 teaspoons gf vanilla extract

1 teaspoon gf almond extract
1/2 cup milk (cow, rice, soy)
1/2 cup butter or oleo or Spectrum™ canola oil spread or 1/3 cup cooking oil
1 large egg or 1/4 cup soft silken tofu
1/2 cup warm (105°) brewed coffee or water
1 can (16 oz.) canned tart cherries, drained
Cooking spray

Preheat oven to 350°. Lightly coat 9-inch, round or square nonstick pan (or use 8-inch springform pan) with cooking spray. Combine flours, cocoa, xanthan gum, baking powder, and salt. Set aside.

In food processor, cream together sugar, vanilla and almond extracts, butter (at room temperature), and egg (or tofu) until very, very smooth. Add warm coffee (or water) and blend until very, very smooth. Add flour mixture and mix at low speed until smooth. Add cherries and pulse until incorporated.

Spoon batter into prepared pan and bake for 25-30 minutes or until top is firm and tester inserted in center comes out clean. Remove from oven. Cool 5 minutes before removing from (springform) pan. Serves 12.

Cupcakes: Bake 12 cupcakes for 20-25 minutes or until tester comes out clean.

Layer Cake: Bake in 9-inch round nonstick pan for 30-35 minutes or two 8-inch round nonstick pans for 25-30 minutes or until toothpick comes out clean. Be sure to line pan(s) with waxed paper or parchment paper and spray with cooking spray for easier cake removal. Frost with desired frosting. (See frosting section.) Serves 12.

Exchanges

Calories	Fat	% Fat Cal	Protein	Carb	Chol	Sodium	Fiber	Carb	Meat	Fat
190	9g	37%	3g	31g	0mg	150mg	2g	1		1.5

Butter and egg add additional 39mg cholesterol per serving.

*Sugar Alternative: 3/4 cup maple sugar. Add 1/4 teaspoon baking soda.

Chocolate Macaroon Tunnel Cake

(can be made without wheat, gluten, dairy, or sugar - see page xi about ingredients)

This cake combines two of the most wonderful flavors on earth—chocolate and coconut.

1 1/4 cups brown rice flour or
    garbfava flour
2/3 cup potato starch
1/3 cup tapioca flour
1 1/2 teaspoons xanthan gum
1 1/2 teaspoons baking soda
1 teaspoon salt
1 1/4 cups granulated sugar*
1 tablespoon gf vanilla extract
1 teaspoon gf coconut extract
2 large eggs**

1/2 cup cooking oil
3/4 cup buttermilk or 1 tablespoon
    cider vinegar with enough non-dairy
    milk to equal 3/4 cup
3/4 cup warm (105°) water
1/2 cup shredded coconut
2 teaspoons gf coconut extract
2/3 cup cocoa powder (not Dutch)
Additional coconut for garnish
Frosting of choice
Cooking spray

Preheat oven to 350°. Coat 10 -inch nonstick Bundt pan with cooking spray. Set aside.

Combine flours, xanthan gum, baking soda, and salt in small bowl. Set aside.

In large bowl, blend sugar, vanilla and coconut extracts, eggs, and oil with electric mixer until thoroughly blended. Add dry ingredients and buttermilk alternately, ending with dry ingredients. Add warm water and mix until thoroughly blended. Remove 2/3 cup batter and combine with coconut and coconut flavoring. Set aside.

To remaining batter, beat in cocoa with electric mixer until thoroughly mixed. Pour 1/2 of chocolate batter into pan, spreading evenly. Carefully spoon coconut batter over center of chocolate batter to form a uniform-sized ring, making sure not to touch sides of pan.

Carefully pour remaining chocolate batter into prepared pan, taking care not to disturb coconut ring. Gently spread chocolate batter to edges of pan as evenly as possible.

Bake for 40-45 minutes or until toothpick placed in center of cake comes out clean. Serves 12.

| | | | | | | | | Exchanges | | |
Calories	Fat	% Fat Cal	Protein	Carb	Chol	Sodium	Fiber	Carb	Meat	Fat
310	13g	37%	4g	47g	32mg	382mg	3g	2		2

*Sugar Alternative: 1 1/4 cups fructose powder in place of 1 1/4 cups granulated sugar

**Chocolate Macaroon Tunnel Cake without Eggs: Use Basic Chocolate Cake without Eggs recipe on page 101.

Double Chocolate Cherry Torte

(can be made without wheat, gluten, dairy, eggs, or sugar - see page xi about ingredients)

For a different flavor twist, try the canned dark (Bing) cherries instead of tart, red cherries. If you can't find chocolate chips to suit your needs, use the Chocolate Syrup on page 136 instead and make it with the reserved cherry juice. Cake will be heavy and dense if tofu is used.

Cake

1 can (16 oz.) canned tart cherries (drain—reserve 1/4 cup juice)
1/3 cup brown rice flour or garbfava flour
1/4 cup potato starch
1/4 cup tapioca flour
1/2 cup cocoa powder (not Dutch)
1 teaspoon xanthan gum
1 teaspoon baking soda
1/2 teaspoon baking powder

3/4 teaspoon salt
1 cup brown sugar or maple sugar
1/3 cup cooking oil
2 teaspoons gf vanilla extract
1 teaspoon gf almond extract
1/2 cup sliced almonds
2 teaspoons water
2 large eggs or 1/2 cup soft silken tofu
Cooking spray

Sauce

1/4 cup reserved cherry juice
1/4 cup cocoa powder (not Dutch)
2 tablespoons almond butter or cooking oil
1/3 cup maple syrup or honey

Filling

1/4 cup milk (cow, rice, soy)
1/2 cup gf/df chocolate chips

Filling: In small saucepan, combine milk and chocolate chips over low heat and stir until smooth. (Or melt in microwave, stirring until smooth.) Set aside.
Cake: Preheat oven to 325°. In blender or food processor, purée drained cherries thoroughly. (Use juice for another purpose.) Set aside.

Spray 8-inch nonstick springform pan with cooking spray. Set aside.

In large bowl, mix flours, cocoa, xanthan gum, baking soda, baking powder, salt, and sugar together with oil and vanilla and almond extracts until thoroughly mixed. Mixture will be dry and crumbly. Set aside 1/2 cup of mixture.

In same large bowl, to dry cake mixture add puréed cherries, and eggs (or tofu) with electric mixer. Mix until very, very smooth. Spread batter in prepared pan. Spoon chocolate filling on top of batter. Stir nuts and water into remaining 1/2 cup dry cake mixture and sprinkle over filling.

Bake for 50 minutes or until top of cake center springs back when touched lightly. Cool in pan on wire rack for 10 minutes. Remove from pan. Cool.
Sauce: Combine ingredients in blender and blend until completely smooth. Store in refrigerator until ready to serve. Drizzle over each serving. Serves 12.

								Exchanges		
Calories	Fat	% Fat Cal	Protein	Carb	Chol	Sodium	Fiber	Carb	Meat	Fat
375	15g	30%	5g	71g	0mg	300mg	5g	3.5	.5	2.5

Eggs add additional 44mg cholesterol per serving.

Ginger Pound Cake with Cardamom Glaze

(can be made without wheat, gluten, dairy, eggs, or sugar - see page xi about ingredients)

Delightfully different, this cake will have your guests clamoring for more. It will be heavier and denser if you use the tofu.

Cake
- 6 tablespoons butter or oleo or Spectrum™ canola spread or 1/4 cup cooking oil
- 1 cup sugar or fructose powder*
- 2 large eggs, or 1/2 cup soft silken tofu
- 1 teaspoon grated lemon peel
- 1 cup white rice flour or brown rice flour
- 6 tablespoons potato starch
- 2 tablespoons tapioca flour
- 1 teaspoon xanthan gum
- 1/2 teaspoon baking powder
- 1/2 teaspoon baking soda
- 1/4 teaspoon salt
- 1 tablespoon ground ginger
- 2/3 cup buttermilk or 2 teaspoons cider vinegar and enough non-dairy milk to equal 2/3 cup
- 1 tablespoon grated fresh ginger
- 1 teaspoon gf vanilla extract
- Cooking spray

Glaze
- 1/4 cup water
- 1/3 cup sugar or 1/4 cup honey
- 1 teaspoon ground cardamom
- 6 whole black peppercorns
- 1 slice fresh ginger root (1/2-inch)

Cake: Preheat oven to 325°. Liberally grease or coat a 6 or 10-cup nonstick Bundt cake pan with cooking spray. Dust with rice flour; shake out excess.

Using electric mixer and large mixer bowl, cream together butter, sugar, eggs, and lemon peel on medium speed until very smooth—about 1 minute.

In medium bowl, sift together flours, xanthan gum, baking powder, baking soda, salt, and ground ginger. In another medium bowl, combine buttermilk, grated fresh ginger, lemon peel, and vanilla. On low speed, beat dry ingredients into butter mixture, alternating with buttermilk, beginning and ending with dry ingredients. Mix just until combined. Spoon batter into prepared pan.

Bake cake for about 50-60 minutes or until top is golden brown and a cake tester inserted in center comes out clean. Cool cake in pan for 5 minutes, then remove from pan and cool on rack.

Glaze: Combine ingredients in small, heavy saucepan. Stir over medium heat until sugar is dissolved. Remove from heat, cover, and let stand for 10 minutes. Strain syrup through sieve into small bowl. Brush syrup all over warm cake. Cool. Sprinkle with powdered sugar or garnish with fruit. Serves 12.

Calories	Fat	% Fat Cal	Protein	Carb	Chol	Sodium	Fiber	Carb	Meat	Fat
								| Exchanges		
215	7g	27%	2g	39g	16mg	148mg	1g	2		1

Eggs and butter add additional 56mg cholesterol.

*Sugar Alternative: 3/4 cup honey instead of 1 cup sugar. Reduce milk to 1/2 cup.

Heart Cake with
Chocolate Covered Strawberries

(can be made without wheat, gluten, dairy, eggs, or sugar - see page xi about ingredients)

Perfect for Valentine's Day or that special occasion where a little romance is appropriate.

Cake
1 prepared Basic Chocolate Cake (page
    100-101) or Basic Cake (page 98-99)
Cooking spray

Frosting
White 7-minute frosting (page 140) or
    preferred egg-free white frosting

Chocolate Drizzle
1 cup gf/df chocolate chips
1 tablespoon butter or oleo or oil

Chocolate Covered Strawberries
    (page 144) or Chocolate Dipped,
    Filled Strawberries (page 144)

Cake: Prepare batter as directed in recipe. Prepare 8 x 2-inch heart-shaped cake pan by greasing it or spraying with cooking spray. Line bottom with waxed paper or parchment paper. Grease or spray again. (If a 2-inch deep heart pan is not available, use 8 x 1 1/4-inch heart pan which holds 3 cups of batter.) Bake remaining batter as cupcakes.

Pour batter into prepared pan. Bake as directed in recipe. Cool in pan on wire rack for 10 minutes. Invert on rack, peel off paper, and let cool completely. Put cake on serving platter. Tuck strips of waxed paper under edges of cake to catch frosting.

Frosting: Prepare frosting. Frost top and sides of cake. Remove waxed paper strips.

Drizzle: Melt chocolate chips and butter and mix thoroughly. Place in small heavy-duty plastic freezer bag and cut off 1/8-inch diagonally on one corner. Drizzle chocolate in zig-zag fashion back and forth across cake.

Strawberries: Just before serving, arrange the strawberries decoratively in the center of the cake. Serves 10.

See each individual recipe for nutritional content. Chocolate Drizzle adds 44 calories per serving.

Irish Apple Cake

(can be made without wheat, gluten, dairy, eggs, or sugar - see page xi about ingredients)

This is an Irish version of the familiar apple cake. Serve it at your next St. Patrick's Day celebration or try it in the fall with Jonathan apples. If nuts aren't appropriate for your diet, use raisins instead.

2 small Granny Smith apples	1 teaspoon xanthan gum
1 tablespoon fresh lemon juice	1 teaspoon baking powder
3/4 cup butter or oleo or Spectrum™	1/2 teaspoon baking soda
canola oil spread or cooking oil	1/2 teaspoon salt
1 tablespoon grated lemon peel	1 teaspoon ground cinnamon
1 cup brown sugar*	1/3 cup raisins or currants
3 large eggs**	1/4 cup chopped pecans
1 cup garbfava flour or	(optional)
brown rice flour	2 tablespoons powdered sugar
1/2 cup potato starch	Cooking spray
1/4 cup tapioca flour	

Preheat oven to 350°. Spray 9-inch springform pan with cooking spray. Set aside. Peel, core, and thinly slice apples. Sprinkle with lemon juice. Set aside.

Cream butter, lemon peel, and sugar. Add eggs, one at a time, and beat thoroughly after each addition. (If using tofu, add all at once and beat until very, very smooth.) Add flours, xanthan gum, baking powder, baking soda, salt, and cinnamon. Beat thoroughly.

Spoon half of mixture into prepared cake pan. Arrange apple slices on top. Scatter raisins and nuts (if using) on top of apples. Spread remaining batter over raisins and nuts.

Bake for 40-45 minutes, or until tester inserted into cake comes out clean. Cool in pan for 15 minutes, then remove sides. Dust with powdered sugar before serving. Serves 12.

								Exchanges		
Calories	Fat	% Fat Cal	Protein	Carb	Chol	Sodium	Fiber	Carb	Meat	Fat
325	15g	42%	5g	42g	0mg	228mg	2g	1	.5	2.5

Butter and eggs add additional 84mg cholesterol.

*Sugar Alternative: 1 cup maple sugar in place of 1 cup brown sugar.

**Irish Apple Cake without Eggs: Omit eggs. Use 3/4 cup soft silken tofu. For best results, use garbfava flour.

Pecan Nut Torte with Chocolate Ganache

(can be made without wheat, gluten, dairy, or sugar - see page xi about ingredients)

Since this cake relies on eggs for leavening, it obviously isn't egg-free.

<u>Torte</u>
1 1/2 cups pecan meal, toasted*
3 tablespoons brown rice or Jowar flour
1 teaspoon xanthan gum
1 teaspoon baking powder
1/4 teaspoon salt
5 large eggs, separated (room temperature)
1/2 cup brown sugar or
   maple sugar, divided
1 teaspoon gf vanilla extract
12 whole pecans for garnish
Cooking spray

<u>Filling</u>
1/2 cup pecan meal, toasted*
1/2 cup Chocolate Ganache
   (page 135)

<u>Frosting</u>
Chocolate Ganache (page
   135)

Torte: Heat oven to 350°. Grease three 8-inch round, nonstick pans or coat with cooking spray. Line with waxed paper or parchment paper. Grease or spray again.

In small bowl, combine pecan meal, flour, xanthan gum, baking powder, and salt. Set aside.

In medium bowl, beat egg whites with electric mixer on medium speed until foamy. Increase speed to high, gradually add 1/4 cup of the sugar, and beat until stiff. Set aside.

In another small bowl, beat egg yolks, remaining 1/4 cup sugar, and vanilla until thick and pale. Whisk yolk mixture into nut mixture and combine thoroughly. Mixture will be fairly thick. Gently whisk nut-egg yolk mixture into egg whites until thoroughly combined. Spread evenly in prepared pans.

Bake 20-25 minutes or until tops spring back when touched lightly. Place on a wire rack to cool completely.

Filling: Combine pecan meal and 1/2 cup Chocolate Ganache. To assemble cake, place first layer on serving plate. Top with 1/2 of the filling and use spatula or knife to spread filling to edges of cake. Repeat with second layer, spreading remaining filling to edges. Place top layer (top side up) on filling.

Frosting: Use Chocolate Ganache. Spread frosting over top of cake and let it run down sides of cake. If mixture is too thick, add water—1 teaspoon at a time to desired consistency. Garnish with reserved whole pecans, placing them toward edge. For best results, serve within 30 minutes or ganache will harden and lose its sheen. Serves 12.

Exchanges

Calories	Fat	% Fat Cal	Protein	Carb	Chol	Sodium	Fiber	Carb	Meat	Fat
450	30g	56%	9g	44g	88mg	140mg	3g	2	1	5

*To toast pecan meal, spread in thin layer on cookie sheet and bake at 350° for 8-10 minutes, stirring frequently. Watch carefully at end of toasting to avoid burning.

Chocolate Raspberry Groom's Cake

(can be made without wheat, gluten, dairy, or sugar - see page xi about ingredients)

This cake makes an excellent bridegroom's cake as well as a wonderful wedding cake for those who prefer chocolate instead of the traditional white wedding cake. To serve larger groups, make another cake rather than doubling this recipe. This can be a two or four layer cake.

1 cup brown rice flour
　or garbfava flour
1 cup potato starch
1/2 cup tapioca flour
1 cup cocoa powder (not Dutch)
2 teaspoons xanthan gum
2 1/2 teaspoons baking soda
1 1/2 teaspoons salt
2 cups brown sugar or maple sugar
1 tablespoon gf vanilla extract
1 cup milk (cow, rice, soy)

1 cup butter or oleo or Spectrum™
　canola oil spread
2 large eggs*
1/4 cup warm (105°) coffee or water
1 cup thoroughly crushed raspberries
Raspberry Filling (page 138)
1/2 cup raspberry jam (fruit-only
　version, slightly warmed)
Chocolate Frosting (pages 136-137)
Cooking spray

Preheat oven to 350°. Coat two 9-inch or four 9-inch nonstick cake pans with cooking spray and line with waxed paper or parchment paper. Spray again. Set aside.

Place all ingredients, except hot water or coffee and raspberries, in large bowl and blend with electric mixer. Add hot water or coffee and raspberries and mix until thoroughly blended. Pour into prepared pans. Bake two layers for 35-40 minutes; four layers for 20 minutes—or until toothpick placed in center of cake comes out clean. Cool for 5 minutes. Turn cakes out of pans onto rack and remove paper. Cool thoroughly.

Slice each layer in half horizontally (if you've baked two rather than four layers). Brush excess crumbs from each layer.

Have Raspberry Filling and Chocolate Frosting ready. To assemble, place first layer on cake stand. Brush with thin layer of raspberry jam. Spread thin layer of Raspberry Filling on top of jam. Top with next cake layer. Repeat process with remaining layers (if using more than two layers). Chill cake for 30 minutes.

Frost with desired chocolate frosting. (See frosting section.) Decorate with fresh flowers and fresh raspberries sprinkled around cake. Serves 16.

| | | | | | | | | Exchanges | | |
Calories	Fat	% Fat Cal	Protein	Carb	Chol	Sodium	Fiber	Carb	Meat	Fat
380	13g	30%	3.5g	66g	58mg	450mg	5g	1		2

Butter adds additional 30mg cholesterol per serving.

*Chocolate Raspberry Groom's Cake without Eggs: Use the Basic Chocolate Cake without Eggs on page 101. Bake as directed, doubling the recipe. Add raspberries with other liquid ingredients.

Coconut Wedding Cake

(can be made without wheat, gluten, dairy, or sugar - see page xi about ingredients)

For large groups, make multiple batches of this small cake instead of doubling it.

6 tablespoons butter or oleo or
    Spectrum™ canola oil spread
1 cup sugar*
2 large eggs**
1 cup white or brown rice flour
6 tablespoons potato starch
2 tablespoons tapioca flour
1 teaspoon xanthan gum
1/2 teaspoon baking powder
1/2 teaspoon baking soda
1/4 teaspoon salt
1/4 cup shredded coconut

3/4 cup buttermilk or 1 tablespoon
     cider vinegar with enough non-dairy
     milk to equal 1 1/2 cups
1 teaspoon gf vanilla extract
1 teaspoon gf coconut extract
1 teaspoon gf almond extract
White 7-Minute Frosting (page 140) or
    preferred white egg-free frosting
1 cup lightly toasted coconut flakes
1/4 cup shredded coconut for
Cooking spray

Preheat oven to 325°. Coat two 8-inch round pans with cooking spray and line with parchment paper. Set aside.

With electric mixer and large mixer bowl, cream together butter (or oleo) and sugar on medium speed until light and fluffy. Mix in eggs on low speed.

In a medium bowl, sift together flours, xanthan gum, baking powder, baking soda, salt, and coconut. In another medium bowl, combine buttermilk and vanilla, almond, and coconut extracts. On low speed, beat dry ingredients into butter mixture, alternating with buttermilk, beginning and ending with dry ingredients. Mix just until combined. Spoon batter into prepared pans.

Bake cakes for about 30 minutes or until tops are golden brown and a cake tester inserted in center comes out clean. Let cakes cool in pans for 5 minutes, then remove from pan, remove parchment paper, and cool on rack.

Prepare 7-minute frosting or white frosting of choice. To make coconut filling, stir 1/4 cup shredded coconut into 1/2 cup frosting. Assemble cakes by placing one layer on cake stand. Using a spatula, spread coconut filling on first layer, working from center out to edges. Add second layer and frost top and edges of cake with a wide knife, using swirls and dips for a pretty effect. Sprinkle toasted coconut on cake. Serves 12.

| | | | | | | | | Exchanges | | |
Calories	Fat	% Fat Cal	Protein	Carb	Chol	Sodium	Fiber	Carb	Meat	Fat
365	10g	25%	4g	67g	52mg	235mg	2g	4		2

Butter adds additional 16mg of cholesterol per serving.

*Sugar Alternative: 1 cup fructose powder in place of granulated sugar. Add 1/4 teaspoon baking soda.

**Coconut Wedding Cake without Eggs: Use Basic Cake on page 99, adding coconut and extracts just before spreading in baking pan. (Coconut adds 30 calories and 3 fat grams per serving.)

Lemon Wedding Cake

(can be made without wheat, gluten, dairy, or sugar - see page xi about ingredients)

Wonderfully lemony, this cake makes a wonderful choice for that special day.

1/2 cup butter or Spectrum™ canola
  oil spread or oleo or cooking oil
2 cups sugar or fructose powder
4 large eggs*
1/2 cup grated lemon peel
2 cups white or brown rice flour
2/3 cup potato starch
1/4 cup tapioca flour
1 1/2 teaspoons xanthan gum
1/2 teaspoon baking powder
1/2 teaspoon baking soda
1/2 teaspoon salt

1 1/2 cups buttermilk or 1 table-
  spoon cider vinegar with enough
  non-dairy milk to equal 1 1/2 cups
2 teaspoon gf vanilla extract
White 7-Minute Frosting (page 140)
  or white egg-free frosting of choice
1/4 cup grated lemon peel
Orange Marmalade (page 39)
Lemon peel strips for garnish**
Fresh mint leaves for garnish
Fresh flowers for garnish
Cooking spray

Preheat oven to 325°. Coat two or four 9-inch round, nonstick cake pans with cooking spray. Line with parchment paper or waxed paper; spray again. Set aside.

Using electric mixer and large mixer bowl, cream together butter (or oil) and sugar on medium speed. Mix in eggs and lemon peel until blended.

In a medium bowl, sift together flours, xanthan gum, baking powder, baking soda, and salt. In another medium bowl, combine buttermilk and vanilla. On low speed, beat dry ingredients into butter mixture, alternating with buttermilk, beginning and ending with dry ingredients. Mix just until combined. Spoon batter into prepared pans and smooth tops.

Bake the two-layer cakes for 30 minutes; four-layer cakes for 20 minutes— or until tops are golden brown and cake tester inserted in center comes out clean. Cool cakes in pans for 5 minutes. Remove from pan and cool on rack.

Slice two-layer cakes in half horizontally. Place first layer on cake stand; brush thin glaze of marmalade. Repeat with remaining layers. Chill.

Stir grated lemon peel into frosting of choice. Frost cake with wide spatula using dips and swirls to create a decorative effect. Garnish. Serves 16.

| | | | | | | | | Exchanges | | |
Calories	Fat	% Fat Cal	Protein	Carb	Chol	Sodium	Fiber	Carb	Meat	Fat
430	9g	18%	5g	87g	54mg	245mg	1.5g	5g		1.5

Butter adds additional 16mg of cholesterol per serving.

Lemon Wedding Cake without Eggs: Use Basic Cake without Eggs on page 99. Double recipe.

****Lemon Peel Strips**: Use potato peeler to remove long strips from lemon. Using sharp knife, cut strips into very thin strips—about 2-3 inches long. To make lemon peel shiny and pliable, boil in mixture of 1 cup water and 1/4 cup honey for 5 minutes. Drain and cool.

Spice Wedding Cake

(can be made without wheat, gluten, dairy, or sugar - see page xi about ingredients)

A spice cake makes a wonderful bridegroom's cake. Or, serve it as the main wedding cake. See egg-free version on next page.

1 1/2 cups brown rice flour or
   garbfava flour
1 cup potato starch
1/2 cup tapioca flour
1 teaspoon xanthan gum
2 teaspoons baking soda
1 teaspoon salt
1 1/2 tablespoons ground ginger
3 teaspoons ground cinnamon
3/4 teaspoon ground nutmeg
1/4 teaspoon ground cloves
2 1/4 cups milk (cow, rice, soy)

2 1/4 cups brown sugar, packed*
1/2 cup cooking oil
1/2 cup molasses (cane or sorghum)
1 1/2 teaspoons gf vanilla extract
3 large eggs
Cooking spray
White 7-Minute Frosting (page 140)
   or egg-free frosting of choice
1 tablespoon gf instant coffee powder
Garnishes of shaved chocolate, Dutch
   cocoa powder, or chopped nuts
Cooking spray

Preheat oven to 325°. Coat two or four 9-inch round, nonstick cake pans with cooking spray. Line bottom with wax paper or parchment paper, then spray again. Set aside.

Sift together flours, xanthan gum, baking soda, salt, ginger, cinnamon, nutmeg, and cloves in a large mixing bowl.

Combine milk and sugar in heavy saucepan and bring just to a boil over medium heat. Remove from heat and add oil, molasses, and vanilla extract.

Add milk mixture to flour mixture in mixing bowl and mix until thoroughly blended. Add eggs and mix until blended. Pour batter into prepared pans.

Bake two-layer cakes for 35-40 minutes; four-layer cakes for 20 minutes—or until toothpick inserted in center of cake comes out clean. Cool cakes in pans for 5 minutes. Invert cakes onto plate or rack to finish cooling. Remove paper.

If using two-layer cakes, slice in half horizontally. Brush excess crumbs from each layer.

Prepare frosting of choice and add 1 tablespoon instant coffee powder dissolved in 1 tablespoon hot water. Place one layer on serving plate. Spread a thin layer of frosting on bottom half. Repeat with remaining layers. Frost sides and top with deep swirls in decorative manner. Garnish. Serves 16.

Without frosting | | | | | | | | Exchanges | |

Calories	Fat	% Fat Cal	Protein	Carb	Chol	Sodium	Fiber	Carb	Meat	Fat
420	12g	30%	4g	73g	370mg	545mg	1g	4		2

Sugar Alternative: 2 1/4 cup maple sugar in place of 2 1/4 cups brown sugar. Add 1/8 teaspoon baking soda.

Spice Wedding Cake without Eggs

(can be made without wheat, gluten, dairy, eggs, or sugar - see page 9 about ingredients)

For an interesting taste, try using brewed coffee as the liquid for the frosting. If you're using it as a wedding cake, make multiple batches rather than doubling recipe.

1 1/2 cup garbfava or
    brown rice flour
1 cup potato starch
3 tablespoons tapioca flour
1 1/2 teaspoons xanthan gum
1 1/2 teaspoons baking powder
1 teaspoon baking soda
1 teaspoon salt
1 tablespoon ground ginger
1 tablespoon ground cinnamon
1/2 teaspoon ground nutmeg
1/2 teaspoon ground cloves
1 1/2 cups boiling water

1 cup brown sugar, packed*
3/4 cup soft silken tofu
3/4 cup molasses (cane or sorghum)
1 1/2 teaspoons gf vanilla extract
1/2 cup cooking oil
Cooking spray
White 7-Minute Frosting (page 140)
    or egg-free frosting of choice
1 tablespoon gf instant coffee powder
Garnishes of shaved chocolate, Dutch
    cocoa powder, or chopped nuts
Cooking spray

Preheat oven to 325°. Spray two or four 9-inch round nonstick pans with cooking spray. Line with waxed paper and spray again. Set aside.

In a large mixing bowl, sift together dry ingredients. Set aside.

Dissolve sugar in 1 cup boiling water (reserve remaining water). Set aside.

In large bowl with electric mixer, blend tofu, dissolved sugar/water mixture, molasses, and vanilla until very smooth. (If using honey, add now.)

Add flour mixture and process just until mixed. Add remaining boiling water and oil. Blend until mixed, scraping sides of food processor bowl with spatula. Batter will be somewhat thick. Pour batter into prepared pan(s).

Bake two-layer cakes for 30-35 minutes; four-layer cakes for 20 minutes—or until toothpick inserted into center comes out clean. Remove from oven. Cool 10 minutes. Remove from pan, remove paper, and cool on wire rack.

Prepare frosting of choice, adding 1 tablespoon instant coffee powder dissolved in 1 tablespoon hot water. Place first layer on serving plate and spread with 1/2 cup frosting. Add top layer and frost sides and top with spatula using deep, decorative swirls. Garnish. Serves 16.

Without frosting								Exchanges		
Calories	Fat	% Fat Cal	Protein	Carb	Chol	Sodium	Fiber	Carb	Meat	Fat
350	8g	20%	4.5g	67g	0mg	475mg	2g	3		1.5

*Sugar Alternative #1: 1 cup dried cane juice or maple sugar in place of 1 cup brown sugar. Increase baking soda to 1 1/4 teaspoons.

*Sugar Alternative #2: 3/4 cup honey or maple syrup in place of 1 cup brown sugar. Reduce boiling water to 1 cup. Increase baking soda to 1 1/4 teaspoons.

White Wedding Cake with Fruit Filling

(can be made without wheat, gluten, dairy, or sugar - see page xi about ingredients)

This cake is especially pretty with the colorful raspberry and apricot layers. It is a small cake, but you can always bake several to feed a larger group.

1/3 cup butter or oleo or
  Spectrum™ canola oil spread or
  1/4 cup cooking oil
1 cup granulated sugar*
3 large egg whites**
1 cup white rice flour
1/3 cup potato starch
3 tablespoons tapioca flour
1 teaspoon xanthan gum
1/2 teaspoon baking powder
1/2 teaspoon baking soda
1/4 teaspoon salt

3/4 cup buttermilk or 2 teaspoons
  cider vinegar with enough
  non-dairy milk to equal 3/4 cup
1 teaspoon gf vanilla extract
1 teaspoon gf almond extract
Raspberry Filling (page 138)
Apricot Filling (page 133)
White 7-Minute Frosting (page 140)
  or preferred egg-free frosting
Fresh raspberries, dried apricot
  slivers, or fresh mint (garnish)
Cooking spray

Preheat oven to 325°. Coat three 8-inch round nonstick pans with cooking spray. Line with parchment paper or waxed paper. Spray again, then set aside.

Using electric mixer and large mixer bowl, cream together butter (or oleo) and sugar (or fructose) on medium speed until blended. Mix in egg whites.

In a medium bowl, sift together flours, xanthan gum, baking powder, baking soda, and salt. In another medium bowl, combine buttermilk and vanilla and almond extracts. On low speed, beat dry ingredients into butter mixture, alternating with buttermilk, beginning and ending with dry ingredients. Mix just until combined. Spoon batter into prepared pans and smooth tops with spatula.

Bake cakes for about 25-30 minutes or until tops are golden brown and cake tester inserted in center comes out clean. Let cakes cool in pans for 5 minutes, then remove from pan, remove paper, and cool on rack.

Assemble cakes by placing one layer on cake stand. Using a spatula, spread Raspberry Filling on first layer. Work from center out to edges. Repeat process for next tier, spreading Apricot Filling from center out to edges. Place third tier on top. Chill cake while preparing frosting. Anchor layers with toothpicks.

Prepare frosting. Frost top layer and edges of cake with wide knife, using swirls and dips for a decorative effect. Garnish. Serves 12.

									Exchanges	
Calories	Fat	% Fat Cal	Protein	Carb	Chol	Sodium	Fiber	Carb	Meat	Fat
288	6g	17%	3g	57g	1mg	150mg	2.5g	2.5		1

Butter adds additional 14mg cholesterol per serving.

*Sugar Alternative: 1 cup fructose powder in place of 1 cup sugar
*White Wedding Cake without Eggs: Use Basic Cake without Eggs on page
  99. See Raspberry Filling and Apricot Filling for nutrient content.

Yellow Tiered Wedding Cake

(can be made without wheat, gluten, dairy, or sugar - see page xi about ingredients)

This is meant to resemble the traditional tiered wedding cake—the kind most of us remember from our own wedding day. However, the use of square rather than round tiers lends a more contemporary note.

1 cup butter or oleo or
   Spectrum™ canola oil spread
   or 3/4 cup cooking oil
3 cups granulated sugar*
6 large eggs**
3 tablespoons grated lemon peel
3 cup white rice flour
1 cup potato starch
1/2 cup tablespoons tapioca flour
1 tablespoon xanthan gum
3/4 teaspoon baking powder

3/4 teaspoon baking soda
1 teaspoon salt
2 1/4 cups buttermilk or 3 tablespoons cider vinegar with enough
   non-dairy milk to equal 2 1/4 cups
1 tablespoon gf vanilla extract
White 7-Minute Frosting (page 140)
   or preferred white egg-free frosting
Fresh flowers for decoration
Cooking spray

Preheat oven to 325°. Coat two 8 x 8 x 2-inch square pans with cooking spray and line with parchment paper. Set aside.

Using electric mixer and large mixer bowl, cream together butter and granulated sugar on medium speed until light and fluffy. Mix in eggs on low speed until blended. Add grated lemon peel.

In medium bowl, sift together flours, xanthan gum, baking powder, baking soda, and salt. In another medium bowl, combine buttermilk and vanilla. On low speed, beat dry ingredients into butter mixture, alternating with buttermilk, beginning and ending with dry ingredients. Mix just until combined. Spoon batter into prepared pans and smooth tops.

Bake cake for about 50 minutes or until top is golden brown and a cake tester inserted in center comes out clean. Let cake cool in pan for 5 minutes, then remove from pan, remove parchment paper, and cool on rack.

If not assembling cake on a sturdy base such as a large cake stand, you'll need a firm base. Make one by cutting 12-inch square of cardboard or foam board (available in art-supply stores) and cover in aluminum foil.

To make wedding cake, cut one of the cakes into a 6 x 6-inch square. Reserve leftover cake for another purpose (see Breakfast Trifle, page 90). Place cake on prepared board.

Cut the second cake into 2 smaller squares, one 3 3/4 x 3 3/4-inches and the other 2 1/4 x 2 1/4-inches. Once again, reserve leftover cake for another use.

With pastry brush, brush excess crumbs from all three pieces. Using a spatula, ice top of 6-inch square cake with thin layer of frosting. Work from center out to edges, then spread frosting around sides of cake. To smooth frosting, dip a wide knife in hot water and dry it before spreading the frosting. (continued on next page)

Repeat the process for remaining tiers. Chill cakes for 30 minutes. Assemble cake by putting two remaining tiers on top of one another in descending order of size. Give entire cake another coating of frosting, again dipping a wide knife in hot water then drying it before spreading the frosting.

Once final coat of frosting sets, (up to 1 hour), fill a pastry bag with reserved frosting. Fit it with a #3 pastry tip and pipe decorative border along edges of each tier. Decorate with fresh flowers as desired. Serves 36. (For more detailed directions on cake decorating, consult a cake decorating book.)

								Exchanges		
Calories	Fat	% Fat Cal	Protein	Carb	Chol	Sodium	Fiber	Carb	Meat	Fat
246	7g	23%	3g	44g	36mg	156mg	1g	1.5		1

Butter adds additional 15mg cholesterol per serving.

*Sugar Alternative: 3 cups fructose powder in place of granulated sugar. Add 1/4 teaspoon baking soda.

**Yellow Tiered Wedding Cake without Eggs: Use yellow cake version of Basic Cake without Eggs on page 99. Make 3 recipes to equal 36 servings.

Butterfly Cake

(can be made without wheat, gluten, dairy, eggs, or sugar - see page xi about ingredients)

Perfect for a little girl's birthday party or a spring luncheon, this pretty cake will delight everyone.

1/3 cup butter or oleo or Spectrum™ canola oil spread or 1/4 cup cooking oil
1 cup sugar*
2 large eggs**
1 cup white rice flour or brown rice flour
1/3 cup potato starch
3 tablespoons tapioca flour
1 teaspoon xanthan gum
1/2 teaspoon baking powder
1/2 teaspoon baking soda

1/4 teaspoon salt
1/2 cup buttermilk or 1 teaspoon cider vinegar and enough non-dairy milk to equal 1/2 cup
1 teaspoon gf vanilla extract
1 teaspoon gf almond extract
Frosting of choice
Fruit leather or Jelly Belly® jelly beans
Cooking spray

Preheat oven to 325°. Coat two 8-inch round pans with cooking spray and line with parchment paper or waxed paper. Set aside.

Using electric mixer and large mixer bowl, cream together butter and granulated sugar on medium speed until completely blended. Mix in eggs on low speed until thoroughly blended.

In a medium bowl, sift together flours, xanthan gum, baking powder, baking soda, and salt. In another medium bowl, combine buttermilk and vanilla and almond extracts.

On low speed, beat dry ingredients into butter mixture, alternating with buttermilk, beginning and ending with dry ingredients. Mix just until combined. Spoon batter into prepared pans and smooth tops.

Bake cakes for about 30-35 minutes or until tops are golden brown and a cake tester inserted in the center comes out clean. Let cakes cool in pans for 5 minutes, then remove from pan, remove paper, and cool on rack.

From each of the cakes, cut a 2-inch triangle and on the opposite side of each cake, cut a 1-inch wedge. Place the two circles together (straight sides together). Put the triangle shapes on either side of "wings" for body of butterfly. (See diagram on next page.) Frost with frosting of choice. Decorate with halved jelly beans. If jelly beans are not appropriate, use small circles cut from pure fruit leather. Use strips of fruit leather for butterfly "antennae". Serves 12.

Without frosting								Exchanges		
Calories	Fat	% Fat Cal	Protein	Carb	Chol	Sodium	Fiber	Carb	Meat	Fat
200	6g	29%	2g	32g	50mg	144mg	1g	2		1

Butter adds additional 14mg of cholesterol per serving.

*Sugar Alternative: 1 cup fructose powder in place of 1 cup granulated sugar. Add 1/4 teaspoon baking soda.

**Butterfly Cake without Eggs: Use Basic Cake without Eggs on page 99.

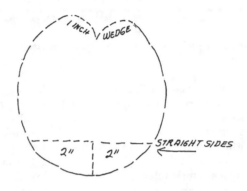

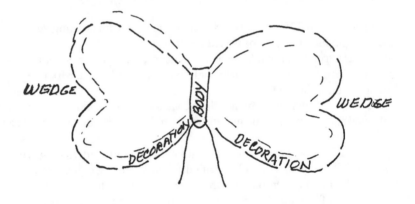

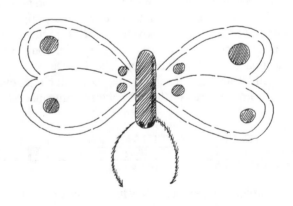

Candle Cake

(can be made without wheat, gluten, dairy, eggs, or sugar - see page xi about ingredients)

This pretty is extremely simple to make and appropriate for any age group. It can be a birthday cake or a first anniversary cake.

1/3 cup butter or oleo or Spectrum™
    canola oil spread or
    1/4 cup cooking oil
1 cup sugar*
2 large eggs**
1 cup white or brown rice flour
1/3 cup potato starch
3 tablespoons tapioca flour
1 teaspoon xanthan gum
1/2 teaspoon baking powder

1/2 teaspoon baking soda
1/4 teaspoon salt
1/2 cup buttermilk or 2 teaspoons
    cider vinegar and enough
    non-dairy milk to equal 1/2 cup
1 teaspoon gf vanilla extract
White Frosting (3-4 cups)
Fruit leather in dark color
Cooking spray

Preheat oven to 325°. Coat 13 x 9-inch nonstick pan with cooking spray. Line with parchment paper or waxed paper. Spray again. Dust with rice flour. Set aside.

Using electric mixer and large mixer bowl, cream together butter and granulated sugar (or fructose) on medium speed until light and fluffy. Mix in eggs on low speed until blended.

In medium bowl, sift together flours, xanthan gum, baking powder, baking soda, and salt. In another medium bowl, combine buttermilk and vanilla extract. On low speed, beat dry ingredients into butter mixture, alternating with buttermilk, beginning and ending with dry ingredients. Mix just until combined. Spoon batter into prepared pan and smooth top.

Bake cake for about 30-35 minutes or until top is golden brown and a cake tester inserted in the center comes out clean. Let cake cool in pan for 5-10 minutes, then invert onto piece of large cardboard covered with aluminum foil.

To make candle, cut cake in half, as shown in diagram on next page, down center of cake. Stack two pieces together, using 1/2 cup frosting between the layers to hold them together. Slice off top right corner, as shown in diagram.

Cut piece into trimmed oval shape to resemble flame. Set flame aside. (Discard scraps of cake or make them disappear with a quick taste-test!)

Tint 1 1/2 to 2 cups of frosting into equal amounts of either light pink, light blue, or light green using commercial food colorings. If these food colorings are not appropriate for your diet, use crushed, strained strawberry or raspberries for the pink frosting, strained blueberry juice for the blue frosting, and crushed, strained kiwis for the green frosting.

Frost entire cake. Put 1 cup white frosting into pastry bag fitted with a basket-weave tip. Or, put frosting in plastic, freezer bag and cut 1/8-inch off one corner. Pipe frosting in diagonal stripes across the candle. With remaining white frosting, arrange on top of candle to resemble melted wax. (continued on next page).

Tint remaining frosting with yellow coloring and frost the flame-shaped piece of cake. Place flame approximately 1/2 to 1-inch from cake and connect with a piece of dark-colored fruit leather (such as grape, raspberry, etc.) to resemble wick. Serves 12.

								Exchanges		
Calories	Fat	% Fat Cal	Protein	Carb	Chol	Sodium	Fiber	Carb	Meat	Fat
200	**6g**	**29%**	**2g**	**32g**	**50mg**	**144mg**	**1g**	**2**		**1**

Butter adds additional 14mg of cholesterol per serving.

*Sugar Alternative: 1 cup fructose powder in place of 1 cup granulated sugar. Add 1/4 teaspoon baking soda.

**Candle Cake without Eggs: Use Basic Cake without Eggs on page 99.

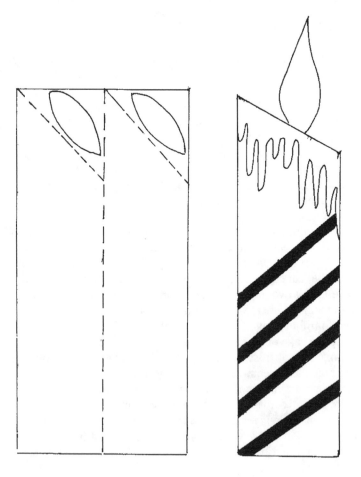

Caterpillar Cake

(can be made without wheat, gluten, dairy, eggs, or sugar - see page xi about ingredients)

Kids seem to love creepy, crawly things so they'll love this cute little caterpillar.

1/3 cup butter or oleo or
  Spectrum™ canola oil spread
  or 1/4 cup cooking oil
1 cup sugar*
2 large eggs, lightly beaten**
1 cup brown rice flour
1/3 cup potato starch
3 tablespoons tapioca flour
1 teaspoon xanthan gum
1/2 teaspoon baking powder
1/2 teaspoon baking soda

1/4 teaspoon salt
1/2 cup buttermilk or 2 teaspoons
  cider vinegar and enough
  non-dairy milk to equal 1/2 cup
1 teaspoon gf vanilla extract
Frosting of choice (tinted green)
Fruit leather or Jelly Belly®
  jelly beans
Coconut
Jet-Puff® miniature marshmallows
Cooking spray

Preheat oven to 325°. Coat a 6 or 10 cup non-stick Bundt pan with cooking spray. Set aside.

Using an electric mixer and a large mixer bowl, cream together butter (or Spectrum™ or oleo or oil) and granulated sugar (or fructose) on medium speed until light and fluffy. Mix in eggs on low speed until blended.

In medium bowl, sift together flours, xanthan gum, baking powder, baking soda, and salt. In another medium bowl, combine buttermilk, and vanilla. On low speed, beat dry ingredients into butter mixture, alternating with buttermilk, beginning and ending with dry ingredients. Mix just until combined.

Spoon batter into prepared pan and smooth top, if necessary. Bake cake for 50-55 minutes or until top is golden brown and a cake tester inserted in the center comes out clean. Let cake cool in pan for 5-10 minutes, then remove from pan, invert, and cool on rack.

To make caterpillar, trim bottom of cake (the top when it's baked) with a sharp, serrated knife so it sits level, without wobbling. Cut into thirds. Arrange on large baking sheet or on cardboard covered with foil (trimmed side down), as shown in diagram on next page.

To make green frosting, add drops of green food coloring to your favorite white frosting. If commercial food coloring is not appropriate for your diet, mash kiwi fruit through a sieve and use juice to tint the frosting. Frost caterpillar, placing frosting between cut ends and filling in crevasses with frosting to hold them together. Use knife or spoon dipped in hot water to smooth "stripes" across the caterpillar's body.

For the head, use a small orange or a lemon sliced in half, lengthwise and covered with frosting and shredded coconut and take a strip of fruit leather, cut in semi-circle, and cut jags across top to form "ruff". (See diagram on next page.) Attach with frosting to neck of caterpillar. Use jelly beans for feet, or oblongs of fruit leather, or cut Jet-Puff® marshmallows. Serves 12.

Calories	Fat	% Fat Cal	Protein	Carb	Chol	Sodium	Fiber	Carb	Meat	Fat
200	6g	29%	2g	32g	50mg	144mg	1g	2		1

Butter adds additional 14mg of cholesterol per serving.

*Sugar Alternative: 1 cup fructose powder in place of 1 cup sugar

**Caterpillar Cake without Eggs: Use Basic Cake without Eggs on page 99.

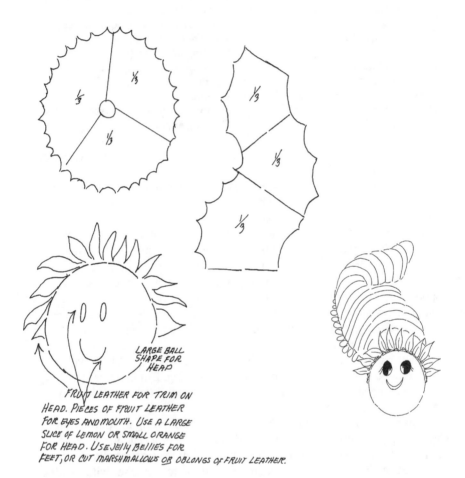

LARGE BALL
SHAPE FOR
HEAD

FRUIT LEATHER FOR TRIM ON
HEAD. PIECES OF FRUIT LEATHER
FOR EYES AND MOUTH. USE A LARGE
SLICE OF LEMON OR SMALL ORANGE
FOR HEAD. USE JELLY BELLIES FOR
FEET, OR CUT MARSHMALLOWS OR OBLONGS OF FRUIT LEATHER.

Down on the Farm Cake

(can be made without wheat, gluten, dairy, eggs, or sugar - see page xi about ingredients)

You'll need a few more "props" with this cake than with some of the others in this section, but if you have them on hand the effect is really worth it.

1/2 cup brown rice flour or
   garbfava flour
1/2 cup potato starch
1/4 cup tapioca flour
1/2 cup cocoa (not Dutch)
1 teaspoon xanthan gum
1 1/4 teaspoons baking soda
3/4 teaspoon salt
1 cup brown sugar
   or maple sugar
2 teaspoons gf vanilla extract

1/2 cup milk (cow, rice, soy)
1/2 cup butter or oleo or Spectrum™
   canola oil spread or 1/3 cup cooking oil
1 large egg*
3/4 cup warm (105°) coffee or water
Coconut
Green food coloring
Cookies (see Basic Cookie, page 157)
Gf (Glutano) pretzels or rice crackers
Toy farm animals and tractors
Cooking spray

Preheat oven to 350°. Coat 11 x 7-inch nonstick pan with cooking spray; line with parchment paper or waxed paper. Spray again. Set aside.

Place all ingredients, except hot water or coffee, in large bowl and blend with electric mixer. Add hot water or coffee and mix until thoroughly blended. Pour into prepared pan and bake for 30-35 minutes or until toothpick placed in center of cake comes out clean. Cool thoroughly. Invert cake onto platter or piece of cardboard covered with aluminum foil.

To make farm, tint frosting green for grass, and color unsweetened coconut with green coloring and lay in "furrows" for crop. (If green food coloring is unacceptable for your diet, use chocolate frosting and dust the coconut with cocoa.) The dark chocolate of the cake becomes the soil. Use clumps of frosting for clumps of grass to anchor fence posts. Use pretzels to make a fence or use rice crackers lined up end to end as a fence.

Make "cow" or "sheep" cookies or other animals using Basic Cookie recipe on page 157. You may also frost the cookies. Or, use miniature toy animals and tractors. Be sure to remove before serving cake to prevent small children from swallowing the toys. Serves 12.

| | | | | | | | | Exchanges | | |
Calories	Fat	% Fat Cal	Protein	Carb	Chol	Sodium	Fiber	Carb	Meat	Fat
210	9g	36%	2g	33g	39mg	300mg	2g	1		1.5

Butter adds additional 20mg cholesterol per serving.

*Down On the Farm Cake without Eggs: Use Basic Chocolate Cake without Eggs on page 99.

Halloween Spider Web Cake

(can be made without wheat, gluten, dairy, eggs, or sugar - see page xi about ingredients)

This cake is so easy and so much fun that the kids can join in the decorating. You may also use a yellow cake or any other cake in this book.

1/2 cup brown rice flour
1/2 cup potato starch
1/4 cup tapioca flour
1/2 cup cocoa (not Dutch)
1 teaspoon xanthan gum
1 1/4 teaspoons baking soda
3/4 teaspoon salt
1 cup brown sugar or maple sugar
2 teaspoons gf vanilla extract

1/2 cup milk (cow, soy, rice)
1/2 cup butter or oleo or Spectrum™
    canola oil spread or
1/3 cup cooking oil
1 large egg*
3/4 cup hot (105°) coffee or water
Frosting, divided (see below)
Cooking spray

Cake: Preheat oven to 350°. Coat 12-inch round nonstick pizza pan (preferably with a 1/2-inch high edge) with cooking spray. Set aside.

Place all ingredients, except hot water or coffee, in large bowl and blend with electric mixer. Add hot water or coffee and mix until thoroughly blended. Pour into prepared pan and bake for 30-35 minutes or until toothpick placed in center of cake comes out clean.

Frosting: Use your favorite white frosting recipe and tint with combination of red and yellow food coloring. Or, use orange or tangerine frozen juice concentrate (thawed) simmered in small, heavy saucepan until syrupy and reduced by half. Reserve 1/4 of frosting and stir in enough cocoa powder to make a brown colored frosting. Set brown frosting aside.

Frost cake with orange frosting. Place brown frosting in small, heavy-duty freezer bag (with 1/4-inch opening cut on corner). Pipe concentric circles around cake, each circle about 1 to 2 inches from the next. Imagine that the cake is a clock. To create spider web, draw line with knife from noon to center circle, 1:30 to center circle, 3:00 and so on. Serves 12. (See diagram below.)

| Without frosting | | | | | | | | Exchanges | | |
Calories	Fat	% Fat Cal	Protein	Carb	Chol	Sodium	Fiber	Carb	Meat	Fat
210	9g	36%	2g	33g	39mg	300mg	2g	1		1.5

Butter adds additional 20mg of cholesterol per serving.

***Halloween Spider Web Cake without Eggs:** Use Basic Chocolate Cake without Eggs on page 101.

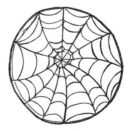

How Old Are You? Birthday Cake

(can be made without wheat, gluten, dairy, eggs, or sugar - see page xi about ingredients)

Sometimes a simple cake in the shape of a child's age is the perfect answer for a birthday party. Directions are given here for ages 1 through 4. Now that you see how simple this is, use your imagination to devise cakes for older age groups.

1/3 cup butter or oleo or Spectrum™ canola oil spread or
  1/4 cup cooking oil
1 cup sugar or fructose powder
2 large eggs, lightly beaten*
1 cup white or brown rice flour
1/3 cup potato starch
3 tablespoons tapioca flour
1 teaspoon xanthan gum
1/2 teaspoon baking powder
1/2 teaspoon baking soda

1/4 teaspoon salt
1/2 cup buttermilk or 2 teaspoons cider vinegar with enough non-dairy milk to equal 1/2 cup
1 teaspoon gf vanilla extract
White frosting of choice
Fruit leather
Jelly Belly® jelly beans
Cooking spray

Preheat oven to 325°. Prepare appropriate pan (see "Ages" below) with cooking spray and parchment paper or waxed paper, if necessary.

Using electric mixer and large mixer bowl, cream together butter (or oleo) and granulated sugar (or fructose) on medium speed until light and fluffy. Mix in eggs on low speed until blended.

In medium bowl, sift together flours, xanthan gum, baking powder, baking soda, and salt. In another medium bowl, combine buttermilk and vanilla extract. On low speed, beat dry ingredients into butter mixture, alternating with buttermilk, beginning and ending with dry ingredients. Mix just until combined. Serves 12. See below for specific instructions.

Age One: Line 13 x 9-inch pan with parchment paper or waxed paper. Pour batter into pan and smooth top with spatula, if necessary. Bake for 20-25 minutes or until cake tester inserted into center comes out clean. Let cake cool in pan for 5-10 minutes, then invert onto large baking sheet or piece of cardboard covered with aluminum foil.

Cut in half down center of cake. Stack one layer on the other. Cut upper right hand corner off with a diagonal cut, as shown in diagram. Cut diagonal piece in half, as shown in diagram below, and place each piece on opposite sides at the base of the cake. Frost as desired.

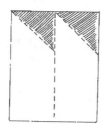 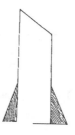

Age Two: Spread batter in 11 x 7-inch nonstick pan coated with cooking spray lined with parchment paper or waxed paper, then sprayed again. Bake for 30-35 minutes or until cake tester inserted into center comes out clean. Let cake cool in pan for 5-10 minutes, then invert onto a large baking sheet or piece of cardboard covered with aluminum foil. Used sharp, serrated knife to carve the number two, following diagram below. Frost as desired.

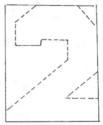

Age Three: Spread batter in 6 or 10-cup Bundt pan that has been sprayed with cooking spray. Bake for 45-50 minutes or until cake tester inserted into center of cake comes clean. Cut cake in half, crosswise, at opposite sides. Cut off end of one piece so that the two pieces fit closer together as shown below.

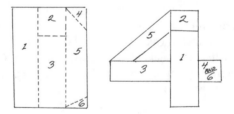

Age Four: Spread batter in 13x9-inch nonstick pan coated with cooking spray, lined with parchment paper or waxed paper, and sprayed again. Bake for 20-25 minutes or until cake tester inserted in center comes out clean. Cool, then invert cake onto cooling rack. Cut cake into pieces using diagram below as a guide. Arrange pieces in shape of 4 on baking sheet (or large piece of cardboard covered with aluminum foil), using diagram as your guide.

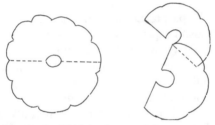

Exchanges

Calories	Fat	% Fat Cal	Protein	Carb	Chol	Sodium	Fiber	Carb	Meat	Fat
200	6g	29%	2g	33g	35mg	144mg	1	1.5		1

Butter adds additional 15mg cholesterol per serving.

*How Old Are You? Birthday Cake without Eggs: Use Basic Cake without Eggs on page 99.

Indy 500 Race Track Cake

(can be made without wheat, gluten, dairy, eggs, or sugar - see page xi about ingredients)

This fabulous cake is sure to delight that youngster with a passion for cars.

Cake
1/2 cup brown rice flour
1/2 cup potato starch
1/4 cup tapioca flour
1/2 cup cocoa powder (not Dutch)
1 teaspoon xanthan gum
1 1/4 teaspoons baking soda
3/4 teaspoon salt
1 cup brown sugar or maple sugar
2 teaspoons gf vanilla extract
1/2 cup milk (cow, rice, soy)
1/2 cup butter or oleo or Spectrum™
   canola oil spread or
   1/3 cup cooking oil
1 large egg**
3/4 cup brewed coffee or hot water
Cooking spray

Decorations
2 1/2 to 3 cups frosting of choice
Cooked gf spaghetti
Gluten® gf pretzels
Rice crackers
Cocoa or carob powder for dusting
Gf crackers (page 202)
Coconut for grass
Miniature flags, cars for race track

Preheat oven to 350°. Coat two 8-inch round cake pan with cooking spray. Line with parchment paper or waxed paper and spray again. Set aside.
Cake: Place all cake ingredients, except coffee (or hot water), in large bowl and blend with electric mixer. Add hot water or coffee and mix until thoroughly blended. Pour into prepared pans and bake for 30-35 minutes or until toothpick placed in center of cake comes out clean.

To assemble cake: Cut 1-inch off one side of both cakes. Place both cakes, cut sides together, to form figure 8 on large jelly-roll pan (or place on large piece of cardboard that has been covered with aluminum foil).

Prepare frosting. Tint 1/2 cup frosting brown by using 1 tablespoon cocoa or carob powder or use a combination of red and blue to achieve a deep purple color. Spread this dark-colored frosting in 2-inch wide strip in figure 8 design around top of cake to form track.

Place cooked spaghetti strands on center of track to form lanes, either in single strands or in 1-inch pieces to resemble the center line on a highway. Tint remainder of frosting green and frost edges of cake and center of each cake (inside race track). Place pretzels, around edge of cakes to form fence. Or, use brown rice crackers (dusted with cocoa or carob powder, if you like) stood on end around the entire perimeter of cake.

Tint 1/2 cup shredded coconut with green food coloring and sprinkle on centers of race track to resemble grass.(If food coloring is not acceptable for your diet, toss coconut with cocoa.) Decorate cake with miniature flags and cars. Serves 12. (continued on next page)

131

Calories	Fat	% Fat Cal	Protein	Carb	Chol	Sodium	Fiber	Carb	Meat	Fat
210	**9g**	**36%**	**33g**	**39mg**	**300mg**	**2g**	**2g**	**1.5**		**1.5**

Butter adds additional 20mg cholesterol per serving.

*Sugar Alternative: 1 cup maple sugar or dried cane juice in place of 1 cup brown sugar. Add 1/4 teaspoon baking soda.

**Indy 500 Race Track Cake without Eggs: Use Basic Chocolate Cake without Eggs on page 101.

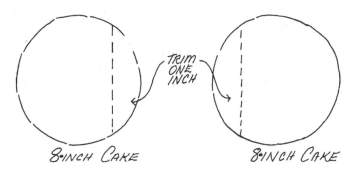

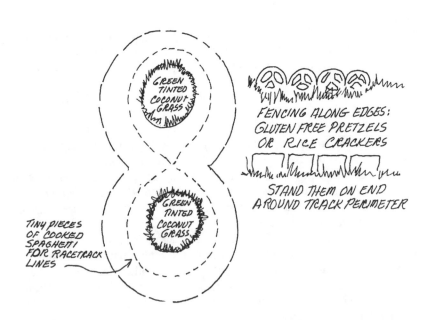

Apricot Filling

(can be made without wheat, gluten, dairy, eggs, or sugar - see page xi about ingredients)

Use this tasty, colorful filling in layer cakes, such as the White Wedding Cake with Fruit Filling on page 118.

2/3 cup dried apricots
1/2 cup fresh orange juice

1/8 teaspoon ground cardamom or nutmeg
1/4 cup sugar or 2 tablespoons honey

Chop dried apricots and combine with orange juice, and cardamom in a 4-cup glass microwave-safe bowl. Bring to boiling in microwave, reduce heat, and simmer, covered, on low power for 10 minutes—or until apricots are tender. Stir in sugar (or honey) and simmer 8-10 minutes more on low power.

Mash mixture with potato masher or fork until smooth. Cover. Chill for 2 hours. Makes about 2/3 cup—enough to cover one layer of cake that serves 12.

| | | | | | | | | Exchanges | | |
Calories	Fat	% Fat Cal	Protein	Carb	Chol	Sodium	Fiber	Carb	Meat	Fat
45	<1g	1%	<1g	11g	0mg	<1g	<1g	.5		

Cherry Pie Filling

(can be made without wheat, gluten, dairy, eggs, or sugar - see page xi about ingredients)

Use this easy recipe when you don't want to use the commercial cherry pie filling, which contains corn syrup, modified food starch, and red food coloring.

1 can (16 oz.) canned tart cherries
1 tablespoon tapioca flour
1/3 cup sugar or fructose powder
1/4 teaspoon salt

1 teaspoon gf vanilla extract
1 teaspoon gf almond extract
Dash red food coloring (optional)

Drain cherries, reserving 1/4 cup juice. Combine 1/4 cup juice with tapioca flour until thoroughly blended.

Place tapioca-cherry juice mixture, cherries, sugar (or fructose), and salt in medium glass or ceramic saucepan. Cook over medium heat until mixture thickens, stirring constantly. Remove from heat and stir in vanilla and almond extracts and red food coloring, if using. Cool completely before using.

Makes approximately 2 cups. Serves 12 (one layer of a 12-serving cake).

| | | | | | | | | Exchanges | | |
Calories	Fat	% Fat Cal	Protein	Carb	Chol	Sodium	Fiber	Carb	Meat	Fat
45	<1g	2%	<1g	11g	0mg	50mg	1g	.5		

Caramel Sauce

(can be made without wheat, gluten, dairy, eggs, or sugar - see page xi about ingredients)

Use this smooth, creamy caramel sauce on your favorite ice cream, drizzled over chocolate cake or brownies, or on fresh fruit.

1 cup sugar or fructose powder	1/2 cup milk (cow, rice, soy)
1/4 cup water	1 teaspoon gf vanilla extract
1 tablespoon butter or oleo	1/8 teaspoon salt

Combine sugar and water in medium-sized, heavy saucepan. Dissolve sugar in water over low-heat. Do not stir. When sugar is completely dissolved, cover saucepan and increase heat to medium. Bring to boil and boil 1 minute. This dissolves any sugar crystals clinging to edge of pan. (Undissolved sugar crystals may crystallize the entire mixture.)

Remove lid and continue to boil, uncovered, over medium heat. Do not stir. It may take up to 8 minutes for any color change to occur. Watch mixture very carefully because it can darken quickly and taste burned.

Continue boiling until mixture becomes amber or golden. Remove from heat. Let stand for one minute. Carefully add butter or oleo with a long-handled wooden spoon. (I wear hot pad mitts to protect my hands because the hot mixture may bubble and spatter.) Gradually add milk, stirring with the long-handled wooden spoon. The mixture will harden and clump on spoon.

Place pan back on medium heat, stirring constantly until caramel sauce is smooth—about three minutes. Stir in vanilla and salt. Makes 1 1/4 cups. Store in refrigerator in sealed container. May need to warm slightly before serving. Serves 10 (2 tablespoons per serving).

								Exchanges		
Calories	Fat	% Fat Cal	Protein	Carb	Chol	Sodium	Fiber	Carb	Meat	Fat
95	1g	13%	<1g	21g	<1mg	36mg	0g	1		.5

Chocolate Cinnamon Cream

(can be made without wheat, gluten, dairy, eggs, or sugar - see page xi about ingredients)

Very, very easy to make and a wonderful dessert topping.

1 tablespoon cocoa powder
1/4 cup sour cream or soft silken tofu
1/4 teaspoon ground cinnamon
1/4 cup pure maple syrup

1 teaspoon gf vanilla extract
1 teaspoon gf butter-flavored
   extract (optional)

Place all ingredients in blender or small bowl of food processor. Purée until very, very smooth. Add water if too thick, 1 tablespoon at a time. Makes 1/2 cup. Serves 4 (2 tablespoons each).

| | | | | | | | | Exchanges | | |
Calories	Fat	% Fat Cal	Protein	Carb	Chol	Sodium	Fiber	Carb	Meat	Fat
70	1g	10%	1g	16g	0mg	3mg	1	1		.5

Sour cream adds additional 20 calories, 2g fat, and 6mg cholesterol.

Chocolate Ganache

(can be made without wheat, gluten, dairy, eggs, or sugar - see page xi about ingredients)

You've seen the lovely, shiny finish on gourmet cakes. Make your own with this easy recipe.

12 ounces gf/df bittersweet chocolate
1/2 cup milk (cow, rice, soy)

1 tablespoon butter or cooking oil
1 tablespoon espresso powder
   (see below)

Break chocolate into pieces and place in heatproof bowl. In a small saucepan, heat milk and butter until bubbles appear around the edge. Remove from heat. (Add espresso, if using—see Espresso Ganache below—and stir to dissolve.) Pour hot milk over chocolate. Let stand for 1 minute. Stir until melted and smooth. Let stand at room temperature for 10 minutes before using. Pour over cake or dessert while lukewarm and spread with spatula. Serve within 30 minutes before ganache loses its sheen and hardens.

| | | | | | | | | Exchanges | | |
Calories	Fat	% Fat Cal	Protein	Carb	Chol	Sodium	Fiber	Carb	Meat	Fat
150	8g	47%	2g	20g	3mg	13mg	‹1g	1		1

Espresso Ganache: Add 1 teaspoon instant espresso powder.

135

Chocolate Syrup

(can be made without wheat, gluten, dairy, eggs, or sugar - see page xi about ingredients)

Use this syrup whenever the recipe calls for chocolate syrup. It's great drizzled on cakes when you don't want to use frosting.

3 tablespoons milk (cow, rice, soy)
2 tablespoons almond butter or
   butter or oleo

1/4 cup cocoa powder (not Dutch)
5 tablespoons maple syrup or honey

Combine in blender and blend until completely smooth. Refrigerate, covered. Serves 8 (about 1 1/2 tablespoons per serving).

Calories	Fat	% Fat Cal	Protein	Carb	Chol	Sodium	Fiber	Exchanges Carb	Meat	Fat
66	3g	34%	1g	11g	<1mg	5mg	1g	.5		.5

Chocolate Chip Frosting

(can be made without wheat, gluten, dairy, eggs, or sugar - see page xi about ingredients)

A very simple frosting that's sure to please your guests.

2 cups gf/df chocolate chips
1/4 cup maple syrup or honey
1/4 cup milk (cow, rice, soy)

1 tablespoon butter or oleo or nut butter
   (almond or cashew)
1 teaspoon gf vanilla extract

Place all ingredients in glass bowl and microwave on medium power for 2 minutes, stopping and stirring after one minute. If you prefer a smooth frosting, process in a food processor until very, very smooth—adding additional milk to reach spreading consistency. Otherwise, use frosting immediately or it will begin to harden. Frosts one double-layer cake to serve 12.

Calories	Fat	% Fat Cal	Protein	Carb	Chol	Sodium	Fiber	Exchanges Carb	Meat	Fat
165	9g	47%	1g	22g	3mg	6mg	2g	1.5		1

Chocolate Frosting

(can be made without wheat, gluten, dairy, eggs, or sugar - see page xi about ingredients)

Another yummy chocolate frosting!

2/3 cup Chocolate Syrup (page 136)   **1/4 cup rice milk**
1 tablespoon arrowroot powder

Place chocolate syrup in small, heavy saucepan. Dissolve arrowroot powder in milk, then stir mixture into chocolate syrup.

Heat mixture over low-medium setting, stirring occasionally, until it starts to thicken—about 8-10 minutes. Remove from heat and cool slightly. Mixture will thicken as it cools.

Frost your favorite single-layer cake to serve 12—or 12 cupcakes. For larger cakes, double or triple the recipe. If frosting thickens too much, stir in a tablespoon of milk at a time to reach desired consistency.

| | | | | | | | | Exchanges | | |
Calories	Fat	% Fat Cal	Protein	Carb	Chol	Sodium	Fiber	Carb	Meat	Fat
50	2g	4%	.5g	12g	0mg	10mg	.5g	1		

Chocolate Tofu Frosting

(can be made without wheat, gluten, dairy, eggs, or sugar - see page xi about ingredients)

This frosting has a very rich, bold chocolate flavor with a very creamy texture.

1/3 cup (3 oz.) extra-firm silken tofu   **2 cups cocoa powder (not Dutch)**
2 cups pure maple syrup   **1 tablespoon gf vanilla extract**

In food processor or blender, blend tofu with maple syrup until completely smooth. Add cocoa and vanilla and blend until very, very smooth. Refrigerate frosting for 15 minutes before using. Frosts a double layer cake that serves 12.

| | | | | | | | | Exchanges | | |
Calories	Fat	% Fat Cal	Protein	Carb	Chol	Sodium	Fiber	Carb	Meat	Fat
180	2g	10%	3g	44g	0mg	8mg	5g	2.5		

Un-chocolate Frosting

(can be made without wheat, gluten, dairy, eggs, or sugar - see page xi about ingredients)

Use this frosting when you don't want to use the traditional powdered sugar frosting––and you want something other than chocolate. Add flavored extracts (e.g. almond or coconut) for additional interest.

1 **package (12 oz.) extra-firm silken tofu**
1/4 **cup sugar or fructose powder**
1 **teaspoon fresh lemon juice**
1 **teaspoon butter or oleo or cooking oil**
1 **teaspoon gf vanilla extract**

1 **teaspoon gf butter-flavored extract**
1/4 **teaspoon salt**
1/4 **teaspoon xanthan gum**

Drain tofu thoroughly in mesh sieve. Discard liquid. Combine all ingredients in food processor. Process until very, very smooth—scraping down sides with spatula. Use immediately. Makes about 1 1/4 cups frosting. Frosts 8 x 8-inch single layer cake. Serves 12.

								Exchanges		
Calories	Fat	% Fat Cal	Protein	Carb	Chol	Sodium	Fiber	Carb	Meat	Fat
35	1g	27%	1g	5g	0mg	50mg	0g	0	0	0

Raspberry Filling

(can be made without wheat, gluten, dairy, eggs, or sugar - see page xi about ingredients)

This is a lovely filling for a white layer cake, but it is also delicious used in chocolate layer cakes.

2 **cups fresh raspberries**
1/2 **cup sugar or fructose powder**

2 **tablespoons cornstarch or arrowroot**
1 **teaspoon gf vanilla or almond extract**

Mash fresh raspberries in small bowl until thoroughly crushed. Press mixture through sieve and discard seeds. Place crushed raspberries and sugar (or fructose) in small saucepan and whisk in cornstarch. Place pan over medium heat, stirring until mixture thickens. Cook and stir two minutes more. Remove from heat. Stir in vanilla or almond extract.

Transfer filling to small bowl, cover, and refrigerate for at least 2 hours. Makes about 1/2 to 2/3 cup, which is enough filling for one layer cake in a two-layer cake that serves 12. Double recipe if you wish to put this filling between two layers. Triple it for cakes with 3 or 4 layers.

								Exchanges		
Calories	Fat	% Fat Cal	Protein	Carb	Chol	Sodium	Fiber	Carb	Meat	Fat
45	<1g	2%	<1g	11g	0mg	<1mg	1g	.5		

Whipped Topping (Soy-based)

(can be made without wheat, gluten, dairy, eggs, or sugar - see page xi about ingredients)

The tofu makes this topping smooth and creamy. Use like any dairy whipped topping.

1/2 cup soft silken tofu
2 tablespoons pure maple syrup or honey
1/2 teaspoon gf vanilla extract

1/4 teaspoon gf butter-flavored
   extract
1/8 teaspoon salt

Combine all ingredients in blender or mini-food processor and blend thoroughly until very, very smooth. Makes about 1/2 cup. Serves 4 (2 tablespoons each).

								Exchanges		
Calories	Fat	% Fat Cal	Protein	Carb	Chol	Sodium	Fiber	Carb	Meat	Fat
45	1g	17%	1.5g	8g	0mg	75mg	0g	.5		

Whipped Topping (Nut-Based)

(can be made without wheat, gluten, dairy, eggs, or sugar - see page xi about ingredients)

Unlike the previous topping, this one uses no soy products. But it does contain nuts.

3/4 cup raw cashews or almonds
1/4 cup honey or maple syrup
2 teaspoons gf vanilla extract

1/2 teaspoon gf butter-flavored extract
1/4 cup water
1/4 teaspoon salt

Place nuts on baking sheet and toast in 350° oven for 5-8 minutes or until lightly toasted, but not browned. In blender, grind nuts finely. Add honey, vanilla and butter extracts, water, and salt. Process again until very, very smooth—about 5-8 minutes. Refrigerate until ready to use. Makes 1 cup. Serves 8 (2 tablespoons each).

								Exchanges		
Calories	Fat	% Fat Cal	Protein	Carb	Chol	Sodium	Fiber	Carb	Meat	Fat
110	5g	36%	2g	17g	0mg	118mg	.5g	1		1

White 7-Minute Frosting

(can be made without wheat, gluten, dairy, or sugar - see page xi about ingredients)

This traditional frosting is usually off-limits for many with food sensitivities because it contains eggs and cane sugar. However, for many of you it will be just fine so use it if you can. If you require an egg-free, cane sugar-free frosting see page 139.

3 large egg whites	1/4 teaspoon cream of tartar
1 1/4 cups granulated sugar or	3 tablespoons cold water
fructose powder	1 teaspoon gf vanilla extract

In double boiler over boiling water, combine egg whites, sugar, cream of tartar, and cold water. Beat with portable electric mixer for 5-7 minutes until glossy and mixture reaches desired spreading consistency. Use immediately. Makes enough frosting to frost a cake double-layer cake for 12.

| | | | | | | | | Exchanges | | |
Calories	Fat	% Fat Cal	Protein	Carb	Chol	Sodium	Fiber	Carb	Meat	Fat
100	0g	0	1g	25g	0mg	17mg	0g	1.5		

Chocolate Pots de Créme

(can be made without wheat, gluten, dairy, eggs, or sugar - see page xi about ingredients)

This is a very simple, yet elegant dessert. Top with a dollop of whipped topping, a dusting of cinnamon, or fresh strawberries. If using rice milk, dissolve 2 teaspoons unflavored gelatin powder in 1/4 cup of the milk for 10 minutes. Add with rest of milk, whisking constantly throughout the cooking process to avoid lumps.

2 tablespoons cocoa powder (not Dutch)	2 cups milk (cow, rice, soy)
	1 ounce gf/df bittersweet chocolate
1/2 cup brown sugar or maple sugar	1/4 teaspoon salt
2 tablespoons + 1 teaspoon cornstarch or arrowroot	1 teaspoon gf vanilla extract
1 teaspoon gf instant coffee or espresso powder	

Combine cocoa powder, sugar, cornstarch, and espresso powder in medium saucepan. Over medium heat, add milk, chocolate, and salt. Whisk constantly until chocolate melts and mixture thickens, about 5-8 minutes.

Remove from heat and add vanilla extract. Pour into individual custard cups or dessert bowls. Chill until firm. Serves 4 (1/2 cup each).

| | | | | | | | | Exchanges | | |
Calories	Fat	% Fat Cal	Protein	Carb	Chol	Sodium	Fiber	Carb	Meat	Fat
200	2g	10%	5g	43g	2mg	222mg	1g	2		.5

Baked Alaska

(can be made without wheat, gluten, dairy, or sugar - see page xi about ingredients)

At first glance, this may seem like lots of work. But, it really isn't. If you have ice cream on hand and don't have to make it from scratch, you're halfway there. And, I sometimes use leftover cake or brownies as the base instead of creating a new cake from scratch. The impact of this dramatic dessert is well worth the effort for that special occasion. Unfortunately for the egg-sensitive, the meringue must be egg-based.

1 prepared cake or brownie recipe (see Brownies, page 156)	1/4 teaspoon cream of tartar
1 pint ice cream or sorbet	1/2 cup granulated sugar or fructose powder
1/3 cup egg whites*	1 cup Chocolate Syrup (page 136) or
1/2 teaspoon gf vanilla extract	preferred sauce

Decide what shape you'll use for the Baked Alaska. Cut a piece of cardboard to fit that dimension and wrap with aluminum foil. Position cake (or brownies) on the cardboard that extends at least 2 inches beyond the cake on all sides.

Freeze cake on aluminum-covered cardboard until firm. Remove cake from freezer and position a block of ice cream or sorbet on top of cake. The ice cream may be softened somewhat so it can be shaped and molded with a spoon or spatula to fit exact dimensions of cake. Return cake to freezer.

To make meringue, preheat oven to 450°. Place egg whites, vanilla extract, and cream of tartar in large bowl. Whip with electric mixer on medium speed until soft peaks form. Increase mixer speed to high and gradually add sugar, a tablespoon at a time. Beat until meringue holds very stiff peaks.

Immediately frost frozen Baked Alaska with meringue, using attractive swirls and dips for added interest.

Preheat broiler in oven. Place Baked Alaska 5 inches from heat (with oven door partially open) for about 3-5 minutes—or until meringue is lightly browned. This depends on several factors so watch carefully to avoid burning. If you wish to further brown meringue, you can use a propane torch (available at cooking stores).

Serve immediately with additional sauce in a flavor that complements the Baked Alaska. For example, provide Chocolate Sauce with chocolate ice cream; berry sauce with strawberry or raspberry sherbet, etc. Serves 8.

* If you have concerns about using meringues due to partially cooked eggs, you may make meringue from Just Whites, a commercial product consisting of dried egg whites.

								Exchanges		
Calories	Fat	% Fat Cal	Protein	Carb	Chol	Sodium	Fiber	Carb	Meat	Fat
420	12	24%	7g	76g	50mg	432mg	2g	5g		

Cantaloupe with Cinnamon

(can be made without wheat, gluten, dairy, eggs, or sugar - see page xi about ingredients)

The riper the cantaloupe, the sweeter this dessert will be. The cinnamon contrasts nicely with the fruit.

1 ripe cantaloupe   **1/2 teaspoon ground cinnamon**

Wash exterior of cantaloupe. Cut into quarters. Remove rind. Cut cantaloupe into bite-size pieces and place in large bowl. Toss with cinnamon. Arrange in large serving bowl or 4 individual dessert bowls or plates. Serve immediately. Serves 4.

								Exchanges		
Calories	Fat	% Fat Cal	Protein	Carb	Chol	Sodium	Fiber	Carb	Meat	Fat
50	.5g	6%	1g	12g	0mg	13mg	1g	1		

Cappuccino Pudding

(can be made without wheat, gluten, dairy, eggs, or sugar - see page xi about ingredients)

Coffee lovers, you'll really enjoy this version that reminds you of a fragrant Cappuccino drink. If using rice milk, dissolve 2 teaspoons unflavored gelatin powder in 1/4 cup of the milk for 10 minutes. Add with rest of the milk.

1/2 cup brown sugar or maple sugar
2 tablespoons arrowroot or
   cornstarch
1 teaspoon ground cinnamon
1/4 teaspoon salt

2 cups milk (cow, rice, soy)
2 tablespoons gf instant coffee
   powder or 1 tablespoon espresso
   powder (Medaglia D'Oro)
1 teaspoon gf vanilla extract

Combine sugar, arrowroot, cinnamon, and salt in medium saucepan. Over medium heat, add milk and instant coffee powder. Stir constantly until mixture thickens, about 5-8 minutes. Do not overcook.

Remove from heat and add vanilla. Pour into individual custard cups or dessert bowls. Chill until firm. Serves 4 (1/2 cup each).

								Exchanges		
Calories	Fat	% Fat Cal	Protein	Carb	Chol	Sodium	Fiber	Carb	Meat	Fat
170	<1g	1%	4g	37g	2mg	220mg	<1g	1.5		

Cherry Cobbler

(can be made without wheat, gluten, dairy, eggs, or sugar - see page xi about ingredients)

This homey dessert is a wonderful way to end a comfort-food meal.

Fruit Filling
2 cans (16 oz. each) tart red cherries
  with 1/4 cup juice reserved
2/3 cup sugar or fructose powder
1 tablespoon quick-cooking tapioca
1 teaspoon grated lemon peel
1 tablespoon fresh lemon juice
1 teaspoon gf vanilla extract
1 teaspoon gf almond extract
Cooking spray

Cobbler Topping
1/2 cup brown rice flour
1/4 cup potato starch
1/4 cup tapioca flour
1/2 teaspoon xanthan gum
1 teaspoon grated lemon peel
1/2 teaspoon baking soda
1/2 teaspoon baking powder
1/4 teaspoon salt
1/4 cup milk (cow, rice, soy)
2 tablespoons fresh lemon juice
2 tablespoons cooking oil
1 teaspoon gf vanilla extract
1 large egg*
1 tablespoon honey or agave nectar

Fruit Filling: Preheat oven to 400°. Spray 8 x 8-inch nonstick pan with cooking spray. Combine fruit filling ingredients (including 1/4 cup reserved juice) in prepared pan and set aside.

Cobbler Topping: In large bowl, combine flours, xanthan gum, lemon peel, baking soda, baking powder, and salt. In another bowl, whisk together milk, lemon juice, oil, vanilla, egg, and honey. Add to dry ingredients, stirring just until dry ingredients are moistened. Drop topping by rounded tablespoons onto fruit filling.

Bake in middle of oven for 20-25 minutes or until filling is bubbly and crust is golden. Serve warm. Serves 6.

| | | | | | | | | Exchanges | | |
Calories	Fat	% Fat Cal	Protein	Carb	Chol	Sodium	Fiber	Carb	Meat	Fat
430	5g	8%	6g	122g	2mg	200mg	6g	6		1

Egg adds additional 26mg cholesterol

*Egg Alternative: In cobbler topping, omit egg and use 1/3 cup milk instead of 1/4 cup milk. Add 2 teaspoons Ener-G® egg replacer powder.

Chocolate Covered Strawberries

(can be made without wheat, gluten, dairy, eggs, or sugar - see page xi about ingredients)

For both of these desserts, choose big strawberries with stems intact.

1 cup gf/df chocolate chips or
   crushed chocolate squares

1 teaspoon butter or oleo or cooking oil
1 pint large strawberries

Melt the chocolate chips (or chocolate squares) and butter (or oil) in microwave or small saucepan over low heat, stirring often. Line cookie sheet or large plate with waxed paper. Dip each whole strawberry into melted chocolate, twist while removing the strawberry from the chocolate, and place on waxed paper—strawberry bottom down. Refrigerate until chocolate sets. Serves 4 (about 2 to 4 strawberries per serving).

								Exchanges		
Calories	Fat	% Fat Cal	Protein	Carb	Chol	Sodium	Fiber	Carb	Meat	Fat
230	14g	48%	2g	32g	0mg	5mg	4g	2		2

Chocolate Dipped, Filled Strawberries

(can be made without wheat, gluten, dairy, eggs, or sugar - see page xi about ingredients)

1 pint large strawberries
1 cup gf/df chocolate chips or
   crushed chocolate squares

1 teaspoon butter or oleo or cooking oil
1 recipe Apricot Filling (page 133)

Wash and thoroughly pat strawberries dry with paper towel. With sharp knife, trim strawberries to make stem end level. Gently hollow out centers, leaving about 1/4-inch-thick shells. Set aside.

Melt chocolate and butter in microwave or small saucepan over low heat, stirring often. (If you have a double boiler, this works well, too.)

Line cookie sheet or large plate with waxed paper. Dip pointed end of each whole strawberry into melted chocolate, twist while removing the strawberry from the chocolate, and place on waxed paper. Refrigerate until chocolate sets.

Using small spoon or knife tip, carefully fill each strawberry with Apricot Filling. Return strawberries to refrigerate until ready to serve. Serves 2 to 4, depending on size of strawberries.

								Exchanges		
Calories	Fat	% Fat Cal	Protein	Carb	Chol	Sodium	Fiber	Carb	Meat	Fat
365	14g	32%	3g	64g	0mg	7mg	6g	4		2

Chocolate Mocha Fudge Trifle

(can be made without wheat, gluten, dairy, eggs, or sugar - see page xi about ingredients)

This recipe is wonderful for a party because 1) it can be prepared ahead of time 2) it looks fabulous on a buffet table with the multi-layered effect, and 3) it is wickedly decadent, especially if you're a chocoholic! For large groups, this recipe can be doubled and even tripled. Just be sure to choose an appropriate-sized container. For this recipe, a 1 1/2-quart container is required. If doubling the recipe, choose a 3-4-quart container. Tripling requires a 6-quart container.

1 recipe Basic Chocolate Cake (pages 100-101)
1/2 cup hot (115°) espresso or strong coffee
2 ounces gf/df chocolate chips or chocolate squares

1 recipe Chocolate Pots de Crème (page 140)
1 recipe Cappuccino Pudding (page 142)
Grated chocolate for garnish
Fresh strawberries for garnish

Cut Chocolate Cake into large strips. Set aside. Melt chocolate in hot coffee. Brush each side of strip with coffee-chocolate mixture. Cut into 1-inch cubes and divide into 3 piles, each pile to be used for a layer. Place first layer of cake cubes in bottom of straight-sided, glass serving bowl that is at least 3 inches deep and 7 to 8 inches in diameter.

Spread 1/3 of Chocolate Pots de Crème over cake. Spread 1/3 of Cappuccino Pudding over Chocolate Pots de Crème. Add second layer of cake cubes. Top with 1/3 of the Chocolate Pots de Crème and 1/3 of the Cappuccino Pudding. Add third layer of cake cubes. Top with final 1/3 of Chocolate Pots de Crème and final 1/3 of the Cappuccino Pudding.

Place in refrigerator. Meanwhile, shave chocolate bar of choice with potato peeler. Place on top of Chocolate Mocha Fudge Trifle. Chill until serving time. To serve, garnish with fresh strawberries. Serves 6.

| | | | | | | | | Exchanges | | |
Calories	Fat	% Fat Cal	Protein	Carb	Chol	Sodium	Fiber	Carb	Meat	Fat
490	12g	21%	10g	91g	38mg	666mg	3g	5		2

Flower Pot Treats

(can be made without wheat, gluten, dairy, eggs, or sugar - see page xi about ingredients)

This is a delightful treat for children. They love to find the hidden treats inside the pudding. And, for some strange reason, children love the idea of eating dirt! One caveat: if using rice milk, dissolve 2 teaspoons unflavored gelatin powder in 1/4 cup of the milk for 10 minutes. Add with rest of the milk. Otherwise, the pudding won't reach desired consistency.

2 tablespoons cocoa powder (not Dutch)
1/2 cup brown sugar or maple sugar
2 tablespoons cornstarch or arrowroot
2 cups milk (cow, soy, rice – see above)
1/4 teaspoon salt

1 ounce gf and df bittersweet chocolate
1 teaspoon gf vanilla extract
1 cup crushed gf Chocolate Wafers (page 153)
4 small terra cotta or plastic plastic flower pots

Combine cocoa powder, sugar, and cornstarch (or arrowroot) in medium saucepan. Over medium heat, add milk and salt. Whisk constantly until mixture thickens, about 5-8 minutes.

Remove from heat and add bittersweet chocolate and vanilla, stirring until chocolate melts. Chill thoroughly in refrigerator.

Assemble flowerpots (which have been cleaned thoroughly.) Lay a piece of aluminum foil over the hole in the bottom.

Layer pudding and crushed chocolate wafers, ending with layer of crushed cookies. You can hide edible surprises inside such as gf gummy worms, fruit leather cut in the shapes of worms, raisins, etc. Just make sure these items are safe for your diet. Top the flowerpot with an edible flower, or an artificial flower (that's been carefully washed and dried.) Serves 4.

Exchanges

Calories	Fat	% Fat Cal	Protein	Carb	Chol	Sodium	Fiber	Carb	Meat	Fat
315	6g	16%	7g	62g	4mg	406mg	2g	3.5		1

Frozen Tiramisu

(can be made without wheat, gluten, dairy, eggs, or sugar - see page xi about ingredients)

This is a great way to use leftover cake. You can slice it in any shape you want as long as it is about 1-inch thick. The amount of ice cream is a matter of personal choice. Some people like lots of ice cream and just a little cake. The overall flavor of the dessert will vary depending on whether you use the espresso coffee or orange juice, but both versions are equally delicious. For maximum flavor, use both!

1 cup brown sugar or maple sugar
1 1/2 cups strong, freshly brewed
espresso or fresh orange juice
2 tablespoons cocoa powder
1 recipe Basic Chocolate Cake
(pages 100-101)
2 pints Chocolate Cappuccino Ice
Cream (page 158) or preferred
ice cream

1/4 cup finely ground espresso or
grated orange peel
1/4 cup Dutch cocoa powder
Garnish with grated chocolate or
crushed gf/df chocolate chips or
Chocolate Cinnamon Cream
(page 135)

Dissolve sugar in freshly brewed espresso (or very strongly brewed coffee.) Bring to boil, reduce heat, and simmer for 1 minute to make espresso syrup. If using orange juice, follow same procedure but boil until mixture is reduced by 1/3, or about 1 cup. Remove from heat and cool.

Slice cake into 1-inch thick pieces with serrated knife. Place one layer in bottom of 9 x 9-inch pan sprayed with cooking spray. Brush cake with espresso or orange syrup. Sprinkle 2 tablespoons of ground espresso over cake. Spread one half of softened ice cream over cake. Top with second layer of cake. Brush with remaining syrup.

Sprinkle with remaining 2 tablespoons espresso powder or orange peel. Top with remaining ice cream, creating decorative dips and swirls with back of spatula.

Return to freezer until completely frozen. At serving time, dust with Dutch cocoa and top with grated chocolate or crushed chocolate chips or Chocolate Cinnamon Cream (page135). Let stand at room temperature for a few minutes before serving. Serves 12.

| | | | | | | | | Exchanges | | |
Calories	Fat	% Fat Cal	Protein	Carb	Chol	Sodium	Fiber	Carb	Meat	Fat
400	15g	31%	6g	68g	35mg	412mg	3g	4		2

Excludes garnishes

Panna Cotta

(can be made without wheat, gluten, dairy, eggs, or sugar - see page xi about ingredients)

Panna Cotta is considered a rather trendy dessert these days but it's actually just creamy gelatin with an Italian name. Of course, the original version is made with heavy cream. Try to use the heaviest, thickest non-dairy milk you can find. Or, perhaps stir in non-dairy milk powder to the liquid milk you're using to boost its density.

1 tablespoon unflavored gelatin powder	1 teaspoon gf almond extract
2 cups milk (cow, rice, soy), divided	1/8 teaspoon salt
1 teaspoon gf vanilla extract	1 cup fresh strawberries or
or 1 vanilla bean	raspberries
1/4 cup honey or agave nectar	Fresh mint for garnish

In small, heavy saucepan sprinkle the gelatin powder over 1/4 cup of the milk to soften, 3-5 minutes. Heat gently over very low heat.

Meanwhile, in another saucepan, heat remaining milk and vanilla bean (opened and scraped) until tiny bubbles form around edges of pan (do not boil.) Remove from heat, remove vanilla bean, and stir in gelatin mixture, honey, vanilla and almond extracts, and salt until thoroughly mixed. (If you're not using the vanilla bean, stir in vanilla extract now.)

Pour into 5-cup, decorative ring mold and refrigerate 6 hours or overnight, until firm. (If you don't have such a mold, a Bundt cake pan will also work.)

Before unmolding panna cotta, hull and slice remaining 2 cups of straw-berries.

To serve, dip mold in lukewarm water and then dry bottom. Loosen edges with knife. Unmold onto serving platter. Spoon sliced strawberries in center of ring and garnish with fresh mint. Serve immediately. Serves 4.

Exchanges

Calories	Fat	% Fat Cal	Protein	Carb	Chol	Sodium	Fiber	Carb	Meat	Fat
130	<1g	2%	6g	26g	2mg	140mg	1g	1		

Peach Melba Ice Cream Pie

(can be made without wheat, gluten, dairy, eggs, or sugar - see page xi about ingredients)

For extra peach flavor and additional texture in the pie, stir in a cup of chopped peaches to the softened peach ice cream before spreading it in the pie plate. For variation, substitute a portion of the coconut—perhaps 1/4 cup—with ground nuts such as pecans, walnuts, or hazelnuts.

Crust
1 1/2 cups shredded coconut
1 tablespoon sweet rice flour
1/4 teaspoon salt
1 teaspoon gf vanilla extract
2 tablespoons butter or oleo or
   Spectrum™ canola oil spread

Pie Filling
1 pint Peach Ice Cream, softened
   (page 160)

Topping
1 cup fresh raspberries
2 tablespoons honey
2 medium ripe peaches, sliced
Fresh mint for garnish

Crust: Spray 9-inch pie plate with cooking spray. Combine ingredients thoroughly and press onto bottom and up sides. Bake at 325° until lightly toasted, approximately 10-15 minutes. Watch carefully so crust doesn't burn. Cool thoroughly.

Pie Filling: Spread softened Peach Ice Cream in crust. Return to freezer for about 4 hours or until firm. Remove from freezer about 15 minutes before serving.

Topping: Wash and pick over fresh raspberries. Combine with sliced peaches and toss with honey. Top each serving with a tablespoon of the peach-raspberry mixture. Garnish with a sprig of fresh mint. Serves 10.

Exchanges

Calories	Fat	% Fat Cal	Protein	Carb	Chol	Sodium	Fiber	Carb	Meat	Fat
210	9g	39%	2g	30g	9mg	161mg	3g	2	.5	2

Theme Cookies for Kids

(can be made without wheat, gluten, dairy, eggs, or sugar - see page xi about ingredients)

Perfect for birthday parties, school treats, or as a rainy-day activity, these cute little creatures are easy and fun to make.

Cookie Monsters: Two Basic Cookies (page 157) or other gf cookies propped open with miniature gf Jet-Puff® marshmallows. Face can be sliced off Jelly Belly® licorice jelly beans for eyes or use pure fruit leather cut in appropriate shapes for facial features.

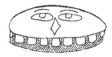

Spider Cookies: Use large gf Jet-Puff® marshmallow decorated with pieces of pure fruit leather for body and use uncooked gf spaghetti strands for legs. For dark legs, spray legs with cooking spray and roll in cocoa powder or carob powder. Or, use small strands of dark-colored fruit leather.

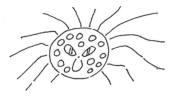

Bug Cookies: Use Basic Cookie (page 157) or other gf cookie for body, with legs made from thin strands of gf spaghetti—or use fruit leather to cut strips.

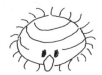

Snakes: 5 Basic Cookies (page 157) or other gf cookie with M&M's, or sliced Jelly Belly® jelly beans, or circles cut from fruit leather for eyes. Fangs of snake can be pasta strands.

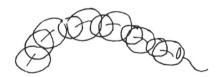

Chocolate Cherry Almond Biscotti

(can be made without wheat, gluten, dairy, eggs, or sugar - see page xi about ingredients)

Biscotti are an elegant treat . . . meant for after-dinner dipping into hot coffee or tea, with morning coffee, or as a treat with cappuccino served any time. Though they are baked twice, they are actually extremely easy to make—especially if you mix them in a food processor.

1 cup brown rice flour or
   garbfava flour
1/2 cup potato starch
1/3 cup tapioca flour
1 1/2 teaspoons xanthan gum
2 teaspoons baking powder
1/2 teaspoon salt
1/2 cup unsweetened cocoa powder
   (not Dutch)
1 teaspoon gf instant coffee powder

3/4 cup brown sugar or maple sugar
2 large eggs or 1/2 cup flax mix
   (page 211)
1/3 cup cooking oil
1 teaspoon gf vanilla extract
1/2 teaspoon gf almond extract
3/4 cup dried tart cherries
1/4 cup gf/df chocolate chips
Cooking spray

Preheat oven to 350°. Spray baking sheet with cooking spray or line with parchment paper. Set aside.

In food processor, combine flours, xanthan gum, baking powder, salt, cocoa powder, coffee powder, and sugar. Whirl until thoroughly mixed. Add eggs (or flax mix), oil, vanilla, and almond extract. Process until mixture forms ball. Break up ball into several pieces, add chopped tart cherries, and process until mixture forms ball again.

Divide dough in half. On baking sheet, shape each half into a log measuring about two inches wide by 12 inches long by 1/2-inch thick. Bake for 20 minutes. Remove from oven, but leave oven on.

Place each log on cutting board. (If using parchment paper, you can carefully slide the parchment paper—logs and all—onto a cutting board.) With electric knife or sharp, serrated knife diagonally cut each log into 3/4 to 1-inch slices. Place each slice on its cut side. Return to oven, reduce heat to 275°, and bake for 10 minutes. Turn slices over and bake another 10 minutes.

To further crisp biscotti, turn oven off but leave baking sheet in oven for another 10-15 minutes with oven door closed.

For chocolate-dipped biscotti, melt chocolate in double boiler or heavy saucepan. Dip each piece halfway into melted chocolate. Dip the end of each biscotti or one of the flat sides into chocolate. Or, use spoon to drizzle melted chocolate over biscotti in zig-zag fashion. Place on waxed paper to cool. Store in airtight container. Makes 24.

Exchanges

Calories	Fat	% Fat Cal	Protein	Carb	Chol	Sodium	Fiber	Carb	Meat	Fat
130	5g	28%	2g	24g	1mg	99mg	1.5g	1		1

Eggs add additional 17mg cholesterol per cookie.

Chocolate Cherry Cookies

(can be made without wheat, gluten, dairy, eggs, or sugar - see page xi about ingredients)

Use cranberries instead of dried tart cherries for a different flavor twist.

1/2 cup brown rice flour or
  garbfava flour
1/4 cup potato starch
2 tablespoons tapioca flour
1 teaspoon xanthan gum
1/2 cup cocoa powder (not Dutch)
1 teaspoon baking soda
1/4 teaspoon salt
1/2 cup butter or oleo or
  Spectrum™ canola oil spread

1/2 cup sugar or fructose powder
1/3 cup brown sugar or maple sugar
1 large egg or 1/4 cup flax mix
  (page 211)
1 teaspoon gf vanilla extract
1/2 cup gf/df chocolate chips
1/4 cup dried tart cherries or
  cranberries
Cooking spray

Preheat oven to 350°. In medium bowl, combine dry ingredients (brown rice flour through salt). Set aside.

With electric mixer, cream butter, sugars, egg (or flax mix), and vanilla until well combined. Add dry ingredients gradually; mix only until moistened. Don't over mix. Fold in chocolate chips and cherries.

With small ice-cream scoop, place balls of dough (about 2 tablespoons each) on cookie sheet lined with nonstick liners or parchment paper—or sprayed with cooking spray. Leave an inch between balls to allow for spreading.

Bake 10-12 minutes until puffed and cracked. (If using canola oil spread, press with spatula after 5 minutes of baking to make flatter cookies.) Cool on baking sheet 5 minutes, then transfer to wire rack to cool. Makes 16.

								Exchanges		
Calories	Fat	% Fat Cal	Protein	Carb	Chol	Sodium	Fiber	Carb	Meat	Fat
165	8g	41%	2g	25g	0mg	124mg	2g	1		1

Egg and butter add additional 29mg cholesterol per cookie.

Celebration Cookies: Add 1/4 cup coconut flakes and 1/4 cup chopped nuts (pecans, walnuts, or almonds). Bake as directed.

								Exchanges		
Calories	Fat	% Fat Cal	Protein	Carb	Chol	Sodium	Fiber	Carb	Meat	Fat
215	10g	37%	2g	34g	0mg	124mg	2g	2		2

Egg and butter add additional 29mg cholesterol per cookie.

Chocolate Ice Cream Sandwiches

(can be made without wheat, gluten, dairy, eggs, or sugar - see page xi about ingredients)

These are so simple that your children or grandchildren can help make them.

Chocolate Wafers
1/4 cup butter or oleo or Spectrum™
  canola oil spread
2 tablespoons honey or maple syrup
1/2 cup brown sugar or maple sugar,
  firmly packed
1 large egg or 1/4 cup flax mix
  (page 211)
1 1/2 teaspoons gf vanilla extract
1 cup brown rice flour
  or garbfava flour
3 tablespoons potato starch
2 tablespoons tapioca flour
1/4 cup cocoa powder (not Dutch)
1/2 teaspoon xanthan gum
1/2 teaspoon salt
1 1/2 teaspoons baking powder
Cooking spray

Filling & Edges
1 pint ice cream of choice
1 cup chopped nuts or crushed
  gf/df chocolate chips or Jowar
  crisps or shredded coconut for
  rolling edges of cookies

Preheat oven to 325°. In a food processor, combine butter, honey, sugar, egg (or flax mix), and vanilla.

Add flours, cocoa powder, xanthan gum, salt, and baking powder and combine thoroughly. Shape batter into soft ball. Batter will be somewhat soft. Cover and refrigerate for 1 hour.

Shape dough into 24 balls measuring 1-inch in diameter. Place balls on nonstick cookie sheet (not insulated) coated with cooking spray. Flatten each ball with spatula to approximately 1 1/2 to 2-inch circle, depending on preferred size of cookie. The cookies will spread more when butter is used and less when oleo or canola oil spread is used.

Bake for about 25-30 minutes or until cookies appear dry on top. Baking time depends on size of cookies, watch carefully so cookies don't burn. Makes about 2 dozen.

To make sandwich cookies, place 2 tablespoons slightly softened ice cream between two cookies. Roll edges in chopped nuts, chopped chocolate chips, or coconut, or Jowar crisp cereal—see Mail-Order Sources. Freeze until ready to eat. Serves 12.

Excluding edges | | | | | | | | Exchanges | |

Calories	Fat	% Fat Cal	Protein	Carb	Chol	Sodium	Fiber	Carb	Meat	Fat
200	7g	32%	3g	32g	38mg	186mg	1g	2		1

Egg and butter add additional 28mg of cholesterol per serving.

Colorado Chocolate Chip Cookies

(can be made without wheat, gluten, dairy, eggs, or sugar - see page xi about ingredients)

You may use the sweetened coconut if you wish, but the unsweetened version works just fine, too.

1/2 cup butter or oleo or Spectrum™ canola oil spread
1/2 cup brown sugar or maple sugar
1 teaspoon gf vanilla extract
1 large egg or 1/4 cup flax mix (page 211)
1/4 cup buttermilk or 1/2 teaspoon cider vinegar plus enough non-dairy milk to equal 1/4 cup
1 cup white or brown rice flour

1/2 cup potato starch
1/4 cup tapioca flour
1/2 teaspoon baking soda
1/2 teaspoon salt
1/2 cup coconut flakes, unsweetened
1/2 cup chopped nuts
1/2 cup dried tart cherries or cranberries
1 1/2 cups gf/df chocolate chips

Preheat oven to 350°. In large mixing bowl, use electric mixer to beat butter (or oleo), sugar, and vanilla extract together until smooth. Beat in egg, then the buttermilk. In separate bowl, combine flours, soda, and salt. Beat into egg mixture on low speed until incorporated.

Stir in coconut, nuts, cranberries, and chocolate chips. Drop by tablespoons (or use a small spring-action ice cream scoop for evenly sized cookies) onto nonstick cookie sheet lined with parchment paper or nonstick liners—or sprayed with nonstick spray.

Bake for 7-10 minutes or until cookies are lightly puffed and slightly browned. Cool on rack. Store in airtight container. Serves 12.

								Exchanges		
Calories	Fat	% Fat Cal	Protein	Carb	Chol	Sodium	Fiber	Carb	Meat	Fat
350	19g	46%	4g	46g	0mg	173mg	3g	2		3

Butter and egg add additional 38mg of cholesterol per serving.

"Oatmeal" Cookies

(can be made without wheat, gluten, dairy, eggs, or sugar - see page xi about ingredients)

Ok, so these aren't REALLY oatmeal cookies, but they taste just as good. You'll find the rolled rice flakes in natural food stores. Be sure to use potato flour—not potato starch or potato starch flour.

1 cup brown rice flour
 or garbfava flour
1/4 cup potato flour
2 tablespoons tapioca flour
1/2 cup brown sugar
 or maple sugar
1/2 teaspoon salt
1/2 teaspoon xanthan gum
1/2 teaspoon baking soda
1/2 teaspoon baking powder
1 teaspoon ground cinnamon

1 large egg or 1/4 cup flax mix
 (page 211)
1/4 cup butter or oleo or Spectrum™
 canola oil spread
1/2 cup applesauce
2 tablespoons molasses
1 teaspoon gf vanilla extract
3/4 cup gf/df chocolate chips or raisins
1/2 cup rolled rice flakes
Cooking spray or parchment paper

Preheat oven to 325°. Coat nonstick cookie sheet with cooking spray or line with parchment paper. Set aside.

Combine dry ingredients (brown rice flour through cinnamon) and set aside.

In food processor, combine egg (or flax mix), butter, applesauce, molasses, and vanilla extract until well blended.

Add dry ingredients and rolled rice flakes. Pulse until thoroughly mixed. Gently stir in chocolate chips (or raisins). Dough will be somewhat stiff.

Drop by tablespoons (or use spring-action ice cream scoop for evenly shaped cookies) onto prepared cookie sheet. Flatten each cookie to 1/2-inch thickness with spatula that has been coated with cooking spray.

Bake for 20-25 minutes or until edges begin to brown. For a flavor twist, add 1/3 cup nut butter of your choice such as almond, cashew, or soy. Makes 12 cookies.

| | | | | | | | | Exchanges | | |
Calories	Fat	% Fat Cal	Protein	Carb	Chol	Sodium	Fiber	Carb	Meat	Fat
200	8g	32%	2g	34g	0mg	192mg	2g	2		1

Egg and butter add additional 29g cholesterol per cookie.

Rocky Road Brownies

(can be made without wheat, gluten, dairy, or sugar - see page xi about ingredients)

Absolutely and completely decadent—chocoholics will love this one. If you can think of anything else to throw in this recipe, do so. It's meant to be truly decadent. If nuts are not appropriate for your diet, omit them or substitute something else.

1/2 cup brown rice flour or garbfava flour
1/2 cup potato starch
1/4 cup tapioca flour
1/2 cup cocoa (not Dutch)
1/2 teaspoon baking powder
1/2 teaspoon salt
1/4 teaspoon xanthan gum
1/4 cup butter or oleo or Spectrum™ canola oil spread or cooking oil
1/2 cup granulated sugar or fructose powder

1/2 cup brown sugar or maple sugar
1 large egg*
2 teaspoons gf vanilla extract
1/4 cup warm (105°) water or coffee
1/2 cup gf/df chocolate chips or chocolate squares, chopped
1/2 cup chopped pecans
1/2 cup gf miniature Jet Puff® marshmallows
1/2 cup dried tart cherries or cranberries
Cooking spray

Preheat oven to 350°. Grease 8-inch square nonstick pan or spray with cooking spray. Stir together the flours, cocoa, baking powder, salt, and xanthan gum (and Egg Replacer, if using—see below). Set aside.

In large mixing bowl, beat the butter (or oleo) and sugars with electric mixer on medium speed until well combined. Add egg and vanilla; beat until well combined.

With mixer on low speed, add dry ingredients. Mix until just blended; a few lumps may remain. Gently stir in chocolate chips, nuts, marshmallows, and cherries or cranberries.

Spread batter in prepared pan and bake for 35 minutes or until a toothpick inserted in center comes out clean. Cool brownies before cutting. Serves 12.

*Rocky Road Brownies without Eggs: Omit egg and add 2 teaspoons Ener-G® Egg Replacer with dry ingredients. Increase water or coffee to 1/2 cup.

Exchanges

Calories	Fat	% Fat Cal	Protein	Carb	Chol	Sodium	Fiber	Carb	Meat	Fat
260	10g	33%	3g	46g	0mg	130mg	3g	2		2

Egg and butter add additional 28mg cholesterol per serving.

Basic Cut-Out Cookies

(can be made without wheat, gluten, dairy, eggs, or sugar - see page xi about ingredients)

You'll find many uses for these versatile cookies—see below for cut-out cookie suggestions.

1/4 cup butter or oleo or
    Spectrum™ canola oil spread
2 tablespoons honey or agave nectar
1/2 cup sugar or fructose powder
1 tablespoon gf vanilla extract
2 teaspoons grated lemon peel
3/4 cup brown rice flour
1/2 cup white rice flour
3 tablespoons potato starch

2 tablespoons tapioca flour
1/2 teaspoon xanthan gum
1/2 teaspoon salt
1 teaspoon baking powder
1/2 teaspoon baking soda
2 tablespoons water (if needed)
Cooking spray or parchment paper
    or non-stick baking liners
Additional rice flour for rolling

In food processor, combine butter (room temperature but not melted), honey, sugar vanilla, and lemon peel and process for 1 minute. Add flours, xanthan gum, salt, baking powder, and baking soda, blending all ingredients until mixture forms large clumps. Scrape down sides or bowl with spatula and blend until mixture forms ball again. Add water only if necessary—1 tablespoon at a time. Refrigerate 1 hour.

Preheat oven to 325°. Using one-half of the dough, roll to 1/4-inch thickness between sheets of waxed paper or plastic wrap which are sprinkled with rice flour. Keep remaining dough chilled until ready to use. Cut into desired shapes (about 2 inches in diameter) and transfer to baking sheet sprayed with cooking spray or lined with parchment paper or non-stick baking liners.

Bake for 10-12 minutes, or until cookies are lightly browned. Remove from cookie sheet and cool on wire rack. Makes 16.

| | | | | | | | | Exchanges | | |
Calories	Fat	% Fat Cal	Protein	Carb	Chol	Sodium	Fiber	Carb	Meat	Fat
88	3g	31%	.5g	15g	0mg	71mg	.5g	1		.5

Butter adds additional 8 mg cholesterol per cookie.

Suggestions for Cut-Out Cookies: Christmas: angel, bell, candy cane, tree, reindeer, star; **Halloween:** cats, half-moon, leaf, owl, pumpkins, witches; **Southwestern:** cactus, howling wolf; **Thanksgiving:** pumpkins, turkey; **Spring/Easter:** bunny, butterfly, chick, tulip; **St. Patrick's Day:** shamrock; **Valentine's Day:** flower, heart

TIPS FOR SUCCESSFUL "CUT-OUT" COOKIES

1. To avoid sticking, use non-stick baking liners or parchment paper.
2. Insulated baking sheets assure even baking and won't buckle.
3. Metal cookie cutters work better than plastic cookie cutters.
4. If the chilled dough is too stiff, leave dough at room temperature for 15-20 minutes. Then knead with hands to make dough more pliable. If dough is too soft after rolling, chill or freeze until firm—then cut into desired shapes. Do not roll dough thinner than 1/4 inch.
5. If you're having trouble transferring the cookies to the baking sheet, try rolling the dough onto parchment paper or nonstick liners, cut desired shapes, remove scraps of dough (leaving cut-out cookies on paper) and transfer paper or liner (cookies and all) to baking sheet.

Chocolate Cappuccino Ice Cream

(can be made without wheat, gluten, dairy, eggs, or sugar - see page xi about ingredients)

The coffee flavor will be more pronounced if you use espresso, rather than regular coffee.

1/2 cup hot brewed espresso or
    very strong brewed coffee
1/2 cup brown sugar or maple sugar
2 packages (12 oz.) soft silken tofu
1 teaspoon gf vanilla extract
1/4 teaspoon xanthan gum

2 tablespoons cocoa powder (not
    Dutch, Ghirardelli is a good brand)
1 teaspoon espresso powder
    (Medaglia D'Oro brand)
1/2 teaspoon ground cinnamon
1/8 teaspoon salt

Dissolve sugar in hot espresso or coffee. Add to food processor, along with remaining ingredients. Purée until very, very smooth.

Cover and chill until mixture reaches 40°. Freeze in ice cream maker according to manufacturer's directions. Makes about 3 cups. Serves 6 (1/2 cup each).

Exchanges

Calories	Fat	% Fat Cal	Protein	Carb	Chol	Sodium	Fiber	Carb	Meat	Fat
130	3g	19%	5g	22g	0mg	63mg	1g	1		.5

Chocolate Sorbet

(can be made without wheat, gluten, dairy, eggs, or sugar - see page xi about ingredients)

Use the very best cocoa you can find for this decadent, yet fat-free dessert.

1 1/2 cups cocoa powder
    (not Dutch)
1 teaspoon xanthan gum
2 cups brown sugar or maple sugar
1/2 teaspoon salt
4 cups water

1 cup brewed espresso or coffee
    (or water)
2 teaspoons gf vanilla extract
1 teaspoon gf rum extract or
    1 tablespoon gf rum (optional)

Stir together cocoa powder, xanthan gum, sugar, and salt in medium, heavy saucepan. Add water and brewed coffee (or water) and whisk to blend. Bring mixture to boil, then reduce heat and simmer for 20 minutes to slightly reduce. Stir occasionally. Add vanilla (and rum or rum extract, if using.) Refrigerate mixture to 40°.

Pour into freezer container of hand-turn or electric freezer. Freeze according to manufacturer's directions. Makes 1 quart. Serves 8.

Exchanges

Calories	Fat	% Fat Cal	Protein	Carb	Chol	Sodium	Fiber	Carb	Meat	Fat
332	3g	7%	4g	84g	0mg	238mg	8g	4		.5

Lemon Sorbet

(can be made without wheat, gluten, dairy, eggs, or sugar - see page xi about ingredients)

For a really special touch, use lemons as the serving dish for this delightful sorbet. Remove the peel from the top 1/3 of the lemons only. Then, slice off the top 1/3 of the lemons and juice them, saving the bottom. Using a spoon, scrape out the remaining pulp from each of the lemons. Slice off the bottom slightly so the shell sits firmly on plate. Refrigerate the empty lemon shells until ready to use. When the sorbet is ready to serve, fill each lemon shell with sorbet and garnish with fresh mint. Serve immediately.

4 large lemons	1 cup granulated sugar or
2 tablespoons grated lemon peel	fructose powder
1 packet (2 1/4 teaspoons) unflavored	3/4 cup fresh lemon juice
gelatin powder	Fresh mint for garnish
2 1/4 cups cold water	

With potato peeler, remove enough peel from lemons to equal 2 tablespoons when grated. Finely mince peel by using either coffee grinder or sharp knife and cutting board. Set peel aside.

Squeeze lemons, extracting enough juice to equal 3/4 cup. Set aside.

In heavy, medium-sized saucepan whisk gelatin into 1/4 cup of the water. Let stand for 5 minutes to dissolve. Add remaining water and sugar. Cook over medium heat until sugar and gelatin are completely dissolved. Remove from heat and stir in lemon juice and lemon peel. Cool to 40°.

Pour mixture into ice cream freezer and follow manufacturer's directions. Remove sorbet by using melon baller or spring-action ice cream scoop. Serve immediately—in dessert goblets or in lemon shells (see above). Garnish with fresh mint. Makes 1 quart. Serves 4.

								Exchanges		
Calories	Fat	% Fat Cal	Protein	Carb	Chol	Sodium	Fiber	Carb	Meat	Fat
105	0g	0	1g	27g	0mg	4mg	0g	1.5		

*Sugar Alternative: Use 2/3 cup honey. Reduce water to 1 3/4 cup.

Peach Ice Cream

(can be made without wheat, gluten, dairy, eggs, or sugar - see page xi about ingredients)

1 box (12 oz.) soft silken tofu
1/2 cup milk (cow, rice, soy)
1/2 cup sugar or fructose powder or 1/3
    cup honey
1 tablespoon butter or oleo or cooking oil
1/4 teaspoon xanthan gum

1/4 cup fresh lemon juice
2 cups sliced fresh peaches
1 teaspoon gf vanilla extract
1 teaspoon gf almond extract
    (optional)
1/4 teaspoon salt

Place all ingredients in food processor and blend until very, very smooth. Chill mixture until it reaches 40°.

Freeze in ice cream maker, according to manufacturer's directions. When ready to serve, use spring-action ice cream scoop or melon baller to remove balls of ice cream. Serve immediately with your favorite sauce. Makes 1 quart. Serves 8 (1/2 cup each).

								Exchanges		
Calories	Fat	% Fat Cal	Protein	Carb	Chol	Sodium	Fiber	Carb	Meat	Fat
110	3g	21%	3g	20g	4mg	47mg	1g	1	.5	.5

Strawberry Sherbet

(can be made without wheat, gluten, dairy, eggs, or sugar - see page xi about ingredients)

1 box (12 oz.) soft silken tofu
2 cups sliced fresh strawberries
1 cup milk (cow, rice, soy)
1/4 cup fresh lemon juice
1/2 teaspoon xanthan gum

2/3 cup sugar or fructose powder or
    1/2 cup honey
1 tablespoon butter or oleo or cooking oil
1 teaspoon gf vanilla extract
1/8 teaspoon salt

Combine all ingredients in food processor. Process until very smooth (or if you like little chunks of fruit, stop before mixture is entirely smooth.)

Chill mixture until it reaches 40°. Place in electric ice cream maker and freeze according to manufacturer's directions. Serve with toppings of your choice. Makes 1 quart. Serves 8 (1/2 cup each).

								Exchanges		
Calories	Fat	% Fat Cal	Protein	Carb	Chol	Sodium	Fiber	Carb	Meat	Fat
125	3g	19%	3g	23g	4mg	55mg	1g	1		.5

Raspberry Sherbet: Use 2 cups fresh raspberries in place of 2 cups strawberries.

Vanilla Frozen Yogurt without Eggs

(can be made without wheat, gluten, dairy, eggs, or sugar - see page xi about ingredients)

If you choose to use goat milk, make sure it's appropriate for your diet.

2 cups vanilla-flavored yogurt (cow, soy, goat)
2 teaspoons unflavored gelatin powder

1 3/4 cups milk (cow, rice, soy)
1/2 cup honey or agave nectar
3 teaspoons gf vanilla extract

Place all ingredients in food processor and blend until very, very smooth. Chill until mixture reaches 40°. Freeze in ice cream maker, according to manufacturer's directions.

To serve, remove from freezer and use spring-action ice cream scoop or melon baller to remove balls of frozen yogurt. Serve immediately with your favorite sauce. Makes 1 quart. Serves 8 (1/2 cup each).

								Exchanges		
Calories	Fat	% Fat Cal	Protein	Carb	Chol	Sodium	Fiber	Carb	Meat	Fat
140	1g	5%	6g	29g	4mg	70mg	0g	2		

Vanilla Ice Cream with Eggs

(can be made without wheat, gluten, dairy, or sugar - see page xi about ingredients)

This delicious frozen treat omits dairy, however, it is the egg yolks that give it a creamy texture. So, it will be perfect for those <u>without</u> egg sensitivities.

1 teaspoon unflavored gelatin powder
4 cups milk (cow, rice, soy), divided
1/2 cup honey or agave nectar

4 large egg yolks, beaten until very smooth (or 2 whole eggs or equivalent gf liquid egg substitute)
3 teaspoons gf vanilla extract

Combine gelatin with 3 tablespoons of the milk and stir until dissolved. Add gelatin mixture, honey (or agave nectar), and remaining milk to small saucepan. Cook over low heat until mixture almost boils. Remove from heat.

Whisk 1/2 cup of the hot mixture into eggs. Add eggs to mixture in saucepan. Return saucepan to low-medium heat and cook, stirring, for another two minutes. Do not boil; mixture may curdle. Remove from heat. Stir in vanilla. Chill until mixture reaches 40°. Freeze in ice cream maker, according to manufacturer's directions.

When ready to serve, use ice cream scoop or melon baller to remove balls of frozen yogurt. Serve immediately. Makes 1 quart. Serves 8 (1/2 cup servings).

								Exchanges		
Calories	Fat	% Fat Cal	Protein	Carb	Chol	Sodium	Fiber	Carb	Meat	Fat
140	3g	17%	6g	24g	109mg	68mg	0g	1		.5

Notes

SALADS

S alads are a marvelous way to add color, texture, and variety to our meals—not to mention that they are a source of important nutrients. And, they can trans-form an ordinary meal into a real showstopper.

For example, a colorful, crunchy, flavorful salad adds "pizzazz" to any meal and shows your guests that this is a special occasion—and they're special, too!

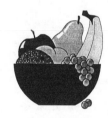

Basic Vinaigrette

(can be made without wheat, gluten, dairy, eggs, or sugar - see page xi about ingredients)

1/4 cup vegetable stock or chicken stock
2 tablespoons apple cider vinegar or
   fresh lemon juice
2 teaspoons Dijonnaise mustard or
   1 teaspoon gf dry mustard

1 tablespoon extra virgin olive oil
1 garlic clove, minced
1/4 teaspoon salt
1/8 teaspoon black pepper

In small bowl, whisk together ingredients until thoroughly mixed. Or, blend in blender or small food processor. Makes about 1/2 cup. Serves 4 (2 tablespoons each.)

| | | | | | | | | Exchanges | | |
Calories	Fat	% Fat Cal	Protein	Carb	Chol	Sodium	Fiber	Carb	Meat	Fat
37	4g	82%	.1g	1g	0mg	400mg	1g			1

Cilantro Citrus Dressing

(can be made without wheat, gluten, dairy, eggs, or sugar - see page xi about ingredients)

3 tablespoons fresh orange juice
1 tablespoon fresh lemon juice
1 tablespoon fresh lime juice
1/2 cup cilantro leaves, packed
1/4 teaspoon cumin powder

1/4 teaspoon dried thyme leaves
1/8 teaspoon cayenne pepper
1/8 teaspoon salt
1/8 teaspoon white pepper
1/4 cup olive oil or cooking oil

Place all ingredients in blender. Process until mixture is very smooth. With motor running, add oil in thin, steady stream. Refrigerate, covered. Bring to room temperature to serve. Makes 1/2 cup. Serves 4 (2 tablespoons each.)

| | | | | | | | | Exchanges | | |
Calories	Fat	% Fat Cal	Protein	Carb	Chol	Sodium	Fiber	Carb	Meat	Fat
130	14g	92%	0g	2g	0mg	76mg	0g			3

Tomato-Basil Vinaigrette

(can be made without wheat, gluten, dairy, eggs, or sugar - see page xi about ingredients)

2 large tomatoes (seeded, chopped)
2 tablespoons fresh lemon or lime juice
   or 2 tablespoons gf red wine vinegar
2 tablespoons fresh basil, packed or
  1 tablespoon dried basil leaves
1/2 teaspoon dried oregano leaves

2 tablespoons extra virgin olive oil
1/2 teaspoon gf garlic powder
   or 1 garlic clove, minced
1/2 teaspoon sugar or honey
1/4 teaspoon salt
1/4 teaspoon black pepper

Combine all ingredients in blender and purée until thoroughly mixed. Refrigerate, covered, for up to 2 days. Makes about 1/2 cup. Serves 4 (2 tablespoons each.)

| | | | | | | | | Exchanges | | |
Calories	Fat	% Fat Cal	Protein	Carb	Chol	Sodium	Fiber	Carb	Meat	Fat
83	7g	72%	1g	6g	0mg	152mg	1g	1		1

Vinegar-Free Herb Dressing

(can be made without wheat, gluten, dairy, eggs, or sugar - see page xi about ingredients)

My favorite herbs are thyme, basil, marjoram, and savory—but use the ones you like.

1/2 cup fresh lemon juice
2 small garlic cloves
1/4 cup extra virgin olive oil
2 teaspoons honey or agave nectar
1/2 cup chopped green onions
  or chives

1/2 teaspoon salt
1/4 cup chopped fresh herbs or
  3 teaspoons dried herbs of choice
1/8 teaspoon xanthan gum (optional)
1/8 teaspoon black pepper

Combine all ingredients in blender and purée until mixture is completely smooth. Makes about 3/4 cup. Serves 6 (about 2 tablespoons each.) Best served immediately.

| | | | | | | | | Exchanges | | |
Calories	Fat	% Fat Cal	Protein	Carb	Chol	Sodium	Fiber	Carb	Meat	Fat
100	9g	79%	0g	5g	0mg	195mg	1g			2

Caesar Salad without Eggs

(can be made without wheat, gluten, dairy, eggs, or sugar - see page xi about ingredients)

Use only half of the garlic-oil mixture to toss with the croutons, adding the remainder to the salad dressing itself.

2 garlic cloves
1/4 cup extra-virgin olive oil
1/2 teaspoon salt
1 cup gf croutons
1 tablespoon fresh lemon juice
1 teaspoon apple cider vinegar
1 teaspoon gf dry mustard

1 teaspoon gf Worcestershire sauce
1 teaspoon Reese gf anchovy paste
   (optional)
1/3 cup grated Parmesan cheese
   (cow, rice, soy)
1 head Romaine lettuce, washed and torn

Use garlic press to mince garlic before mashing with salt and olive oil. Brown croutons in 350° oven for 10 minutes. Toss them with half of the garlic-oil mixture and return to oven for another 3-5 minutes, or until golden. Remove from oven. Set aside until cool.

In large salad bowl, whisk together remaining garlic-oil mixture, lemon juice, vinegar, mustard, Worcestershire sauce, and anchovy paste (if using). Add Romaine lettuce and toss thoroughly. Sprinkle with Parmesan cheese and croutons, toss again, and serve immediately. Serves 4.

| | | | | | | | | Exchanges | | |
Calories	Fat	% Fat Cal	Protein	Carb	Chol	Sodium	Fiber	Carb	Meat	Fat
230	18g	71%	7g	10g	11mg	999mg	2g	.5	.5	3

Fruit Salad with Balsamic Dressing

(can be made without wheat, gluten, dairy, eggs, or sugar - see page xi about ingredients

Dressing
1 tablespoon balsamic vinegar
2 tablespoons cooking oil
1/4 cup fresh orange juice
1 teaspoon grated lemon peel
1/8 teaspoon black pepper

Fruit
1 pink or red grapefruit
1 orange
1 red pear, cored and halved
1/2 cup red or green seedless grapes
4 large lettuce leaves

Dressing: In screw-top jar, combine ingredients and shake vigorously to blend.
Fruit: Using sharp knife, remove peel and all of white membrane from grapefruit and orange. Section the grapefruit and slice orange crosswise into 8 slices.
Cut pear in 1/4-inch thick slices lengthwise. Dip slices in reserved juices from
grapefruit and orange.

Cover large platter or 4 individual serving plates with lettuce leaves.
Decoratively arrange fruit over lettuce. Drizzle with dressing. Serves 4.

								Exchanges		
Calories	Fat	% Fat Cal	Protein	Carb	Chol	Sodium	Fiber	Carb	Meat	Fat
140	7g	40%	1g	20g	0mg	4mg	3g	2		1

Grapefruit & Avocado Salad

(can be made without wheat, gluten, dairy, eggs, or sugar - see page xi about ingredients)

Dressing
1/4 cup each olive oil and water
3 tablespoons red wine vinegar
2 teaspoons honey or agave nectar
1/2 teaspoon dried tarragon leaves
1 teaspoon Dijonnaise mustard
1 garlic clove, minced
1/4 teaspoon each salt and white pepper

Fruit
1 head red leaf lettuce
1 avocado, peeled and sliced
1 red grapefruit (peeled, sectioned)
1/2 cup toasted almonds

In screw-top jar, combine dressing ingredients by shaking vigorously to
emulsify. In large salad bowl, toss lettuce with dressing. Add avocado,
grapefruit, and toasted almonds. Toss gently. Drizzle with dressing. Serve
chilled. Serves 4.

								Exchanges		
Calories	Fat	% Fat Cal	Protein	Carb	Chol	Sodium	Fiber	Carb	Meat	Fat
345	30g	74%	5g	18g	0mg	322mg	7g	.5		6

Jicama & Mandarin Orange Salad

(can be made without wheat, gluten, dairy, eggs, or sugar - see page xi about ingredients)

1 medium jicama
(peeled, shredded)
1 cup cilantro, coarsely chopped
2 tablespoons fresh lime juice

2 tablespoons red wine vinegar or rice
vinegar
1 can (11 oz.) mandarin oranges,
drained

Combine jicama, cilantro, lime juice, and vinegar in medium bowl and mix well. Gently stir in oranges. Serve slightly chilled. Makes 3 cups. Serves 4.

| | | | | | | | | Exchanges | | |
Calories	Fat	% Fat Cal	Protein	Carb	Chol	Sodium	Fiber	Carb	Meat	Fat
150	.5g	3%	3g	36g	0mg	19ng	17g	6		

Jicama, Orange, & Avocado Salad

(can be made without wheat, gluten, dairy, eggs, or sugar - see page xi about ingredients)

2 tablespoons olive oil
2 tablespoons fresh lime
or lemon juice
2 tablespoons fresh orange juice
1 teaspoon sugar or honey
1/4 teaspoon chili powder
1 teaspoon red wine vinegar
1/8 teaspoon salt

1/8 teaspoon cayenne pepper
1 head red leaf lettuce, torn in pieces
2 medium oranges (peeled, sectioned)
2 chopped green onions
1 cup jicama, peeled and cubed
1 large avocado, peeled and slice

In screw-top jar, combine olive oil, lime juice, orange juice, sugar, chili powder, vinegar, salt, and cayenne pepper. Shake vigorously to blend. Set dressing aside.

Wash and dry lettuce. Place in large serving bowl. Add oranges, green onions and jicama. Toss with dressing to coat evenly. Add avocado and toss gently. Serve chilled. Makes about 4 cups. Serves 4.

| | | | | | | | | Exchanges | | |
Calories	Fat	% Fat Cal	Protein	Carb	Chol	Sodium	Fiber	Carb	Meat	Fat
200	15g	61%	3g	19g	0mg	85mg	7g	2		3

Potato Salad

(can be made without wheat, gluten, dairy, eggs, or sugar - see page xi about ingredients)

If eggs are not appropriate for your diet, omit them and use another potato instead.

3 cups cooked potatoes (peeled, diced)
4 hard-boiled eggs(peeled, chopped)
1/2 cup finely chopped celery
1/4 cup finely chopped green onion
2 tablespoons gf sweet pickle relish
   or 2 teaspoons dried dill weed
1/2 cup gf Mayonnaise (page 217)

1 tablespoon cider vinegar
1 teaspoon sugar
1/2 teaspoon celery salt or plain salt
1/2 teaspoon celery seed
1/4 teaspoon white pepper
1/2 teaspoon gf dry mustard
Paprika for garnish

Combine chopped potatoes, eggs, celery, onion, and relish (or dill) in large bowl. In small bowl, combine remaining ingredients (except paprika) until smooth. Pour over potato mixture and toss until thoroughly coated. Turn into serving bowl and garnish with paprika. Chill until serving time. Makes about 5 cups. Serves 6.

								Exchanges		
Calories	Fat	% Fat Cal	Protein	Carb	Chol	Sodium	Fiber	Carb	Meat	Fat
165	7g	40%	6g	19g	146mg	280mg	2g	2		1

Lettuce Salad with Pears & Feta Cheese

(can be made without wheat, gluten, dairy, eggs, or sugar - see page xi about ingredients)

3 cups red leaf lettuce, torn in pieces
2 tablespoons gf balsamic vinegar
2 teaspoons Dijonnaise mustard or 1
   teaspoon gf dry mustard
2 teaspoons vegetable or walnut oil
2 teaspoons water

1 garlic clove, minced
1/2 teaspoon dried thyme leaves
1 red pear, thinly sliced
3 tablespoons feta cheese, crumbled
1/2 cup toasted pecans

Place washed, dried, torn lettuce into large bowl. Set aside.
In screw-top jar, combine vinegar, mustard, oil, water, garlic, and thyme. Shake vigorously to blend. Toss with greens. Arrange on salad plates. Place red pear slices decoratively in pin-wheel design on each salad. Top with crumbled feta cheese and toasted pecans. Serves 4.

								Exchanges		
Calories	Fat	% Fat Cal	Protein	Carb	Chol	Sodium	Fiber	Carb	Meat	Fat
178	14g	68%	3g	12g	6mg	147mg	3g	1		3

Spinach Salad with Strawberries

(can be made without wheat, gluten, dairy, eggs, or sugar - see page xi about ingredients)

Next time try mixing in a few green or red grapes for added interest.

3 tablespoons fresh orange juice
1 tablespoon fresh lemon juice
1 tablespoon honey
2 tablespoons dried basil leaves
  or 1/2 cup chopped fresh basil
1/4 teaspoon dried thyme leaves
1/4 teaspoon xanthan gum
1/8 teaspoon cayenne pepper

1/8 teaspoon salt
1/8 teaspoon white pepper
1/4 cup olive oil or cooking oil
1 package (10 oz.) baby spinach leaves,
  (rinsed, dried)
1 pint hulled strawberries, halved
1 cup toasted pecan halves
1/4 cup feta cheese, crumbled

In small jar, whisk together orange juice, lemon juice, honey, basil, thyme, xanthan gum, cayenne pepper, salt, white pepper, and oil until smooth. You may chill dressing at this point or proceed directly to making the salad.

Place cleaned spinach leaves in large bowl. Add strawberries and pecans. Add enough dressing to coat leaves and toss gently. Just before serving, sprinkle crumbled feta cheese on top. Serves 10.

| | | | | | | | | Exchanges | | |
Calories	Fat	% Fat Cal	Protein	Carb	Chol	Sodium	Fiber	Carb	Meat	Fat
160	15g	78%	2g	7g	3mg	71mg	2g	.5		3

Waldorf Salad

(can be made without wheat, gluten, dairy, eggs, or sugar - see page xi about ingredients)

2 red delicious apples, chopped
2 stalks celery, chopped
1/2 cup toasted pecan halves
1/2 cup golden raisins

1 teaspoon fresh lemon juice
2 tablespoons gf Mayonnaise (page 217)
1/8 teaspoon salt
1/2 teaspoon sugar or honey

Combine apples, celery, pecans, and raisins in small bowl. In another bowl, stir together lemon juice, mayonnaise, salt, and sugar. Pour mayonnaise mixture over apple mixture and toss thoroughly. Serve immediately. Serves 4.

| | | | | | | | | Exchanges | | |
Calories	Fat	% Fat Cal	Protein	Carb	Chol	Sodium	Fiber	Carb	Meat	Fat
225	12g	44%	2g	32g	2mg	130mg	4g	2		2

Fruit-Sweetened Gelatin Salad

(can be made without wheat, gluten, dairy, eggs, or sugar - see page xi about ingredients)

Gelatin salads (or jello as we usually say) are almost a staple in American culture. Yet, the sugar and artificial color can be a problem for some of us. You can make this gelatin as sweet as you like, either by adding a sweetener that you tolerate—or intensifying the juice.

Juices that work especially well include pure white grape or pure apple juice, because they produce a lovely translucent look that allows fruits and vegetables to show through nicely. However, orange juice or tomato juice also work. Use whatever fruits or vegetables you prefer (but don't use fresh pineapple or it won't gel properly). Vary the colors of the fruit to achieve a pretty effect. For a festive touch, replace 1/4 cup of the cold fruit juice with your favorite gf champagne or gf white wine.

You can halve this recipe so it fits nicely into a 6-cup Bundt pan to serve 8.

1/4 cup unflavored gelatin powder	1 cup mandarin oranges
2 cups fruit juice, cold	1/2 cup fresh raspberries
6 cups fruit juice, hot	1/2 cup chopped celery
1/2 cup fresh blueberries	Cooking spray

Dissolve gelatin powder in 2 cups cold fruit juice in large bowl. Add hot fruit juice, stirring thoroughly until dissolved. For a sweeter salad, simmer juice until it is reduced by 1/3. Remember you'll still need 6 cups of hot juice, so if you're reducing the juice you must start with 8 cups.

Chill gelatin in refrigerator until it just begins to set (it will begin to resist when you try to stir it). Stir in fruit or vegetables until thoroughly distributed. Pour mixture into 10-cup pan that has been sprayed with cooking spray. Chill all day or overnight.

To unmold, place pan in room-temperature water for 2 to 3 minutes. Remove from water, dry bottom of pan, and invert onto serving plate. If it won't release, try pressing a hot, wet towel on the pan for a few minutes. Serves 16.

								Exchanges		
Calories	Fat	% Fat Cal	Protein	Carb	Chol	Sodium	Fiber	Carb	Meat	Fat
70	0g	0	2g	15g	0mg	12mg	1g	1		

SIDE DISHES

S ide dishes are often taken for granted, but they can also be the touch that transforms an ordinary meal into a spectacular event. Think of them as playing "supporting roles" alongside the main dish. As such, they should complement the main dish yet stand on their own in terms of color, texture, and eye appeal.

I've tried to make each side dish in this chapter worthy of an "Oscar" nomination for supporting role. Instead of ordinary baked potatoes try baking them into crispy rounds (Potatoes Anna) or combine them other vegetables and grill or roast them over hot coals on the grill (Roasted or Grilled Vegetables). Two different taste and texture sensations from a simple vegetable.

Side dishes, especially fruits and vegetables, also add important nutrients and fiber. But, instead of simply steaming vegetables, try sautéing them for a completely different taste sensation. Or, try cooking pineapple slices or peaches on the grill. Fabulous and so easy

For additional side dishes, see **Wheat-Free Recipes & Menus: Delicious Dining Without Wheat & Gluten, 1997 (Savory Palate, Inc.)**

Brown Rice Pilaf

(can be made without wheat, gluten, dairy, eggs, or sugar - see page xi about ingredients)

See Mail Order Sources about Jowar pearled grain.

1/2 cup brown rice or
   Jowar pearled grain
1/2 cup Wehani rice or brown rice
1 tablespoon cooking oil, divided
1/2 cup chopped onion
1/4 cup chopped celery
1/4 cup chopped carrots
1 medium garlic clove, minced

1/4 cup currants or raisins
1/2 teaspoon dried sage leaves
1/2 teaspoon dried thyme leaves
1/4 teaspoon black pepper
2 1/2 cups low-sodium chicken
   broth
1 bay leaf

Place first two ingredients and half of the oil in heavy saucepan. Sauté over medium heat stirring frequently, until lightly browned—about 5 minutes. Remove rice from pan. Place remaining oil in saucepan and sauté onions, celery, and carrots over medium heat until tender—about 5-8 minutes.

Add remaining ingredients and bring to boil. Cover, reduce heat, and simmer mixture for 50 minutes or until liquid is absorbed. Discard bay leaf before serving. Serves 4 (1/2 cup servings).

| | | | | | | | | Exchanges | | |
Calories	Fat	% Fat Cal	Protein	Carb	Chol	Sodium	Fiber	Carb	Meat	Fat
240	6g	22%	6g	41g	2mg	80mg	3g	3		1

Cabbage Coleslaw

(can be made without wheat, gluten, dairy, eggs, or sugar - see page xi about ingredients)

1 small cabbage, shredded
1 medium carrot, coarsely grated
2 celery stalks (1/4-inch diagonals)
1 bunch green onions (1/4-inch
   diagonals)
2 tablespoons apple cider vinegar
3 tablespoons fresh lemon juice
1 teaspoon honey

1/2 tablespoon Dijonnaise mustard
1/3 cup cooking oil
1/2 teaspoon celery seed
1/2 teaspoon salt
1/4 teaspoon ground white pepper
1/4 teaspoon paprika

In large bowl, toss together cabbage, carrots, celery, and onions. In blender or food processor, blend remaining ingredients—except paprika. Toss vegetables with dressing. Garnish with paprika. Serve chilled. Serves 4.

| | | | | | | | | Exchanges | | |
Calories	Fat	% Fat Cal	Protein	Carb	Chol	Sodium	Fiber	Carb	Meat	Fat
250	19g	64%	4g	20mg	0mg	410mg	8g	3		4

Couscous

(can be made without wheat, gluten, dairy, eggs, or sugar - see page xi about ingredients)

The flavor is deeper and richer using basmati rice (available at your grocery store), but you can use plain white, long-grain rice if you prefer. If you're using commercial vegetable broth, you may not need the 1 teaspoon salt.

1 cup long-grain basmati rice or
long-grain white rice

2 cups vegetable or chicken stock
1 teaspoon salt

Place half of rice in blender or food processor. Pulse machine until rice kernels are broken into smaller pieces—similar to the size of couscous. Continue with remaining rice.

Spread rice in thin layer on baking sheet and toast at 350° oven until lightly browned, about 25-30 minutes, stirring occasionally for even browning.

Place rice and remaining ingredients in medium, heavy saucepan, bring to boil and reduce heat. Simmer, covered, until mixture has absorbed water—about 30 minutes. Fluff with fork and serve at once. Serves 4.

								Exchanges		
Calories	Fat	% Fat Cal	Protein	Carb	Chol	Sodium	Fiber	Carb	Meat	Fat
188	1g	5%	5g	41g	0mg	639mg	1g	2.5		

Couscous Salad

(can be made without wheat, gluten, dairy, eggs, or sugar - see page xi about ingredients)

A great salad for picnics since it can be made ahead of time and tastes great whether it's cold or at room temperature.

2 cups cooked Couscous (see above)
1/2 cup diced celery
1 tablespoon grated lemon or lime peel
1 tablespoon chopped fresh mint
1 tablespoon chopped fresh cilantro or
parsley, packed

1/4 cup olive oil
1/4 cup fresh lemon juice
1/2 teaspoon gf onion powder
1/2 teaspoon salt
1/4 teaspoon black pepper
Paprika for garnish

Combine couscous, celery, lemon or lime peel, mint, and cilantro (or parsley) in medium bowl. To make salad dressing, whisk together olive oil, lemon juice, onion powder, salt, and black pepper. Mix with rice. Serve chilled. Garnish with paprika before serving. Serves 4 (1/2 cup each).

								Exchanges		
Calories	Fat	% Fat Cal	Protein	Carb	Chol	Sodium	Fiber	Carb	Meat	Fat
322	15g	41%	6g	42g	2mg	999mg	2g	2.5g		3

Handmade Egg Pasta

(can be made without wheat, gluten, dairy, or sugar - see page xi about ingredients)

Despite the fact that we have lots of wonderful wheat-free/gluten-free commercial pasta to choose from, sometimes it's nice to have the hearty, handmade version. For those times when you want the real thing, try this recipe. It's not hard. In fact, with an electric pasta machine it is extremely easy. Please note that this recipe contains eggs.

1/2 cup brown or white rice flour	1/2 teaspoon salt
1/2 cup tapioca flour	2 large eggs
1/4 cup potato starch	1/4 cup water
1/2 cup cornstarch	Cooking oil (see below)
4 teaspoons xanthan gum	Additional rice flour for rolling
1 teaspoon unflavored gelatin powder	

Hand Shaped Pasta: Combine all ingredients in food processor, using **1 tablespoon** oil. Process until mixture forms a ball. Place half of dough on a board or firm surface that is lightly floured with rice flour. (Cover remaining half with plastic wrap to prevent drying out.)

Roll dough as thin as possible. Cut into desired shapes, very thin for spaghetti or fettuccine; slightly wider for noodles. A rolling slicer is excellent for making uniformly shaped noodles. For lasagna, cut in 1 1/2 wide strips. Repeat with remaining half of dough.

Electric Machine Shaped Pasta: Follow machine directions. Reduce oil to **1 teaspoon**. Whisk eggs and water thoroughly until no egg membranes are visible. When adding liquid, withhold last 2 tablespoons (add only if mixture seems very, very dry.) Usually, pasta dough can be drier when using an electric machine, so don't add the additional liquid until you're sure it is needed. Serves 4.

Exchanges

Calories	Fat	% Fat Cal	Protein	Carb	Chol	Sodium	Fiber	Carb	Meat	Fat
295	7g	21%	6g	54g	138mg	340mg	5g	2	1	1

Herbed Rice Salad

(can be made without wheat, gluten, dairy, eggs, or sugar - see page xi about ingredients)

Perfect for informal parties such as picnics, or elegant enough for a wedding reception.

1 1/2 cups white long grain rice	1/2 cup chopped fresh cilantro or parsley
3 cups water	1/2 cup chopped green onions
1 teaspoon salt	1/2 cup fresh or frozen green peas
2 tablespoons fresh lemon juice	2 tablespoons diced red bell pepper
2 tablespoons rice vinegar	1 teaspoon salt
2 teaspoons Dijonnaise mustard	1/4 teaspoon black pepper
2 tablespoons olive oil	Paprika, cilantro, and red bell pepper
2 tablespoons minced fresh dill	strips or circles for garnish

In a medium saucepan, combine rice, water, and 1 teaspoon salt. Cover, bring to boil, reduce heat, and simmer until rice is done—about 18 minutes. Remove from heat, let stand for 5 minutes, then fluff rice with fork.

Chill cooked rice. Meanwhile, to make dressing combine lemon juice, vinegar, mustard, olive oil, and dill weed. Set aside.

When rice is cool, toss thoroughly with dressing in large bowl. Stir in cilantro (or parsley), onions, peas, and red bell pepper. Season with salt and pepper. Garnish. Serves 6.

								Exchanges		
Calories	Fat	% Fat Cal	Protein	Carb	Chol	Sodium	Fiber	Carb	Meat	Fat
228	5g	20%	4g	41g	0mg	630mg	2g	2.5		1

Pineapple Fruit Boats

(can be made without wheat, gluten, dairy, eggs, or sugar - see page xi about ingredients)

Use this colorful dish as a centerpiece on the table.

1 whole fresh pineapple	1 pint fresh hulled strawberries, halved
3 kiwi fruit, peeled and quartered	Fresh mint leaves for garnish

Slice pineapple in half lengthwise, leaving leafy crown attached to each half. Use grapefruit knife to slice around perimeter of each half to separate fruit from the skin. The skin forms two boats.

Remove core, then slice pineapple into bite-size pieces. Combine with kiwi and strawberries. Place mixture in two boats. Refrigerate. Garnish. Serves 6.

								Exchanges		
Calories	Fat	% Fat Cal	Protein	Carb	Chol	Sodium	Fiber	Carb	Meat	Fat
75	1g	7%	1g	19g	0mg	3mg	3g	1		

Rice Pilaf with Dill

(can be made without wheat, gluten, dairy, eggs, or sugar - see page xi about ingredients)

For a really special presentation, grease small custard cups, timbale forms, or a single large Bundt pan. Gently press the hot rice mixture into the mold(s). Invert the mold(s) onto the serving plate or platter and serve.

1 tablespoon olive oil	2 cups vegetable broth
3 green onions, finely chopped	1/2 teaspoon salt
2 tablespoons chopped fresh dill weed	1/8 teaspoon ground nutmeg
or 2 teaspoons dried dill weed	1 tablespoon fresh lemon juice
1 teaspoon grated lemon peel	Dill weed for garnish
1 cup long-grain white rice	

In large saucepan, combine oil, onions, dill, lemon peel, and rice. Cook, stirring constantly, for 1 minute to slightly cook vegetables and brown rice. Add broth, salt, and nutmeg. Bring to boil, reduce heat to low. Cover and simmer until rice is absorbed—about 15-20 minutes.

Stir in lemon juice. Garnish with dill weed. Serves 4 (1/2 cup servings).

								Exchanges		
Calories	Fat	% Fat Cal	Protein	Carb	Chol	Sodium	Fiber	Carb	Meat	Fat
220	5g	19%	5g	39g	2mg	346mg	1g	2.5		1

Tomatillo Rice

Tomatillos are those funny-looking green things with papery skins. They belong to the nightshade family and are related to tomatoes, peppers, potatoes, and so on. Wear rubber gloves when chopping the jalapeño.

3 large tomatillos (husked, washed)	1 large garlic clove
1 small plum tomato (seeded, chopped)	1/2 cup long grain white rice
2 tablespoons chopped fresh cilantro	1 1/4 cups low-sodium chicken
1 small chopped jalapeño (optional)	broth
1/4 teaspoon salt	Additional cilantro for garnish

Chop tomatillos coarsely. Combine chopped tomatillos and remaining ingredients in medium, heavy saucepan. Bring to boil, reduce heat, and simmer until liquid is absorbed—about 20 minutes. Let stand, covered, for 5 minutes. Garnish with cilantro. Serves 4 (1/3 cup each).

								Exchanges		
Calories	Fat	% Fat Cal	Protein	Carb	Chol	Sodium	Fiber	Carb	Meat	Fat
110	1g	8%	3g	22g	1mg	180mg	1g	2		

Dilled Baby Carrots

(can be made without wheat, gluten, dairy, eggs, or sugar - see page xi about ingredients)

My guests always enjoy these carrots, but inevitably ask me about the recipe. They are usually surprised to learn how easy it is to make this delicious vegetable.

1 pound baby carrots (washed, trimmed)
1/2 teaspoon salt

2 tablespoons pure maple syrup
2 teaspoons dill weed

Combine baby carrots and salt with enough water to cover in a medium saucepan. Bring to boil and simmer, covered, for 6-8 minutes. Drain thoroughly. Toss carrots with maple syrup and dill weed. Serve immediately. Serves 4.

| | | | | | | | | Exchanges | | |
Calories	Fat	% Fat Cal	Protein	Carb	Chol	Sodium	Fiber	Carb	Meat	Fat
70	1g	8%	1g	16g	0mg	330mg	2g	2		

Green Onion Pancakes

(can be made without wheat, gluten, dairy, eggs, or sugar - see page xi about ingredients)

Serve these tasty pancakes in place of potatoes or rice. Roll into cylinders and garnish with paprika and chives. Or, top with your favorite creamed sauce for a special brunch.

2/3 cup milk (cow, rice, soy)
1/4 cup brown rice flour
** or garbfava flour**
1/4 cup potato starch
1 tablespoon tapioca flour
2 tablespoons chopped toasted
** nuts or sesame seeds**
1 1/4 teaspoons baking powder

3/4 teaspoon baking soda
1 teaspoon olive oil
1/4 teaspoon gf onion salt
1/4 teaspoon ground white pepper
1/4 cup finely chopped green onions
Additional oil for frying
Paprika and chopped chives (garnish)

In medium mixing bowl, whisk together all ingredients. Lightly coat small non-stick skillet with cooking oil and warm over medium heat. Add 2 tablespoons of batter to skillet. Cook until edges are golden—about 1 minute. Flip carefully. Cook another 30 seconds or until browned.

Transfer to plate and keep warm. Repeat with remaining batter. Serve as a side dish with fish or chicken. Serves 4 (2 pancakes each).

| | | | | | | | | Exchanges | | |
Calories	Fat	% Fat Cal	Protein	Carb	Chol	Sodium	Fiber	Carb	Meat	Fat
170	7g	38%	8g	19g	138mg	178mg	2g	1		1

Pineapple Coconut Rice

(can be made without wheat, gluten, dairy, eggs, or sugar - see page xi about ingredients)

1 tablespoon olive oil
1 small onion, finely chopped
1 teaspoon dried thyme leaves
1/2 teaspoon dried savory leaves
1/2 teaspoon salt
1/4 teaspoon ground white pepper

3/4 cup long grain white rice
1 can (8 oz.) crushed pineapple
2 tablespoons coconut flakes
1/2 cup chopped chives or cilantro
1/3 cup minced red bell pepper
Paprika for garnish

In large saucepan over medium heat, sauté onions, thyme, savory, salt, pepper, and rice in oil until onion is translucent and rice is browned, stirring constantly—about 2 minutes.

Drain pineapple thoroughly, reserving juice. To pineapple juice, add enough water to equal 1 1/2 cups. Add juice to rice in pan, along with pineapple and coconut flakes. Cover, reduce heat, and simmer 20 minutes or until liquid is absorbed. Stir in chives and red bell pepper. Garnish with paprika at serving time. Serve warm or chilled. Serves 4.

| | | | | | | | | Exchanges | | |
Calories	Fat	% Fat Cal	Protein	Carb	Chol	Sodium	Fiber	Carb	Meat	Fat
200	5g	20%	3g	37g	0mg	295mg	2g	3		1

Polenta

(can be made without wheat, gluten, dairy, eggs, or sugar - see page xi about ingredients)

1 small onion, grated
1 tablespoon olive oil
1/2 teaspoon dried oregano leaves
1/4 teaspoon black pepper
3/4 teaspoon salt
3/4 cup low sodium chicken broth

1 cup milk (cow, rice, soy)
1/2 cup yellow cornmeal
2 tablespoons grated Parmesan cheese
(cow, rice, soy - optional)
1 tablespoon cooking oil

In large saucepan over high heat, combine all ingredients except cornmeal and cheese. Bring to boil. Reduce heat to low; gradually whisk in cornmeal. Cook, whisking constantly, for 3-5 minutes or until very thick. Remove from heat. Stir in cheese, if using

Pour into greased 11 x 7-inch dish and refrigerate, covered, until firm. Cut into wedges or squares. Heat oil in large, heavy skillet and fry polenta over medium-heat until very crisp on both sides. Serve immediately. Serves 4.

| | | | | | | | | Exchanges | | |
Calories	Fat	% Fat Cal	Protein	Carb	Chol	Sodium	Fiber	Carb	Meat	Fat
165	9g	46%	6g	18g	4mg	548mg	2g	1		1

Roasted Asparagus

(can be made without wheat, gluten, dairy, eggs, or sugar - see page xi about ingredients)

Roasted asparagus has a fuller flavor and more interesting texture than simply steaming or boiling it. Use the bigger asparagus spears for this dish.

1 1/2 pounds fresh large asparagus spears	1/4 teaspoon salt
2 tablespoons olive oil	1/4 teaspoon black pepper

Preheat oven to 450°. Rinse spears, then snap off ends (the stalks will break naturally at the point where they start to get tough). Peel asparagus stalks with potato peeler to remove stringy skin, if desired.

Place asparagus in single layer on baking sheet. Drizzle with oil and shake to coat thoroughly. Season with salt and pepper. Roast until tender and lightly browned, about 10-15 minutes. Serve immediately. Serves 4.

| | | | | | | | | Exchanges | | |
Calories	Fat	% Fat Cal	Protein	Carb	Chol	Sodium	Fiber	Carb	Meat	Fat
75	7g	77%	2g	3g	0mg	150mg	1g	1		1

Roasted Fennel

(can be made without wheat, gluten, dairy, eggs, or sugar - see page xi about ingredients)

An unusual vegetable, most people are not well acquainted with fennel. But it adds lots of interest to a winter meal.

2 fennel bulbs	1/2 teaspoon salt
1/4 cup olive oil	1/4 teaspoon black pepper
2 tablespoons fresh lemon juice	

Preheat oven to 400°. Wash fennel and trim tops and outer leaves. Reserve leafy fronds. Cut through fennel lengthwise into 1/4-inch slices. Toss pieces with 3 tablespoons olive oil, making sure that all pieces are thoroughly coated.

Place on nonstick baking sheet and roast for 15-20 minutes. Turn pieces with spatula and roast another 15-20 minutes, or until pieces are caramelized. Drizzle with lemon juice and remaining olive oil. Add salt and pepper and chopped, reserved fronds and serve immediately. Serves 4.

| | | | | | | | | Exchanges | | |
Calories	Fat	% Fat Cal	Protein	Carb	Chol	Sodium	Fiber	Carb	Meat	Fat
155	14g	74%	2g	9g	0mg	348mg	4g	1		3

Roasted (Grilled) Vegetables

(can be made without wheat, gluten, dairy, eggs, or sugar - see page xi about ingredients)

The flavor of vegetables cooked on a grill is much fuller than if they're just steamed. In this recipe, the marinade introduces even more flavor. See next page for tips on roasting vegetables.

2 tablespoons olive oil
1/3 cup gf balsamic vinegar
1/2 teaspoon dried oregano leaves
1 large garlic clove, minced
1/2 teaspoon ground coriander
1/4 teaspoon ground cumin
1/4 teaspoon salt
1/4 teaspoon pepper
2 teaspoons molasses
(cane or sorghum)

1 large yellow onion, quartered
4 large carrots, halved lengthwise
1 large red pepper, quartered
1 large yellow pepper, quartered
4 small red new potatoes, halved
2 medium zucchini, halved
1 large onion, halved
2 small yellow squash, halved
Cooking spray

Combine first 9 ingredients (olive oil through molasses) in large bowl. Marinate vegetables in mixture for about 30-45 minutes. Stir occasionally.

Drain vegetables, reserving marinade, and arrange in grill basket liberally coated with cooking spray. (Withhold the more delicate vegetables such as red and yellow bell pepper until final 10 minutes so they don't overcook.)

Cook on grill over medium-hot coals with lid down about 15-20 minutes or until done, turning every 5 minutes. The type and thickness of vegetables determines cooking time. Add remaining vegetables during last 10 minutes. Meanwhile, warm the marinade over low-medium heat. Remove vegetables from grill basket and toss with marinade. Serve warm. Makes about 6 cups. Serves 6 (1 cup each).

As an alternative to grilling, roast the vegetables (uncovered) in a 400° oven, turning occasionally, until they reach desired degree of doneness.

| | | | | | | | | Exchanges | | |
Calories	Fat	% Fat Cal	Protein	Carb	Chol	Sodium	Fiber	Carb	Meat	Fat
135	5g	31%	2g	23g	0mg	122mg	4g	3		

Tips on Roasting & Grilling Vegetables

Since so many of the recipes in this chapter involve roasting, it seems appropriate to discuss this important method of cooking a little further.

There are two ways to roast vegetables: in the oven and on the grill. While the oven routine is fairly straightforward, using a grill is a little more involved.

Roasting On the Grill
Roasting on the grill brings out the flavor, introduces color, and usually introduces a crispy exterior on vegetables that is pleasing to the palate. You can purchase inexpensive grill pans in kitchen stores. For the most successful grilling, here are some tips:

(1) Wash and trim the vegetables, then pat dry with a paper towel so that the heat grills the vegetables instead of steaming them.

(2) Experts advise against marinades or basting sauces to avoid flare-ups. However, I like to coat the vegetables in olive oil first. Then sprinkle with dry spices before grilling. You may salt and pepper before or after the vegetables are cooked.

(3) Into what shapes should the vegetables be cut? Halve vegetables such as onions and bell peppers. Leave mushrooms and carrots whole. Slicing potatoes in half lengthwise gives a broad, flat surface for more complete cooking. Cut the vegetables in similar-size pieces for uniform cooking. For example, a medium-sized potato slices lengthwise into four equal pieces that are a good size for grilling.

(4) Close the lid for hard, dense vegetables. Leave it open for softer, more tender ones. Or, use a closed lid for the first half of the cooking period, then leave the lid open for the remainder. Experiment a little to see what you like.

(5) Turn vegetables when one side shows grill marks. Avoid overcooking vegetables because this blackens and toughens them. Vegetables with higher sugar content, such as sweet potatoes, cook faster as do those with high water content such as zucchini or tomatoes. Put these high-water-content vegetables on the grill toward the end.

Roasting In the Oven
Save your old, darkened, battered cake pans and cookie sheets for this task. Toss the vegetables in your favorite marinade or salad dressing and roast at high temperatures until done. I prefer temperatures between 400° and 425°.

Sautéed Brussels Sprouts

(can be made without wheat, gluten, dairy, eggs, or sugar - see page xi about ingredients)

Enjoy a change of pace with this tasty version of brussels sprouts. Sauté at the last minute so you can serve them fresh from the hot skillet.

1 pound brussels sprouts	1/4 teaspoon black pepper
1 tablespoon olive oil	1/4 teaspoon ground nutmeg or mace
1/2 teaspoon salt	2 limes, juiced

Cut off ends and trim brussels sprouts. Cut each in half, lengthwise, then lay each half flat on cutting board and cut in narrow strips.

In small skillet, sauté brussels sprouts in olive oil over low-medium heat for 3-5 minutes. Add salt, pepper, ground nutmeg (or mace), and lime juice to skillet and toss thoroughly. Serve immediately. Serves 4.

								Exchanges		
Calories	Fat	% Fat Cal	Protein	Carb	Chol	Sodium	Fiber	Carb	Meat	Fat
85	4g	35%	4g	12g	0mg	316mg	4g	2		1

Colcannon

(can be made without wheat, gluten, dairy, eggs, or sugar - see page xi about ingredients)

This is a traditional dish in Ireland. If Savoy cabbage is not available, use regular cabbage instead. It will be a little different than the real thing, but it will still be great.

2 pounds potatoes	2 tablespoons chopped fresh
1 head savoy cabbage (remove outer leaves)	parsley
1/4 cup butter or cooking oil	1/2 teaspoon salt
1 small onion	1/4 teaspoon black pepper

Peel potatoes and cut into equal-size chunks. Place in medium-size saucepan and cover with cold water. Bring to boil. Cook for 20-25 minutes or until fork tender. Drain thoroughly, then mash.

Meanwhile, while potatoes are cooking, bring another pan of water to boil and cook savoy cabbage for 15 minutes or until just tender. Drain thoroughly.

Melt butter in large, heavy skillet. Add onion and cook until soft, about 3-5 minutes. Add mashed potato and cabbage and fry for 5 minutes over medium heat, stirring occasionally, until it browns around the edges. Stir in the chopped parsley and salt and pepper. Serve hot. Serves 4.

								Exchanges		
Calories	Fat	% Fat Cal	Protein	Carb	Chol	Sodium	Fiber	Carb	Meat	Fat
350	14g	35%	6g	54g	0mg	310mg	5g	4		3

Duchess Potatoes

(can be made without wheat, gluten, dairy, eggs, or sugar - see page xi about ingredients)

These potatoes are especially pretty when placed around the perimeter of a platter of roast beef or chicken. If you don't have the pastry tips, don't despair. Just use a heavy-duty plastic freezer bag with the corner cut off.

1 1/2 pounds russet potatoes	1/4 teaspoon ground nutmeg
3 cups chicken broth	Salt & white pepper to taste
1/4 cup butter or oleo or Spectrum™ canola oil spread	1/2 cup hot (115°) milk (cow, rice, soy)

Wash, peel and slice potatoes into chunks. Place potatoes and chicken broth in large saucepan, bring to boil, then cover and simmer until potatoes are done—about 20-30 minutes. Remove pan from heat and turn off heat. Drain potatoes thoroughly. Return potatoes to hot pan and place on burner for 5-10 seconds to thoroughly dry.

Put potatoes through potato ricer (or mash thoroughly by hand with potato masher). Add nutmeg and salt and pepper to taste. Stir in enough of the 1/2 cup hot milk to reach consistency of mashed potatoes. Use more milk, if necessary.

Preheat oven to 350°. Place potatoes in pastry bag fitted with a large decorative tip (or use heavy duty, plastic freezer bag). Coat baking sheet with oleo or cooking spray and pipe 4 large rosettes (or 8 smaller ones) onto sheet.

Bake rosettes in the middle of oven for 10-15 minutes or until lightly browned. (If you've previously prepared the rosettes and chilled them, bake until they're heated through, about 15-20 minutes.) Then place under the broiler to finish browning. Serve immediately. Serves 4.

								Exchanges		
Calories	Fat	% Fat Cal	Protein	Carb	Chol	Sodium	Fiber	Carb	Meat	Fat
295	13g	39%	7g	40g	35mg	106mg	3g	2.5		2

Garlic Mashed Potatoes

(can be made without wheat, gluten, dairy, eggs, or sugar - see page xi about ingredients)

Garlic mashed potatoes are a trendy dish in many restaurants. However, they're nothing more than down-home mashed potatoes with roasted garlic. Easy, yet delicious. You may double this recipe to serve 8. If you'd rather not roast the garlic, try a teaspoon of gf garlic powder or bottled gf minced garlic instead—or just add the minced garlic to the boiling water.

2 large whole garlic cloves   Chicken broth to cover potatoes
1 teaspoon olive oil   1/4 teaspoon white pepper
2 pounds Idaho potatoes, peeled   3 cups water
1/4 teaspoon salt   1 cup hot (115°) milk (cow, rice, soy)

Preheat oven to 350°. Place garlic cloves on a small piece of aluminum foil, drizzle with 1 teaspoon olive oil (or spray with cooking spray), and sprinkle with salt and pepper. Close foil loosely and bake in a small baking pan or cooking sheet until garlic is done, about 30 minutes. Remove garlic from oven and loosen foil to allow garlic to cool.

Meanwhile, cut the potatoes into large chunks. Place them in a large pot with enough chicken broth to cover. Bring to boil, reduce the heat, and gently boil until potatoes are done—about 20–30 minutes.

Drain the cooked potatoes and return them to the cooking pot. Shake gently over low heat a few times to remove all moisture. Press through a potato ricer (or blend with electric mixer.) Squeeze roasted garlic into potatoes and blend thoroughly. Add hot milk to potatoes, 1/4 cup at a time, until desired consistency is reached. (You can do this with the electric mixer or mash with a hand-masher.)

Serve immediately. Drizzle with extra butter or oleo. Serves 4.

Garlic Mashed Potatoes with Spinach: Add 1 cup blanched spinach.
Horseradish Mashed Potatoes: Add 1 tablespoon grated fresh horseradish or add to taste.

| | | | | | | | | Exchanges | | |
Calories	Fat	% Fat Cal	Protein	Carb	Chol	Sodium	Fiber	Carb	Meat	Fat
245	2g	5%	7g	53g	1mg	192mg	3.5g	3		

New Potatoes & Peas in Lemon-Dill Sauce

(can be made without wheat, gluten, dairy, eggs, or sugar - see page xi about ingredients)

Especially tasty in the spring and summer, this colorful, innovative way to serve potatoes and peas together will delight your family and guests.

16 small new red potatoes, unpeeled	3 tablespoons chopped onion
1 teaspoon salt	1/2 teaspoon salt
3 tablespoons fresh lemon juice	2 tablespoons fresh dill weed
1 small garlic clove, minced	1/4 teaspoon xanthan gum
2 tablespoons extra virgin olive oil	1/8 teaspoon black pepper
1/2 teaspoon honey or agave nectar	1 cup cooked green peas

Scrub potatoes well. In large saucepan, place potatoes in enough water to cover. Add salt and cook, covered, until tender. Quarter potatoes while hot.

Meanwhile purée remaining ingredients (except peas) in blender until very smooth. Toss potatoes and peas with lemon-dill sauce. Serve hot. Serves 4.

								Exchanges		
Calories	Fat	% Fat Cal	Protein	Carb	Chol	Sodium	Fiber	Carb	Meat	Fat
240	7g	25%	5g	42g	0mg	874mg	5g	2.5		1

Roasted Potatoes

(can be made without wheat, gluten, dairy, eggs, or sugar - see page xi about ingredients)

The first four ingredients combine to make a tasty gremolata.

3 tablespoons minced fresh parsley	1/2 teaspoon salt
1 tablespoon grated lemon peel	1/4 teaspoon black pepper
2 teaspoons minced garlic	1 teaspoon chopped fresh rosemary
1 teaspoon extra-virgin olive oil	1 teaspoon chopped fresh thyme
1 1/2 pounds small red potatoes, halved	1/4 cup chopped flat-leaf parsley
2 tablespoons extra-virgin olive oil	1/4 cup chopped fresh basil

Combine first four ingredients. Set aside. Preheat oven to 400°. In large shallow baking pan, toss potatoes with olive oil. Toss with remaining ingredients.

Bake for 30 minutes, shaking pan occasionally. Then reduce temperature to 350° and bake another 15-20 minutes or until potatoes are fork-tender. Combine 2/3 of the parsley-lemon mixture and toss with potatoes. Serve vegetables sprinkled with remaining 1/3 parsley mixture. Serves 4.

								Exchanges		
Calories	Fat	% Fat Cal	Protein	Carb	Chol	Sodium	Fiber	Carb	Meat	Fat
225	8g	32%	4g	36g	0mg	300mg	3g	2		1.5

Potatoes Anna

(can be made without wheat, gluten, dairy, eggs, or sugar - see page xi about ingredients)

Try this easy dish for a special occasion. Your guests will appreciate the added touch, but you'll know how very easy it is. Be sure to use a deep enough cast-iron skillet or the excess juices will run over into your oven. For added flavor, sprinkle 1 teaspoon crushed rosemary leaves between the potato layers.

1/4 cup butter or oleo or cooking oil	1/2 teaspoon black pepper or to taste
2 pounds red potatoes	Chopped parsley or rosemary
1/2 teaspoon salt or to taste	

Heat oven to 450°. Peel and slice potatoes in 3/8-inch slices. Heat 9 or 10-inch cast-iron skillet over medium-high heat and add 1 tablespoon of the butter (or oleo or oil). Quickly arrange layer of sliced potatoes in overlapping, concentric circles. Drizzle with more butter and sprinkle with salt and pepper (and rosemary, if using).

Continue making layers of concentric circles drizzled with butter and salt and pepper. Top with aluminum foil and press down with heavy object to compress slices. Remove foil and bake in oven for 30 minutes. Remove from oven, press again with foil and heavy object. Remove foil and return to oven to bake for another 30-40 minutes or until potatoes are golden brown and tender when pierced with fork.

Remove skillet from oven and invert onto plate (be careful—it's hot). If potatoes won't come out, slide metal spatula under potatoes to loosen them. Serve immediately. Garnish with sprinkle of parsley or crushed rosemary leaves. Serves 4.

								Exchanges		
Calories	Fat	% Fat Cal	Protein	Carb	Chol	Sodium	Fiber	Carb	Meat	Fat
315	12g	33%	5g	49g	0mg	300mg	4g	3		2

Butter adds additional 31mg cholesterol per serving.

APPETIZERS, SNACKS, & BEVERAGES

A ppetizers are designed to take the edge off your hunger . . . or to whet your appetite for the main course. At other times, appetizers can be a meal in themselves. Sort of like understudies in a play—ready at any moment to take center stage, if necessary.

Finger foods, dips, crackers, beverages—you'll find a wide range of tasty tidbits to delight your family and guests at any special occasion.

Hearty Appetizers
Appetizer Meatballs 190
Buffalo Wings 191
Falafel 192
Miniature Focaccia Sandwiches 193
Focaccia Sandwich Fillings 194
Grilled Quesadillas 195
Grilled Shrimp with Wraps 195
Oven-Baked Crab Cakes 196
Pizza Crust & Pizza Sauce 51
Shrimp with Cocktail Sauce 196

Dips & Spreads
Avocado Bean Salsa 197
Chutney Appetizer Spread 198
Hot Seafood Dip 199
Mexican Tomato Salsa Dip 200
Sunny Tomato-Basil Dip 201
Tuscan Bean Spread 198

Miscellaneous
Savory Crackers 202
Dried Apple Rings 197
Rosemary-Thyme Pecan 203
Spicy "Nuts" 203

Beverages
Cranberry Grapefruit Punch 204
Iced Coffee Lattes 204
Fruit Punch 205
Fruity Mint Punch 205
Iced Coffee 206
Lemon Mint Punch with Raspberries 206
Minty Ginger Iced Tea 207
Simple Syrup for Beverages 207

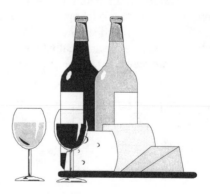

Appetizer Meatballs

(can be made without wheat, gluten, dairy, eggs, or sugar —see page xi about ingredients)

I like to use this recipe when I want something hot on the buffet table, yet can be prepared ahead of time. A heated chafing dish works just great, but I've also served the meatballs in a crock pot.

Meatballs
1 pound lean ground beef
1/2 cup gf crushed corn flakes
   or gf cracker crumbs
2 tablespoons gf ketchup
1 teaspoon dried thyme leaves
1 teaspoon salt
1/4 teaspoon black pepper
1/4 teaspoon gf chili powder
1/4 cup finely chopped onion
Cooking spray or parchment
   paper

Sauce
2 tablespoons gf sweet pickle relish
8 ounces gf tomato sauce
2 tablespoons finely chopped onion
2 tablespoons brown sugar
   or maple sugar
1 tablespoon cider vinegar
1/4 cup gf ketchup
1 tablespoon gf Worcestershire sauce
1/2 teaspoon salt
1/4 teaspoon black pepper
1/4 teaspoon ground allspice
1/4 cup water

Preheat oven to 400°. Coat baking sheet with cooking spray or parchment paper.

Meatballs: In large bowl, thoroughly combine beef, crumbs, ketchup, thyme, salt, pepper, chili powder, and onion. Shape into 36 small meatballs (about 1 tablespoon each). Place on prepared baking sheet and bake until nicely browned, about15-20 minutes.

Sauce: Meanwhile, in medium saucepan combine pickle relish, tomato sauce, onion, sugar, vinegar, ketchup, Worcestershire sauce, salt, pepper, allspice, and water. Bring to boil and simmer for 15 minutes. Add meatballs and simmer another 15 minutes. Spear meatballs with toothpicks. Serves 12 (3 meatballs each). Double recipe for larger groups.

| | | | | | | | | Exchanges | | |
Calories	Fat	% Fat Cal	Protein	Carb	Chol	Sodium	Fiber	Carb	Meat	Fat
100	4g	32%	8g	9g	14mg	470mg	1g	1	1	

Buffalo Wings

(can be made without wheat, gluten, dairy, eggs, or sugar —see page xi about ingredients)

You can eat these tasty wings plain or dip in your favorite dipping sauce. Have plenty of napkins handy. These wings are a little bit messy—but definitely worth it!

4 pounds chicken wings
   or drummettes
1 tablespoon olive oil
1 tablespoon paprika
1 tablespoon black pepper
1 tablespoon ground white pepper
1 teaspoon gf garlic powder
1 teaspoon gf onion powder

1 teaspoon sugar or fructose powder
2 teaspoons gf celery salt
1 teaspoon dried oregano leaves
1 teaspoon dried thyme leaves
1/2 teaspoon cayenne pepper
1 teaspoon gf dry mustard

Wash chicken wings and pat dry with paper towel. If they're not drummettes, cut off wings at first joint and reserve discarded pieces for another use (such as chicken stock).

In large bowl or plastic freezer bag, toss wings with olive oil. Combine remaining ingredients. Then toss wings with spice mixture until thoroughly coated.

Refrigerate for at least two hours or overnight. Arrange wings on shallow baking pan or cookie sheet. Preheat oven to 450°. Bake wings for 12-15 minutes on middle rack of oven. Turn wings and continue baking another 12-15 minutes or until crispy. As an alternative, you may grill the wings on a barbecue grill until done. Serve with dipping sauce of your choice. Serves 16 as appetizers (1/4 pound each).

| | | | | | | | | Exchanges | | |
Calories	Fat	% Fat Cal	Protein	Carb	Chol	Sodium	Fiber	Carb	Meat	Fat
300	20g	62%	26g	1g	79mg	77mg	.5g		4	2

Falafel

(can be made without wheat, gluten, dairy, eggs, or sugar —see page xi about ingredients)

If you're using rice crackers instead of bread crumbs, add a tablespoon of olive oil to make sure the mixture sticks together. If tahini paste or soy nut butter are not available or appropriate, omit them.

<u>Falafel Patties</u>
1 can (19 oz.) canned chickpeas (rinsed, drained)
1/2 cup chopped onions
1/3 cup bread crumbs
2 tablespoons fresh chopped parsley or cilantro
1 teaspoon ground cumin
1/2 teaspoon ground coriander
1/4 teaspoon baking soda
1/8 teaspoon cayenne pepper
2 garlic cloves, minced
1/4 teaspoon salt
1/4 teaspoon black pepper
1 tablespoon olive oil for frying

<u>Dressing</u>
1 cup yogurt (cow, soy) or soft silken tofu
1/4 cup tahini paste or soy nut butter
2 tablespoons fresh lemon juice
1 small garlic clove, minced
1/4 teaspoon salt
1/8 teaspoon black pepper
1 small cucumber(peeled, diced)

Combine chickpeas, onion, bread crumbs, parsley, cumin, coriander, baking soda, cayenne pepper, garlic, salt, and pepper in food processor. Purée until well blended. Divide into 12 portions and shape into patty, flattening slightly.

In large skillet coated with cooking spray and 1 tablespoon olive oil, brown falafel patties on both sides (about 2-3 minutes per side).

For dressing, combine yogurt, tahini (if using), lemon juice, garlic, salt, and pepper and purée until smooth. Stir in diced cucumbers. Serve with falafel in bread, buns, or with crackers or vegetables. Serves 12 (1 patty each).

| | | | | | | | | Exchanges | | |
Calories	Fat	% Fat Cal	Protein	Carb	Chol	Sodium	Fiber	Carb	Meat	Fat
110	4g	34%	5g	14g	1mg	282mg	3g	1		1

Miniature Focaccia Sandwiches

(can be made without wheat, gluten, dairy, eggs, or sugar —see page xi about ingredients)

Focaccia is so simple to make. And, it makes extremely flavorful sandwiches. Try these at your next party or reserve them for a truly special occasion such as a wedding or shower. Arrange them decoratively on a large platter, garnished with sprigs of fresh parsley or your favorite herbs.

Bread
3/4 cup warm milk (105°)
1 teaspoon sugar or honey
2 large eggs*
2 tablespoons olive oil
1/2 teaspoon cider vinegar
1 1/2 teaspoons gf active dry yeast
1 cup brown rice flour or
    garbfava flour
1/2 cup tapioca flour
1 1/2 teaspoons xanthan gum

1 teaspoon unflavored gelatin powder
1 teaspoon dried rosemary leaves
1/2 teaspoon gf onion powder
3/4 teaspoon salt

Topping
1 1/4 teaspoons Italian Seasoning
1/4 teaspoon salt
1 tablespoon olive oil
Cooking spray

Bread: Combine warm milk, sugar (or honey), eggs (or tofu—see below), olive oil, and vinegar in mixer bowl. Beat with electric mixer until very, very smooth—about 1 minute. Add yeast, flours, xanthan gum, gelatin powder, rosemary, onion powder, and salt. Beat dough for 2 minutes. The dough will be soft and sticky—like thick cake batter.

Transfer dough to 11 x 7-inch nonstick pan that has been coated with cooking spray. Cover with aluminum foil and let rise in warm place for 30 minutes or until desired height.

Topping: Preheat oven to 400°. Sprinkle Focaccia with Italian seasoning, salt, and olive oil (or to taste). Bake for 15 minutes or until top is golden brown. Cool completely before slicing. Makes 11 x 7-inch loaf.

Sandwiches: To make Miniature Focaccia Sandwiches, cut Focaccia into 12 equal pieces. Using a sharp, serrated knife, carefully slice each piece horizontally. Spread filling of choice (see next page) between slices. Serve immediately or cover tightly and refrigerate up to 4 hours. Serves 6.

Without fillings   Exchanges

Calories	Fat	% Fat Cal	Protein	Carb	Chol	Sodium	Fiber	Carb	Meat	Fat
230	9g	35%	5g	32g	52mg	410mg	2.5g	1	.5	1.5

*Egg Alternative: Omit eggs. Use 1/2 cup soft silken tofu.

Focaccia Sandwich Fillings

(can be made without wheat, gluten, dairy, eggs, or sugar —see page xi about ingredients)

Choose from this wide variety of savory fillings for the Miniature Focaccia Sandwiches on the previous page.

Chicken Salad or Tuna Salad Filling

2 cups ground cooked chicken (about 2 whole chicken breasts) or 2 cups low-salt canned tuna (about 4 small cans)

1/2 cup gf Mayonnaise (page 217)

1 teaspoon dried thyme leaves

1 teaspoon dried dill weed

1 teaspoon gf onion powder

1/2 teaspoon gf celery salt

1/4 teaspoon black pepper

Combine all ingredients in a bowl and mash together with fork. Chill until serving time. Serves 16 (2 tablespoons per sandwich).

| | | | | | | | | Exchanges | | |
Calories	Fat	% Fat Cal	Protein	Carb	Chol	Sodium	Fiber	Carb	Meat	Fat
60	2g	33%	3g	7g	8mg	205mg	<1g	.5		.5

Additional Fillings (recipes for italicized ingredients are in this book)

• Paper-thin slices of cucumber and red onion, *Sunny Tomato-Basil Dip*, lettuce

• Paper-thin slices of proscuitto and Granny Smith apples, fresh basil leaves, gf mayonnaise, lettuce

• Softened goat cheese with raisins, *Orange Marmalade* or *Apricot Ketchup*, whole mint leaves, lettuce. (Make sure goat cheese is approved for you.)

• Paper-thin slices of roast beef and red onion, gf horseradish sauce, butter or Spectrum™ canola oil spread, lettuce

• Paper-thin slices of plum tomatoes and red onion, guacamole dip, lettuce

• Paper-thin slices of smoked turkey and red onion, Dijonnaise mustard, lettuce

• Paper-thin slices of smoked ham, *Tuscan Bean Spread*, lettuce

• Crumbled crisp bacon, finely chopped *Oven-Dried Tomatoes*, *Tuscan Bean Spread*, lettuce

Grilled Shrimp with Wraps

(can be made without wheat, gluten, dairy, eggs, or sugar —see page xi about ingredients)

1 cup olive oil	20 whole large basil leaves
1/4 cup rice vinegar	20 Oven-Dried Tomatoes
1/2 cup fresh lemon juice	(page 214)
1/2 cup finely chopped fresh basil or	20 fresh cilantro sprigs
2 tablespoons dried basil leaves	20 proscuitto strips (2-inches wide)
20 jumbo shrimp (cleaned, de-veined)	Toothpicks

Mix together the oil, vinegar, lemon juice, and chopped basil. Set aside.

Wrap each shrimp, first with basil leaf, then sun-dried tomato, then a sprig of cilantro, then a strip of proscuitto. Use toothpicks to fasten proscuitto in place. Pour marinade over shrimp in large, shallow container. Refrigerate, covered, for 4 hours.

Remove shrimp from marinade (reserving marinade) and place shrimp in a fish basket or lay carefully on grate. Grill shrimp, basting often with reserved marinade, for about 5 minutes on each side—or until desired doneness. They will turn pink and curl up when done. Serve immediately. Serves 10 (2 each).

								Exchanges		
Calories	Fat	% Fat Cal	Protein	Carb	Chol	Sodium	Fiber	Carb	Meat	Fat
251	25g	88%	5g	3g	37mg	207mg	1g	.5	.5	5

Grilled Quesadillas

(can be made without wheat, gluten, dairy, eggs, or sugar —see page xi about ingredients)

2 corn tortillas	3 tomatillos (grilled, smashed flat*)
2 teaspoons olive oil	1/4 cup finely chopped green onion
1/4 cup shredded cheese	1/4 cup chopped fresh cilantro
(cow, rice, soy)	

Brush one side of tortilla with oil. Place oil-side down on cutting board. Top tortilla with half of cheese—then smashed tomatillos, onion, and cilantro. Top with remaining half of cheese and remaining tortilla, coated with olive oil on top side. Carefully slide quesadilla onto grill, 4-5 inches from heat. Grill until browned on underside, about 5 minutes. Turn and grill other side. Remove, cut into wedges with kitchen shears. Makes 1 quesadilla, Serves 4 (1/4 each).

								Exchanges		
Calories	Fat	% Fat Cal	Protein	Carb	Chol	Sodium	Fiber	Carb	Meat	Fat
160	10g	54%	5g	14g	13mg	84mg	1.5g	2		1

*Grill tomatillos, 5 inches from heat until soft. Remove from heat and smash.

Oven-Baked Crab Cakes

(can be made without wheat, gluten, dairy, eggs, or sugar —see page xi about ingredients)

Crab cakes are featured here as an appetizer; make them larger for a main course.

1 pound shelled crabmeat, picked over
1 celery stalk, finely chopped
1 tablespoon gf onion flakes or 2
  tablespoons grated fresh onion
2 teaspoons gf Seafood Seasoning
  or use recipe on page 221
1 tablespoon chopped fresh parsley
1 tablespoon gf Worcestershire sauce

1 teaspoon Italian Seasoning or
  use recipe on page 221
1/2 cup gf Mayonnaise or use
  recipe on page 217
1 tablespoon baking powder
1 cup gf bread crumbs
Cooking spray or parchment paper
Cocktail Sauce (see below)

Preheat oven to 400°. Combine all ingredients in food processor. Process until ingredients are thoroughly mixed. Shape mixture into 16 small crab cakes. Arrange on cookie sheet coated with cooking spray or parchment paper.

Bake on lower rack in oven for about 10 minutes per side, or until both sides are gently browned. Serves 8 (2 crab cakes each).

								Exchanges		
Calories	Fat	% Fat Cal	Protein	Carb	Chol	Sodium	Fiber	Carb	Meat	Fat
265	4g	14%	30g	26g	115mg	999mg	1g	1.5	4	

Shrimp with Cocktail Sauce

(can be made without wheat, gluten, dairy, eggs, or sugar —see page xi about ingredients)

This simple sauce is moderately spicy; add more horseradish to jazz it up.

2 pounds large cooked shrimp
1 teaspoon gf horseradish sauce
  or grated fresh horseradish
1 teaspoon fresh lemon juice

2 tablespoons Dijonnaise mustard
  or 1 tablespoon gf dry mustard
3 tablespoons gf ketchup or use recipe
  on page 218

Peel and de-vein shrimp. Chill until ready to use. Thoroughly combine all remaining ingredients in small bowl or blender. Serve with shrimp. Serves 8 (about 1/4 pound each).

								Exchanges		
Calories	Fat	% Fat Cal	Protein	Carb	Chol	Sodium	Fiber	Carb	Meat	Fat
130	2g	16%	24g	3g	170mg	330mg	0g		3	

Avocado Bean Salsa

(can be made without wheat, gluten, dairy, eggs, or sugar —see page xi about ingredients)

Serve this great dip to complement a Southwestern meal.

1 firm ripe avocado, diced
1 medium tomato (seeded, diced)
1 small red onion, finely chopped
2 tablespoons fresh lime juice
1/4 cup chopped fresh cilantro,
  packed

1/2 small jalapeño, finely chopped
1 tablespoon olive oil
1 small garlic clove, minced
1/4 teaspoon black pepper
1 can (16 oz.) white beans, drained

Combine all ingredients in small bowl and toss thoroughly. Serve with tortilla chips, crackers, or fresh vegetables. Or, serve on lettuce leaf as side salad to a Southwestern-inspired meal. If cooking your own beans, you may want to add salt to taste. Serves 4.

| | | | | | | | | Exchanges | | |
Calories	Fat	% Fat Cal	Protein	Carb	Chol	Sodium	Fiber	Carb	Meat	Fat
210	12g	45%	9g	24g	0mg	25mg	8g	4		2

Dried Apple Rings

(can be made without wheat, gluten, dairy, eggs, or sugar —see page xi about ingredients)

Dried apples are great in a "survival" kit. But if you who don't want the sulfites found in the commercial variety, here's an easy version you can make yourself—and they're completely natural. You can also omit the sweetener, if you wish.

4 large Granny Smith apples,
  cored and sliced in 1/8-inch slices
4 cups water

1/4 cup sugar or honey
1/4 teaspoon ground cinnamon
Juice of 1 lemon

Preheat oven to 200°. In large saucepan, bring the water, sugar (or honey), cinnamon (if using), and lemon juice to boil. Stir until sweetener is dissolved.
Reduce heat to low, add apple slices, and simmer until just tender, for about 2-5 minutes. Transfer to baking sheet lined with parchment paper. Bake apples for 1 hour. Reduce heat to 150° and bake until apples are dry. Watch carefully because apples will dry quickly toward end of baking. Serves 4.

| | | | | | | | | Exchanges | | |
Calories	Fat	% Fat Cal	Protein	Carb	Chol	Sodium	Fiber	Carb	Meat	Fat
160	0g	0	0g	44g	0mg	2mg	3g	3		

Chutney Appetizer Spread

(can be made without wheat, gluten, dairy, eggs, or sugar —see page xi about ingredients)

The sweet, yet spicy flavor of chutney melds wonderfully with creamy, mellow cream cheese (or tofu.) This duo seems unlikely, yet produces a wonderful taste sensation. And, if you have the chutney on hand you can whip this dish up in seconds. If you're not using cream cheese, add a teaspoon of gf butter-flavored extract to lend a "dairy" taste.

8 ounces cream cheese
   or soft silken tofu
1/4 cup chopped fresh cilantro,
   packed
2 tablespoons grated fresh onion
	1/4 teaspoon salt
	1/4 teaspoon white pepper
	2/3 cup Mango Chutney (page 22)
	   or your favorite gf chutney
	1/4 teaspoon crushed red pepper

In a food processor, blend together cream cheese (or tofu), cilantro, onion, salt, and pepper. Stir in chutney and red pepper flakes. Makes slightly less than 2 cups. Serves 6 (about 1/3 cup each).

Exchanges

Calories	Fat	% Fat Cal	Protein	Carb	Chol	Sodium	Fiber	Carb	Meat	Fat
76	15g	71%	3g	11g	0mg	415mg	.5g	.5		3

Cream cheese adds additional 90 calories and 42mg cholesterol per serving.

Tuscan Bean Spread

(can be made without wheat, gluten, dairy, eggs, or sugar —see page xi about ingredients)

Even the trendiest restaurants are now serving little bowls of bean spread like this one, instead of the traditional butter. It's far lower in calories and, of course—no dairy. For a dramatic, colorful presentation, serve in a hollowed out red cabbage half that nestles in a bed of greens.

1 can (16 oz.) garbanzo beans 1 garlic cloves, minced 3 tablespoons olive oil 1/4 cup fresh lemon juice 1 teaspoon salt 1 teaspoon ground cumin	1 teaspoon dried dill weed or 1 table- spoon fresh chopped dill weed 2 tablespoons fresh cilantro 1/2 teaspoon black pepper 1/4 teaspoon crushed red pepper

Place beans (undrained) and remaining ingredients in food processor and purée until smooth. Scrape down sides of bowl often. If mixture is too thick, add water, 1 tablespoon at a time. Makes 1 1/2 cups. Serves 6 (1/4 cup each).

Exchanges

Calories	Fat	% Fat Cal	Protein	Carb	Chol	Sodium	Fiber	Carb	Meat	Fat
135	8g	54%	3g	13g	0mg	547mg	4g	1	.5	2

Hot Seafood Dip

(can be made without wheat, gluten, dairy, eggs, or sugar —see page xi about ingredients)

If you don't use cream cheese, yet want to replicate the dairy taste, try adding a teaspoon of gf butter flavored extract. Whether you use 1 or 2 teaspoons of the seafood seasoning is up to you. You might 1 teaspoon at first and add more later.

1 **cup cooked crab meat**
8 **ounces cream cheese (cow, soy)**
   or soft silken tofu
2 **tablespoons Dijonnaise mustard**
   or 1 tablespoon gf dry mustard
1 **tablespoon fresh lemon juice**
1 **teaspoon gf horseradish sauce or**
   1/2 teaspoon fresh grated horse-
   radish

2 **tablespoons finely chopped onion**
1-2 **teaspoons gf Seafood Seasoning**
   or use recipe on page 221
1 **stalk finely chopped celery**
2 **tablespoons fresh chopped**
   parsley for garnish
1 **teaspoon paprika for garnish**

Prepare seafood by discarding any cartilage or bones. If seafood has been previously frozen or contains a lot of water, drain in sieve by pushing meat firmly with paper towel. Chop finely. Set aside.

Combine cream cheese (or tofu), mustard, milk, lemon juice, horseradish sauce, and onion in food processor. Purée until very, very smooth. Stir in celery and prepared seafood.

Spoon mixture into oven-proof bowl and heat to serving temperature, either by baking in 350° oven for 15-20 minutes or in microwave oven at low-medium setting until mixture reaches desired temperature.

Garnish with chopped parsley and dash of paprika. Serve hot with crackers or crisp bread. Makes about 2 cups. Serves 8 (not quite 1/4 cup each).

Calories	Fat	% Fat Cal	Protein	Carb	Chol	Sodium	Fiber	Exchanges Carb	Meat	Fat
125	11g	75%	6g	2g	46mg	342mg	.5g		1	2

Mexican Tomato Salsa Dip

(can be made without wheat, gluten, dairy, eggs, or sugar —see page xi about ingredients)

I've been making this salsa for at least 20 years. Although I usually serve it with corn chips or vegetables, I've also thickened it slightly with cornstarch or arrowroot and used it as a sauce for Southwestern main dishes. If you prefer a less spicy version, reduce the chiles to 2 tablespoons.

4 medium tomatoes or 10 plum
   tomatoes
1/2 cup chopped onion
1/2 cup chopped celery
1/4 cup green pepper
2 tablespoons olive oil
1 can (4 oz.) green chiles or 1/4 cup
   finely chopped fresh chiles

2 tablespoons red wine vinegar
1 tablespoon mustard seeds
1 teaspoon crushed coriander seed
   or 1/2 teaspoon dried coriander
1 teaspoon salt
1/4 teaspoon black pepper
1/4 teaspoon sugar or honey

Combine all ingredients in food processor or blender and whirl until mixture reaches desired texture.

I prefer a slightly chunky texture, so here's what I do. Reserve half of the onion, celery, and green pepper until you have blended the other ingredients. Add reserved onion, celery, and green pepper and whirl or pulse just a few times to incorporate them into salsa. Refrigerate in a glass container for up to one week. Makes 2 pints. Serves 16 (1/4 cup each).

Exchanges

Calories	Fat	% Fat Cal	Protein	Carb	Chol	Sodium	Fiber	Carb	Meat	Fat
60	4g	55%	1g	6g	0mg	310mg	1g	1		1

Sunny Tomato-Basil Dip

(can be made without wheat, gluten, dairy, eggs, or sugar —see page xi about ingredients)

You can use sun-dried tomatoes packed in oil (be sure to drain them well). However, they may contain unacceptable ingredients. In that event, use the sun-dried tomatoes that are dry. Reconstitute by simmering in 1/3 cup hot water. Let stand for 15 minutes. Drain thoroughly before using. Or make your own using the recipe on page 214. If using tofu but you really like the taste of cream cheese, add a teaspoon of gf butter-flavored extract to help replicate that "dairy" taste.

8 ounces cream cheese
  or soft silken tofu
1/2 cup sun-dried tomatoes
1/3 cup chopped fresh basil or 2
  tablespoons dried basil leaves
1 teaspoon grated lemon peel

1 small garlic clove, minced
2 tablespoons Parmesan cheese
  (cow, rice, soy)
1/4 teaspoon gf onion salt

Combine all ingredients in food processor and purée until smooth. Transfer to serving bowl and chill for at least 2 hours. Return to room temperature before serving. Serve with crackers, French bread, or fresh vegetables. Makes 1 cup. Serves 4 (1/4 cup each).

| | | | | | | | | Exchanges | | |
Calories	Fat	% Fat Cal	Protein	Carb	Chol	Sodium	Fiber	Carb	Meat	Fat
65	3g	34%	7g	6g	2mg	316mg	1g	1	1	.5

Cream cheese adds 100 calories, 12g fat, and 41mg cholesterol per serving.

Savory Crackers

(can be made without wheat, gluten, dairy, eggs, or sugar —see page xi about ingredients)

These crackers are very easy to make and also travel well. Try adding your favorite dried herbs for variety.

1/4 cup garbfava flour or
   brown rice flour
1/4 cup potato starch
1/4 cup sweet rice flour
1/2 teaspoon xanthan gum
1/4 teaspoon baking soda
1/2 teaspoon salt
2 tablespoons Parmesan cheese
   (cow, rice, soy)

1 teaspoon gf onion powder or 1
   tablespoon grated fresh onion
2 tablespoons butter or cooking oil
1 tablespoon honey
3 tablespoons toasted sesame seeds
2 tablespoons milk
1 teaspoon cider vinegar

Preheat oven to 350°. Spray baking sheet with cooking spray. Set aside.

In medium-size mixing bowl, combine flours, xanthan gum, baking soda, salt, Parmesan cheese, and onion powder. Add butter and honey and mix until dough resembles coarse crumbs. Stir in sesame seeds. Add milk and vinegar. Shape dough into soft ball. (You may also mix all ingredients together in a food processor.)

Shape dough into 20 balls, each 1-inch in diameter, and place on baking sheet at least 2 inches apart. Using bottom of drinking glass or a rolling pin, flatten balls to approximately 1/8-inch thick. Use your fingers to smooth edges of circle.

If you prefer not to hand-shape the crackers, roll dough to 1/8-inch thickness on cookie sheet. Then, using a cookie cutter or biscuit cutter, cut cookies to desired shapes. Peel off unused dough and hand shape these scraps into crackers.

Bake for 12-15 minutes, or until crackers look firm and slightly toasted. Turn each cracker and bake another 5-7 minutes or until golden brown. (You may sprinkle with additional sesame seeds and salt, if desired). Makes about 20 crackers. Serves 10 (2 crackers each).

								Exchanges		
Calories	Fat	% Fat Cal	Protein	Carb	Chol	Sodium	Fiber	Carb	Meat	Fat
95	5g	44%	2g	11g	1mg	175mg	1g	.5		1

Rosemary-Thyme Pecans

(can be made without wheat, gluten, dairy, eggs, or sugar —see page xi about ingredients)

If you love rosemary, you'll be absolutely intoxicated by the aroma of these delicacies toasting in the oven. Serve them warm. If you prefer less salt, just reduce it to your liking. And, you may substitute walnuts or cashews for the pecans.

2 cups pecan halves
2 tablespoons olive oil
2 teaspoons dried rosemary leaves

3/4 teaspoon salt
1/2 teaspoon dried thyme leaves
1/2 teaspoon cayenne pepper

Preheat oven to 300°. Sort nuts to remove any hulls or debris. Pulverize rosemary leaves with mortar and pestle or use coffee grinder to crush leaves to coarse powder. In large bowl, toss nuts and rosemary with remaining ingredients until nuts are thoroughly coated.

Spread nuts in single layer on large baking sheet or pan. Bake 10-15 minutes or until lightly toasted. Serve warm. Makes 2 cups. Serves 16 (1/8 cup or about 6 whole pecans).

| | | | | | | | | Exchanges | | |
Calories	Fat	% Fat Cal	Protein	Carb	Chol	Sodium	Fiber	Carb	Meat	Fat
210	22g	87%	2g	5g	0mg	216mg	0g			4

Spicy "Nuts"

(can be made without wheat, gluten, dairy, eggs, or sugar —see page xi about ingredients)

These spicy "nuts" are excellent for traveling or place some in a pretty glass jar, tie with a ribbon, and give them to someone who can't eat regular nuts.

1 can (16 oz.) garbanzo beans, drained
2 teaspoons olive oil
1 teaspoon gf chili powder
1/4 teaspoon ground cumin

1/2 teaspoon gf garlic powder or
1 garlic clove, minced
1/2 teaspoon salt

Preheat oven to 325°. If using canned garbanzos, rinse and drain thoroughly. (Or cook your own garbanzo beans, but add more salt to taste.)

In large bowl, toss olive oil with remaining ingredients. Add beans and toss until thoroughly coated. Bake on large baking sheet or pan for approximately 1 hour, shaking pan occasionally to promote even browning. Store in airtight container. Serves 4 (1/4 cup each).

| | | | | | | | | Exchanges | | |
Calories	Fat	% Fat Cal	Protein	Carb	Chol	Sodium	Fiber	Carb	Meat	Fat
125	5g	31%	5g	18g	0mg	538mg	6g	1	1	1

Cranberry Grapefruit Punch

(can be made without wheat, gluten, dairy, eggs, or sugar —see page xi about ingredients)

If you have cranberry juice cocktail on hand, it is most likely already sweetened—probably with sugar. If that works for your diet, fine. You can omit the white grape juice, which provides sweetness, and substitute carbonated mineral water, instead. If not, look for unsweetened cranberry juice. It will be very, very tart and will need the sweetness provided by the white grape juice.

2 cups cranberry juice, unsweetened
3 cups grapefruit juice, unsweetened

2 cups pure white grape juice, reconstituted
Lime wedges for garnish

Mix ingredients together and serve over ice, garnished with fresh lime wedges. You may halve or double this recipe, depending on the number of guests. Serves 12 (1/2 cup each).

Exchanges

Calories	Fat	% Fat Cal	Protein	Carb	Chol	Sodium	Fiber	Carb	Meat	Fat
50	0g	0	1g	12g	0mg	2mg	0g	1		

Frozen Coffee Slush

(can be made without wheat, gluten, dairy, eggs, or sugar —see page xi about ingredients)

This comes pretty close to the frozen drinks you buy at popular coffee houses. If you can't use sweetened condensed milk, then use 2/3 cup non-dairy milk, plus 1/4 cup sweetener of choice, plus 1 tablespoon cooking oil.

1/4 cup brewed espresso or 3 tablespoons gf instant coffee powder dissolved in 1/4 cup hot water
1 cup ice cubes

2 tablespoons gf chocolate syrup or use Chocolate Syrup (page 136)
1 cup fat-free sweetened condensed milk (or see note above)

Place all ingredients in blender and blend until very smooth. Serve immediately. Serves 4 (1/2 cup each).

Exchanges

Calories	Fat	% Fat Cal	Protein	Carb	Chol	Sodium	Fiber	Carb	Meat	Fat
330	4g	11%	9g	65g	0mg	108mg	0g	4.5		.5

Sweetened condensed milk adds additional 15mg cholesterol per serving.

Fruit Punch

(can be made without wheat, gluten, dairy, eggs, or sugar —see page xi about ingredients)

Non-alcoholic and light, this is the perfect drink for a luncheon, shower, or wedding. If you prefer, you may add your favorite alcohol such as gf rum or vodka. For a pretty ice ring in the punch bowl, combine pineapple and orange juice in a small Bundt pan and add pineapple rings, mandarin oranges, and sprigs of mint. Freeze overnight.

2 cups Simple Syrup for Beverages   2 cups fresh orange juice
    (page 207)   Fresh mint leaves for garnish
3/4 cup fresh lemon juice   Strips of fresh lemon peels for garnish
1 quart pineapple juice

Combine ingredients in large pitcher or punch bowl, stir, and chill. Serve chilled with ice. Serves 10 (about 3/4 cup each).

| | | | | | | | | Exchanges | | |
Calories	Fat	% Fat Cal	Protein	Carb	Chol	Sodium	Fiber	Carb	Meat	Fat
270	0g	0	1g	71g	0mg	81mg	0g	4		

Fruity Mint Punch

(can be made without wheat, gluten, dairy, eggs, or sugar —see page xi about ingredients)

Jazz up ordinary tea (such as orange pekoe and pekoe) with fruit and spices and you have a drink appropriate for the finest occasion. Vary the fruit juice as you wish— perhaps pineapple or orange juice. Best of all, it's alcohol-free—but you could always add a dash of your favorite gluten-free spirits!

4 cups hot brewed lemon herb tea   1 bunch fresh mint sprigs (bunch
6 cups apple or pure white grape juice   measures 1-inch in diameter)
1/4 cup sugar or honey   Fresh mint leaves for garnish

In pitcher, combine hot brewed tea, fruit juice, sugar, and mint leaves (that have been tied together with kitchen string or dental floss). Cover and chill until ready to serve.

Serve over ice, garnished with fresh mint leaves. Serves 10 (1 cup each).

| | | | | | | | | Exchanges | | |
Calories	Fat	% Fat Cal	Protein	Carb	Chol	Sodium	Fiber	Carb	Meat	Fat
100	0g	0	0g	26g	0mg	4mg	0g	2		

Iced Coffee

(can be made without wheat, gluten, dairy, eggs, or sugar —see page xi about ingredients)

Refreshing and distinctively different. If you can't use dairy topping, try one of the many Whipped Toppings in the Dessert chapter. You may add sweetener to taste. If your ice cubes dilute the coffee taste, use ice cubes made of brewed coffee.

6 cups water	1/2 teaspoon ground cinnamon or
1/3 cup ground coffee	a 2-inch stick
1/2 teaspoon ground cardamom	1/4 teaspoon ground nutmeg

Place the coffee, cardamon, and cinnamon in brew basket of coffee maker. Add water and brew coffee according to manufacturer's directions. Chill brewed coffee for at least 1 hour. Divide among 4 ice-filled glasses. Garnish with dash of ground nutmeg. Serves 6 (1 cup each).

								Exchanges		
Calories	Fat	% Fat Cal	Protein	Carb	Chol	Sodium	Fiber	Carb	Meat	Fat
6	<1g	8%	<1g	1g	0mg	5mg	0g			

Lemon Mint Punch with Raspberries

(can be made without wheat, gluten, dairy, eggs, or sugar —see page xi about ingredients)

Pretty as a picture, this lightly-sweetened lemon punch is accented with fresh raspberries. You may increase the size of this recipe for larger groups. Add a dash of your favorite gf liquor (gin or vodka), if you wish.

2 cups fresh lemon juice	2 cups seltzer water or club soda
1 1/2 cups Simple Syrup	1/2 cup fresh raspberries
for Beverages (page 207)	Lemon slices and fresh mint for garnish
1/4 cup fresh mint leaves, packed	

Combine lemon juice, syrup, and mint in pitcher and stir until completely smooth. Add seltzer water and ice cubes. Place a few raspberries in each glass of punch (or float several in a large punch bowl.). Garnish each glass with lemon slices or fresh mint leaves. Serves 6 (about 1 cup each).

								Exchanges		
Calories	Fat	% Fat Cal	Protein	Carb	Chol	Sodium	Fiber	Carb	Meat	Fat
200	0g	0	0g	71g	0mg	115mg	1g	4		

Minty Ginger Iced Tea

(can be made without wheat, gluten, dairy, eggs, or sugar —see page xi about ingredients)

Even plain old black tea (known as Orange Pekoe & Pekoe) takes on new life in this refreshing drink. For an alcoholic version, try adding your favorite gf gin, vodka, or rum.

6 cups boiling water
3 tablespoons loose tea of choice
1/2 cup honey or liquid fructose

1 bunch fresh mint leaves
(about 1/2 cup)
1 piece fresh ginger (1/2-inch thick)

Bring water to boil. Remove from heat. Add tea, honey, mint, and fresh ginger. Steep for 3-5 minutes, or to taste. Strain. Serve over ice. You may halve or double this recipe, as you wish. Serves 6 (1 cup each).

| | | | | | | | | Exchanges | | |
Calories	Fat	% Fat Cal	Protein	Carb	Chol	Sodium	Fiber	Carb	Meat	Fat
88	0g	0	0g	24g	0mg	8mg	0g	1		

Simple Syrup for Beverages

(can be made without wheat, gluten, dairy, eggs, or sugar —see page xi about ingredients)

This syrup is used in several beverages and punches but you'll see several different variations of this syrup, depending on which cookbook you consult. This version is decidedly less sweet than others. If you prefer a sweeter syrup, simply increase the sweetener accordingly.

2 cups honey or agave nectar or
2 1/4 cups sugar
or 2 1/4 cups fructose powder

5 cups water

Combine ingredients in small saucepan. Bring to boil. Reduce to medium heat and cook for 5-8 minutes. Remove from heat and cool thoroughly before using. Refrigerate, covered, for up to 1 month. Serves 14 (1/2 cup each).

| | | | | | | | | Exchanges | | |
Calories	Fat	% Fat Cal	Protein	Carb	Chol	Sodium	Fiber	Carb	Meat	Fat
170	0g	0	0g	47g	0mg	5mg	0g	3		

Notes

INGREDIENTS & CONDIMENTS

Ever notice how some of the minor actors in a play or movie are critical to its success? So it is with condiments and other ingredients that play "bit parts". Their role is small, but their impact is mighty.

The recipes in this chapter play "bit parts" in a meal. They are designed to help you with other recipes in this book. For example, condiments play a very important role in several recipes but many commercially prepared condiments have forbidden components.

So . . . make your own ketchup, mustard, or mayonnaise. Or maybe simple things such as chicken stock, rice milk, or baking powder. If you love to use spice mixes such as Italian (Herb) Seasoning, Seafood Seasoning, Asian Seasoning, or Curry Powder but fear the unknown in commercial varieties—make your own using dried herbs from commercial sources you trust. Or, grow your own herbs and dry them yourself.

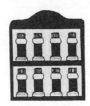

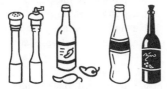

Applesauce

(can be made without wheat, gluten, dairy, eggs, or sugar - see page xi about ingredients)

I prefer using Granny Smith apples because of their tart flavor, but you can use any apples you happen to have on hand. Applesauce can be used to sweeten hot cereal, as a binder in baking, or as a spread on toast or rolls.

1 pound apples (3 medium apples)	1/8 teaspoon ground cinnamon
1 cup apple juice or apple cider	1/8 teaspoon ground allspice
2 tablespoons fresh lemon juice	1/2 teaspoon gf vanilla extract
2 tablespoons fresh orange juice	1/8 teaspoon salt
2 tablespoons maple sugar	1 strip orange peel (3 inches long)
or date sugar	1 strip lemon peel (3 inches long)

Core, peel, and chop apples. Place all ingredients in medium sized, heavy saucepan and bring to boil. Reduce heat, cover, and simmer for 15-20 minutes or until apples are done. Remove cover and mash apples with potato masher.

Continue simmering until applesauce reaches desired consistency. Cool. Refrigerate, tightly covered, for up to 1 week. Makes about 2 cups. Serves 8 (1/2 cup each).

								Exchanges		
Calories	Fat	% Fat Cal	Protein	Carb	Chol	Sodium	Fiber	Carb	Meat	Fat
44	0g	0	0g	11g	0mg	42mg	2g	1		

Vegetable Spice Rub

(can be made without wheat, gluten, dairy, eggs, or sugar - see page xi about ingredients)

Sprinkle this boldly flavored mix on your favorite vegetables before you roast them. Or, sprinkle after steaming them.

1 tablespoon paprika	1 teaspoon cayenne pepper
2 teaspoons salt	1 teaspoon gf onion powder
2 teaspoons gf garlic powder	1 teaspoon dried oregano leaves
1 teaspoon black pepper	1 teaspoon dried thyme leaves
1 teaspoon white pepper	

Combine all ingredients and store, tightly covered, in cool, dark place. Sprinkle on vegetables. Serves 4 (1 tablespoon each).

Baking Powder with Corn

(can be made without wheat, gluten, dairy, eggs, or sugar - see page xi about ingredients)

If you can't eat corn, try the grain-free version below.

1/4 cup cream of tartar   **2 tablespoons baking soda**
3 tablespoons cornstarch

Mix together in glass jar and store in cool, dark place for up to 1 month. Use in same proportions as baking powder. Makes about 1/2 cup.

Baking Powder without Corn

(can be made without wheat, gluten, dairy, eggs, or sugar - see page xi about ingredients)

When the recipe calls for 1 teaspoon baking powder, you may use 1 1/2 teaspoons of this corn-free version. Make this frequently rather than doubling it—it loses potency over time.

3 tablespoons baking soda   **1/3 cup arrowroot**
1/3 cup cream of tartar

Mix together in glass jar and store in cool, dark place for up to1 month. Makes about 3/4 cup.

Flax (Flaxseed) Mix

(can be made without wheat, gluten, dairy, eggs, or sugar - see page xi about ingredients)

This egg substitute works best in recipes with a darker color where you are replacing 1 egg rather than two. It works best as a binder and moisturizer, but it is not a leavening agent—as are eggs. Therefore, baked goods will be heavier and denser.

3 teaspoons flaxseeds or flaxseed meal   **1 cup boiling water**

Grind seeds into fine powder with coffee grinder or use flaxseed meal. Whisk into boiling water, remove from heat, and let stand for 5 minutes. Use as substitute for eggs—1/4 cup flax mix equals 1 large egg.

Calories	Fat	% Fat Cal	Protein	Carb	Chol	Sodium	Fiber	Carb	Meat	Fat
								Exchanges		
12	1g	59%	<1g	0mg	0mg	3mg	1g			

Beef Stock

(can be made without wheat, gluten, dairy, eggs, or sugar - see page xi about ingredients)

This version produces a deeper, more fully flavored beef stock because the beef and vegetables are roasted. If you don't have time to roast the ingredients—or prefer a milder stock—simply simmer the ingredients together for a couple of hours. I prefer to use an ovenproof Dutch oven that goes from oven to stove top, thus eliminating an extra pan. For chicken or vegetable stock, see next page.

1 **pound beef stew meat (1-inch cubes)**	1 **teaspoon dried thyme leaves**
1 **large onion, peeled and quartered**	1/4 **teaspoon dill seeds**
1 **large carrot, sliced lengthwise**	1 **teaspoon salt**
1 **large celery ribs, halved**	6 **whole black peppercorns**
2 **large garlic cloves, peeled**	1 **large bay leaf**
4 **quarts cold water**	1 **large tomato, halved**
1 **bunch parsley**	

Place beef, onions, and carrot in large baking pan and roast for 20-30 minutes in 400° oven until nicely browned. Transfer vegetables to large stockpot and add remaining ingredients. Pour off any extra fat from roasting pan and add just enough water to cover bottom of pan. De-glaze pan over medium-high heat, scraping up browned bits. Add this mixture to stockpot.

Bring mixture in stockpot slowly to a simmer, cover, and continue to simmer for 3 hours. (Avoid bringing to a boil rapidly since this produces foam that you'll have to skim off.)

Strain stock through sieve. Chill stock and remove fat that rises to top. If you're not using all the stock immediately, freeze for up to 3 months. Makes about 4 quarts. Serves 16 (1 cup each).

								Exchanges		
Calories	Fat	% Fat Cal	Protein	Carb	Chol	Sodium	Fiber	Carb	Meat	Fat
8	1g	7%	0g	2g	0mg	156mg	1g			

Chicken Stock

(can be made without wheat, gluten, dairy, eggs, or sugar - see page xi about ingredients)

Save the bones from Sunday's roast chicken and use them to flavor this stock. If you refrigerate the stock, the fat can easily be skimmed off the following day and frozen in containers. For beef stock, see the previous page. For vegetable stock, see below.

3 quarts water
2 pounds chicken pieces or bones
1 tablespoon salt
1 small onion, halved
4 ribs celery, leaves left on
4 large peeled carrots
2 small parsnips (optional)

6 dill seeds
6 whole black peppercorns
1 large tomato, halved
1 bunch fresh herbs (thyme, savory, marjoram, etc.) or 2 teaspoons dried herbs of choice

Combine all ingredients in large stockpot. Bring to simmer slowly, cover tightly, and let cook for 2-3 hours. Let stock cool in refrigerator. Skim off fat. Strain stock through fine mesh sieve and discard solids. Store in tightly covered containers in freezer. Makes 3 quarts. Serves 12 (1 cup each).

Exchanges

Calories	Fat	% Fat Cal	Protein	Carb	Chol	Sodium	Fiber	Carb	Meat	Fat
40	<1g	4%	1g	9g	0mg	670mg	2g	2		

Vegetable Stock

(can be made without wheat, gluten, dairy, eggs, or sugar - see page xi about ingredients)

Keep jars of this flavorful stock in your freezer and you'll always be prepared.

3 quarts water
1 tablespoon salt
1 small onion, halved
4 ribs celery, leaves left on
4 large carrots, peeled
2 small parsnips (optional)

6 dill seeds
6 whole black peppercorns
1 large tomato, halved
1 bunch fresh herbs (thyme, marjoram, savory, etc.) or 2 teaspoons dried herbs of choice

Combine all ingredients in large stockpot. Bring to simmer slowly, cover tightly, and let cook for 2-3 hours. Let stock cool in refrigerator. Strain stock through fine mesh sieve and discard solids. Store in tightly covered containers in freezer until ready to use. Makes 3 quarts. Serves 12 (1 cup each).

Exchanges

Calories	Fat	% Fat Cal	Protein	Carb	Chol	Sodium	Fiber	Carb	Meat	Fat
40	0g	0	0g	9g	0mg	670mg	2g	2		

Oven-Dried Cherries

(can be made without wheat, gluten, dairy, eggs, or sugar - see page xi about ingredients)

If you love dried cherries but don't want to use the commercial variety, then dry your own. It is really quite simple. You can use either fresh or canned tart cherries.

2 cans (16 oz. each) red tart cherries, drained or 4 cups fresh tart cherries	**1 tablespoon honey or agave nectar Parchment paper**

Heat oven to 250° Line large baking sheet with parchment paper. Set aside.

Check each cherry for stones. Toss cherries with honey (or agave nectar) and arrange on prepared baking sheets.

Bake for 1 hour or until cherries appear wrinkled but still moist. As cherries bake, remove those that dry faster than others. If cherries are still not dry after 1 hour, turn oven off—but leave cherries in oven for another 30 minutes or until desired degree of dryness. Serves 8 (about 1/2 cup each).

								Exchanges		
Calories	Fat	% Fat Cal	Protein	Carb	Chol	Sodium	Fiber	Carb	Meat	Fat
257	1g	1%	3g	89g	1mg	1mg	5g	5		

Oven-Dried Tomatoes

(can be made without wheat, gluten, dairy, eggs, or sugar - see page xi about ingredients)

Plum tomatoes dry thoroughly and evenly and have a wonderful flavor. Use these flavorful little morsels in tossed salads or salad dressings—or any dish you choose.

12 plum or cherry tomatoes	**Parchment paper**
1 tablespoon olive oil	**1/2 teaspoon dried basil**
1/4 teaspoon salt—or to taste	

Wash and pat tomatoes dry with paper towel. Remove stems and slice in half, lengthwise (from stem to bottom of tomato). Remove seeds and pulp. A melon baller works especially well. (If you wish, you may leave seeds and pulp intact, but tomatoes dry faster and more thoroughly when the pulp is removed.)

Toss with olive oil. Place on baking sheet lined with parchment paper or silicone liners. Sprinkle with salt (and basil, if using).

Bake at 200° for 2 to 4 hours or to desired degree of dryness. Store in refrigerator. Makes 24 dried tomatoes. Serves 4 (6 tomato halves each).

								Exchanges		
Calories	Fat	% Fat Cal	Protein	Carb	Chol	Sodium	Fiber	Carb	Meat	Fat
68	4g	47%	2g	9g	0mg	160mg	2g	2		1

Nut Milk

(can be made without wheat, gluten, dairy, eggs, or sugar - see page xi about ingredients)

The nice thing about making your own nut milk is that you can vary the ingredients to achieve the desired result. For example, for a sweeter version simply increase the sweetener. Likewise, for a less sweet version to be used for savory dishes, omit the sweetener altogether. Vary the density of the milk by increasing the nuts and/or decreasing the amount of water.

| 1/2 cup raw cashews or almonds | 1 teaspoon honey or agave nectar |
| 2 cups water | 1/2 teaspoon gf vanilla extract (optional) |

Combine ingredients in blender and blend until completely smooth, about 10 minutes. Strain through cheesecloth to remove any remaining nuts. Refrigerate, covered, for up to 1 week. Use in dishes as you would use any non-dairy milk substitute. Makes about 2 cups. Serves 4 (1/2 cup each).

| | | | | | | | | Exchanges | | |
Calories	Fat	% Fat Cal	Protein	Carb	Chol	Sodium	Fiber	Carb	Meat	Fat
105	8g	65%	3g	7g	0mg	6mg	1g		.5	2

Rice Milk

(can be made without wheat, gluten, dairy, eggs, or sugar - see page xi about ingredients)

The advantage to making your own rice milk is that you can vary the density of the milk by increasing the rice and/or decreasing the amount of water. The cashews add flavor and body, but they can be omitted. I prefer using basmati rice, but you can use plain white or brown rice, also.

2/3 cup hot cooked rice	1 teaspoon gf vanilla extract
3 cups warm water	1 tablespoon honey—or to taste
1/3 cup raw cashews (optional)	1/8 teaspoon xanthan gum

Blend all ingredients in blender until very, very smooth. Strain through cheesecloth to remove any remaining rice particles. Refrigerate, covered, for up to 1 week. Makes about 3 cups. Serves 12 (1/4 cup each).

| | | | | | | | | Exchanges | | |
Calories	Fat	% Fat Cal	Protein	Carb	Chol	Sodium	Fiber	Carb	Meat	Fat
23	0g	0	0g	5g	0mg	3mg	0g	.5		

Tomato Sauce

(can be made without wheat, gluten, dairy, eggs, or sugar - see page xi about ingredients)

If you can't eat commercial canned tomato sauce (it often contains several other ingredients), make your own with this easy recipe.

2 tablespoons chopped onion	1/4 teaspoon salt
1 small garlic clove, minced	1/2 teaspoon sugar or honey
1 can (14.5 oz) whole peeled tomatoes	(optional)
or 4 large peeled fresh tomatoes	1/8 teaspoon black pepper

Purée all ingredients in blender until very, very smooth. Place in small saucepan and cook over low-medium heat for 20-25 minutes or until desired consistency. Makes 1 cup, which is equivalent to 1 can (8 oz.) of commercial canned tomato sauce. Serves 4 (1/4 cup each).

								Exchanges		
Calories	Fat	% Fat Cal	Protein	Carb	Chol	Sodium	Fiber	Carb	Meat	Fat
40	.5g	11%	2g	8g	0mg	158mg	1g	2		

Apricot Ketchup

(can be made without wheat, gluten, dairy, eggs, or sugar - see page xi about ingredients)

Experts on food trends say that exotic-flavored ketchup will be very popular.

1 can (16 oz.) apricots in fruit juice, undrained	1/4 teaspoon ground cloves
1/2 cup finely chopped onion	1/4 teaspoon ground allspice
1/2 cup white wine vinegar	1/2 teaspoon salt
1 small garlic clove, minced	1/8 teaspoon cayenne pepper
1/2 teaspoon ground cinnamon	1/8 teaspoon ground nutmeg
	1/8 teaspoon ground white pepper

Drain apricots, reserving juice in small saucepan. Set apricots aside.

Cook juice over low-medium heat, stirring occasionally, for 7-10 minutes—or until reduced to 1/2 cup.

Add apricots and remaining ingredients. Mash apricots slightly. Bring to boil, reduce heat, and simmer for 40-50 minutes—or until thickened. Cool thoroughly.

In food processor, purée apricot mixture until very, very smooth. Refrigerate in glass container, covered, for 1 day before serving. Keeps in refrigerator for 1 week. Makes 1 cup. Serves 8 (2 tablespoons each).

								Exchanges		
Calories	Fat	% Fat Cal	Protein	Carb	Chol	Sodium	Fiber	Carb	Meat	Fat
32	0g	0	1g	8g	0mg	148mg	1g	1		

Egg-Free Mayonnaise

(can be made without wheat, gluten, dairy, eggs, or sugar - see page xi about ingredients)

Use this easy mayonnaise as you would use ordinary mayonnaise. See below for an egg-free, dairy-free mayonnaise. Ask your physician about using goat yogurt.

1 cup plain yogurt (cow, soy, goat)	1/4 teaspoon salt
1 teaspoon gf dry mustard	1/8 teaspoon cayenne pepper
1/2 teaspoon grated lemon peel	1/8 teaspoon white pepper
1/4 teaspoon sugar or honey	

Place the yogurt in strainer lined with coffee filter or cheesecloth. Place strainer over bowl, cover the entire thing with large plastic bag or foil and refrigerate for 24 hours. Discard liquid (whey). (You may use goat yogurt or soy yogurt, if your diet allows them, but soy yogurt won't drain as well.)

In small bowl, whisk together yogurt and remaining ingredients until thoroughly blended. Makes 1 cup. Store in refrigerator for 1 week. Serves 8 (2 tablespoons each).

								Exchanges		
Calories	Fat	% Fat Cal	Protein	Carb	Chol	Sodium	Fiber	Carb	Meat	Fat
22	1g	25%	2g	2g	2mg	94mg	0g			

Egg-Free, Dairy-Free Mayonnaise

(can be made without wheat, gluten, dairy, eggs, or sugar - see page xi about ingredients)

2 teaspoons sweet rice flour	1/8 teaspoon paprika
1/4 teaspoon gf dry mustard	1/4 cup fresh lemon juice
1/4 teaspoon salt	1/4 cup water
1/4 teaspoon sugar or honey	1 teaspoon cider vinegar
1/8 teaspoon white pepper	1/4 cup cooking oil
1/8 teaspoon cayenne pepper	

Combine flour, mustard, salt, sugar (or honey), peppers, paprika, lemon juice, and water in small, heavy pan. Over low-medium heat, bring to boil and whisk until thickened.

Remove from heat and cool for 2-3 minutes. Combine vinegar and oil and slowly pour into flour mixture, whisking constantly until completely blended. Refrigerate in airtight container for up to 1 week. Makes about 1 cup. Store in refrigerator for up to 1 week. Serves 8 (2 tablespoons each).

								Exchanges		
Calories	Fat	% Fat Cal	Protein	Carb	Chol	Sodium	Fiber	Carb	Meat	Fat
65	7g	90%	0g	2g	0mg	72mg	0g			1

Mustard

(can be made without wheat, gluten, dairy, eggs, or sugar - see page xi about ingredients)

This recipe makes the traditional yellow version of mustard.

3 tablespoons tapioca flour
2/3 cup water, divided
1/4 cup gf dry mustard
1/3 cup cider vinegar
2 tablespoons honey

1/2 teaspoon salt
2 tablespoons fresh grated horseradish
   or gf horseradish sauce
1/4 teaspoon ground turmeric
1/8 teaspoon paprika

Mix tapioca flour in 1/4 cup of the water until paste forms. Set aside. In small saucepan over low-medium heat, mix together dry mustard, vinegar, honey, salt, and remainder of water. Gradually whisk in tapioca flour paste until well blended. Bring to boil, stirring constantly, until mixture thickens.

Remove from heat and stir in horseradish, turmeric, and paprika. Refrigerate in airtight container up to1 week. Makes 1 cup. Serves 8 (2 tablespoons each).

								Exchanges		
Calories	Fat	% Fat Cal	Protein	Carb	Chol	Sodium	Fiber	Carb	Meat	Fat
30	0g	0	0g	8g	0mg	145mg	0g	.5		

Tomato Ketchup

(can be made without wheat, gluten, dairy, eggs, or sugar - see page xi about ingredients)

After you have made this recipe once, check to see whether you want to reduce or increase the spices to suit your family's tastes. You may halve the recipe, if you wish.

1 can (35 oz.) canned tomatoes
2 garlic cloves, minced
2 tablespoons grated fresh ginger
1/4 cup cider vinegar
1/2 teaspoon ground cinnamon
1/4 cup brown sugar or maple sugar

1 teaspoon ground cumin
1/4 teaspoon cayenne pepper
1/8 teaspoon ground allspice
1/8 teaspoon ground cloves
1/2 teaspoon salt
1/4 teaspoon black pepper

Place all ingredients in medium, heavy saucepan and bring to boil. Reduce to low and simmer, uncovered, for 1 hour or until liquid has evaporated. Stir occasionally to avoid scorching and sticking. Let mixture cool for 15 minutes.

Transfer mixture to food processor and purée until very, very smooth. Refrigerate, covered, for up to 2 weeks. Makes 4 cups. Serves 32 (2 tablespoons each).

								Exchanges		
Calories	Fat	% Fat Cal	Protein	Carb	Chol	Sodium	Fiber	Carb	Meat	Fat
11	0g	0	0g	3g	0mg	39mg	.5g	.5		

Asian Seasoning

(can be made without wheat, gluten, dairy, eggs, or sugar - see page xi about ingredients)

Combine with oil and rub on seafood or other meat. One of the easiest ways to crush the toasted sesame seeds is to use a small coffee grinder used only for grinding spices.

- 2 tablespoons toasted sesame seeds, crushed
- 1 teaspoon ground coriander
- 1 teaspoon ground allspice
- 1 teaspoon gf onion powder
- 1/2 teaspoon ground cumin
- 1/2 teaspoon dried thyme leaves
- 1/4 teaspoon ground cinnamon
- 1/4 teaspoon ground nutmeg
- 1/4 teaspoon cayenne pepper
- 1/4 teaspoon salt

Combine ingredients in tightly closed glass container. Store in cool, dark place for up to 3 months. Best if used quickly. Makes 1/4 cup. Serves 12 (1 teaspoon each).

Curry Powder

(can be made without wheat, gluten, dairy, eggs, or sugar - see page xi about ingredients)

If you can't find the whole seed versions of coriander and cumin you can also use the powdered versions—which don't need to be toasted. The flavors won't be as intense, but the final product will work. Fenugreek and whole curry leaves are unusual and sometimes hard to find—you can omit them, if necessary, with some loss of flavor.

- 2 teaspoons whole coriander seeds
- 1 teaspoon whole cumin seeds
- 1/2 teaspoon whole mustard seeds
- 1 teaspoon whole fenugreek seeds
- 4 whole red chiles (or 1 teaspoon crushed red peppers—not cayenne pepper)
- 1 teaspoon whole black peppercorns
- 10 dried curry leaves (optional)
- 1 teaspoon ground turmeric
- 1/2 teaspoon ground ginger

In a small frying pan, toast coriander, cumin, mustard, and fenugreek seeds over medium heat until spices become fragrant. Watch carefully and shake pan frequently to prevent burning. This should take anywhere from 2-3 minutes, depending on your range and your skillet.

Put toasted spices in spice grinder (or small coffee grinder reserved just for spices) and add the chiles, peppercorns, curry leaves, turmeric, and ginger. Grind until spices are smooth. Store in airtight glass container in cool, dark place for up to 3 months. Makes 3 tablespoons Serves 8 (1 teaspoon each).

Fines Herbes

(can be made without wheat, gluten, dairy, eggs, or sugar - see page xi about ingredients)

Keep this flavorful seasoning on hand to sprinkle on meat, vegetable, or salads.

1 teaspoon dried chervil
1 teaspoon chives, freeze-dried
1 teaspoon dried parsley

1/4 teaspoon dried tarragon
1/4 teaspoon salt

Combine all ingredients in airtight, glass container. Store in cool, dark place for up to 3 months. Makes 1 1/2 tablespoons.

Herbes de Provence

(can be made without wheat, gluten, dairy, eggs, or sugar - see page xi about ingredients)

This is excellent sprinkled on roasted chicken, steamed vegetables, or in salad dressings.

1 teaspoon dried basil leaves
1/2 teaspoon fennel seed, crushed
1 teaspoon dried marjoram leaves
1 teaspoon dried rosemary, crushed

1/2 teaspoon dried sage leaves
1/2 teaspoon dried thyme leaves
1/2 teaspoon dried lavender
   (optional)

Combine all ingredients in glass, airtight container. Store in cool, dark place for up to 3 months. Makes about 2 tablespoons.

Italian Bread Crumbs

(can be made without wheat, gluten, dairy, eggs, or sugar - see page xi about ingredients)

Italian bread crumbs are so easy to make and add so much flavor to our dining. If you prefer them dry, toast them in a slow oven to desired degree of dryness.

4 cups gf bread torn in small pieces
1 teaspoon gf onion powder

4 teaspoons Italian seasoning or
1 teaspoon each dried basil, oregano, rosemary, and marjoram or thyme

Place bread in food processor and pulse on/off until crumbs reach desired consistency. Toss with remaining ingredients. Store tightly covered, in refrigerator, for up to 2 weeks. Makes 2 cups. Serves 16 (1/2 cup each).

| | | | | | | | | Exchanges | | |
Calories	Fat	% Fat Cal	Protein	Carb	Chol	Sodium	Fiber	Carb	Meat	Fat
63	1g	14%	2g	12g	1mg	114mg	1g	1		

Italian (Herb) Seasoning

(can be made without wheat, gluten, dairy, eggs, or sugar - see page xi about ingredients)

The advantage of making your own spice mixes is that you know they're safe. If any of these spices disagree with you or your family, omit them—or substitute a similar one.

1 tablespoon dried basil leaves	1 teaspoon dried sage leaves
1 tablespoon rosemary, crushed	1 teaspoon gf onion powder
2 teaspoons dried majoram leaves	1/4 teaspoon black pepper
2 teaspoons dried thyme leaves	1/4 teaspoon cayenne pepper
2 teaspoons dried oregano leaves	1/8 teaspoon ground nutmeg

Combine all ingredients and store, covered, in dark, dry place. Use within 3 months. Makes 5 tablespoons.

Seafood Seasoning

(can be made without wheat, gluten, dairy, eggs, or sugar - see page xi about ingredients)

Use this seasoning on your favorite seafood by rubbing it on all sides of the fish and then refrigerate for at least 1 hour. Cook as directed.

1 tablespoon dried thyme leaves	1/2 teaspoon gf mustard powder
1 tablespoon dried sage leaves	1/2 teaspoon gf onion powder
1 tablespoon dried marjoram leaves	1/4 teaspoon ground ginger
1 tablespoon dried savory leaves	1/4 teaspoon ground nutmeg
2 teaspoons freeze-dried chives	1/4 teaspoon ground cardamom
1 small bay leaf, crushed	1/4 teaspoon cayenne pepper
1 teaspoon paprika	1/8 teaspoon ground cloves
1 teaspoon gf celery salt	

Combine all ingredients in glass jar with tightly sealed lid. Store in dark, cool place for up to 3 months. Makes about 6 tablespoons.

Notes

APPENDICES

Baking with Alternative Sweeteners

This section presents information for those who prefer to use sweeteners other than white sugar. Recipes may require some experimentation to achieve desired results.

Liquid Sweeteners

SWEETENER	AMOUNT TO USE	WHEN TO USE/TIPS
Brown Rice Syrup Made from brown rice (and maybe barley enzymes). Half as sweet as sugar. Refrigerate.	Use 1 1/3 cups for 1 cup sugar. Reduce liquid 1/4 cup per cup rice syrup. Add 1/4 tsp. baking soda per cup of syrup.	Cookies, pies, puddings. Use with other sweeteners in cakes. Makes baked goods crisp. Lundberg is gf.
Honey From bees. Color and taste depend on flower source. 20- 60% sweeter than sugar.	Use 2/3 - 3/4 cup for 1 cup sugar. Reduce liquid 1/4 cup per cup honey. Add 1/4 tsp. baking soda per cup honey. Reduce oven 25°.	All baked goods. Don't give honey to children under age 2, because of possible botulism.
Maple Syrup (pure) From maple tree sap. Grade B best for flavor in baking. Dark brown.	Use 2/3 - 3/4 cup for 1 cup white sugar. Reduce liquid by 3 Tbsp. per cup syrup. Add 1/4 tsp. baking soda per cup syrup.	All baked goods, especially cakes. Use organic to avoid formaldehyde and other additives. Refrigerate.
Mixed Fruit Juice Concentrate (liquid) Peach, pear, grape, pineapple juices, rice syrup. **(Fruit Source™)**. Fruit-tasting. Refrigerate.	Use 2/3 cup for 1 cup white sugar. Reduce liquid 1/3 cup per cup concentrate. Add 1/4 tsp. baking soda per cup concentrate. Reduce oven 25°; adjust baking time.	All baked goods, except white cakes and chocolate dishes. Drain canned fruit thoroughly to avoid soggy pie crust. Company verifies product as gf.
Frozen Fruit Juice Concentrate (e.g., apple, white grape, orange, pineapple) Look for *pure* concentrate.	Same as mixed fruit juice concentrate, but 25% less. Add 1/4 tsp. baking soda per recipe. Reduce liquid 1/4 cup per cup concentrate.	Applesauce, cakes, cookies, bars. For stronger, sweeter flavor, simmer the juice over low heat until it is reduced by 1/3. Cool.
Fruit Purée Use baby food fruits or purée fruits in blender.	Prune, apple, apricot, banana, pear. Best as substitute for 1/2 (not all) sugar/fat.	Baked goods, e.g., prunes in "dark" colored foods, pears in light foods, etc.
Molasses Made from concentrated sugar cane juice. Strong flavor.	Use 1/2 cup molasses for 1 cup sugar. Reduce liquid by 1/4 cup per cup molasses.	All baked goods, especially with spiced cakes, muffins, cookies.

Note: Ask your health professional if these alternative sweeteners are safe for your diet.

Baking with Alternative Sweeteners

(continued)

Granular Sweeteners

SWEETENER	AMOUNT TO USE	WHEN TO USE/TIPS
Date Sugar Ground, dehydrated dates. Coarse, brown granules. Very sweet.	Use 2/3 as much as sugar. Good when used in combination with other sweeteners. Store in dry, cool place. Sift.	Dissolve in hot liquid before adding to recipe. Use as topping for fruit dessert. Burns if baked long time.
Dried Cane Juice (Sucanat®) - *Sugar Cane Natural*) Sugar cane with water removed. Coarse, amber grains.. Mild molasses taste.	Use same amount as sugar. Add 1/4 tsp. baking soda per cup of dried cane juice. Sift before using. Store in dry, cool place.	Cookies, cakes, pies, and puddings, but not white cakes. May be a bit grainy in baked goods unless dissolved in warmed liquid ingredient first.
Granulated Fruit Sweetener (FruitSource™). Grape juice concentrate and rice syrup Light brown; like brown sugar but not as sweet.	Use 1 1/4 cups for 1 cup sugar. Reduce salt 30- 50%. Use cooking spray or parchment paper on pans. Don't over-mix batter. Keep oven at ≤350°; adjust baking time.	Cookies, cakes, and puddings. Works better when dissolved in warmed liquid before adding to recipe. Company sources verify that the rice syrup is gf.
Maple Sugar From maple syrup boiled down to light brown granules.	Use 1 cup maple sugar for 1 cup sugar. Add 1/8 tsp. baking soda for each cup maple sugar.	Dissolve in warmed liquid from recipe before using in batters, if possible.
Stevia (leaf, powder, tincture) Sweet-leafed herb from Paraguay.	30 to 40 times sweeter than sugar. Slight licorice after-taste.	Recipes need total change to successfully use stevia. Best for low-sugar recipes.

Sweeteners for Diabetics: You may use your favorite sweetener in these recipes, but make sure the sweetener is designed for baking if you use it in baked goods. You may need to experiment a bit to achieve desired results. NutraSweet (aspartame) will not work in baking.

FOS (Fructooligosaccharides). White, low-calorie powder—about half as sweet as sugar. Derived from fruit carbohydrates. Best used in combination with caloric sweeteners in baking, but can be used alone to sweeten cereals, beverages, sauces. May cause gas.

Agave Nectar: Honey-like liquid derived from agave plant. Gluten-free, 90% fructose. Experimentation with this new sweetener continues in my kitchen.

Note: Ask your health professional if these alternative sweeteners are safe for your diet.

Baking with Alternative Sweeteners

(continued)

The following sweeteners are believed to be more highly refined than those on the previous pages. Nonetheless, they work quite well in baking. Here are some guidelines to assure successful results.

More Highly Refined Sweeteners

SWEETENER	AMOUNT TO USE	WHEN TO USE/TIPS
Brown Sugar Actually white sugar with molasses added for heartier flavor and color. May use light or dark version.	Use 1 cup brown sugar in place of 1 cup white sugar.	Lends heartier flavor and darker color in baked goods.
Corn Syrup Produced by action of enzymes on cornstarch. Used in many commercial products.	Use 1 cup corn syrup in place of 1 cup white sugar. Reduce liquid by 1/4 to 1/3 cup per cup syrup.	Use in any baked item that can use honey. **NOTE:** High fructose corn syrup <u>may</u> contain gluten from a brewer's yeast extract used in processing.
Fructose Granular version usually refined from corn syrup or from fruit sources. Bit sweeter than white sugar.	Use 1 cup of fructose in place of 1 cup white sugar.	Use in cakes, cookies, bars, breads, muffins, or any baked item where honey is also appropriate.
Liquid version also derived from corn.	Use 1 cup liquid fructose in place of 1 cup white sugar. Reduce liquid 1/4 - 1/3 cup.	Use liquid fructose in same way as corn syrup.
Turbinado Actually just raw sugar with the impurities removed.	Use 1 cup turbinado in place of 1 cup white sugar.	Use in any recipe, but works better in darker colored baked goods.

Note: Ask your health professional if these alternative sweeteners are safe for your diet.

Baking with Dairy Substitutes

Milk is one of the easiest ingredients to make substitutions for in baking, although some milk substitutes lend a subtle flavor to baked goods and may affect the degree of browning while baking. In addition, read labels to avoid problem ingredients such as casein or barley malt. Choose low-sugar versions when making savory dishes.

In place of 1 cup of cow's milk, use:

SUBSTITUTE	AMOUNT TO USE	WHEN TO USE/TIPS
Rice Milk (rice beverage) Buy fortified brands.	1 cup. Mild flavor, white color. Looks like skim milk from cows.	In any recipe, but slightly sweet-tasting. Check gf status. Reduce by 2 tablespoons per cup if used as buttermilk substitute.
Soy Milk (soy beverage) Be sure to buy brands that are vitamin-fortified and gf.	1 cup. Slight soy flavor, light tan in color. Buy in liquid or powder form (to mix with water.) Powdered version makes lighter color milk.	Best in recipes with stronger flavors to mask soy and in baked goods with darker colors since soy milk darkens with heat.
Nut Milk (usually almond) Persons with allergies to nuts should use caution. Ener-G ® NutQuik is made of almond meal, guar gum.	1 cup. Mild, slightly nutty flavor. Light brown color.	Best in dessert recipes. Tastes slightly "off" in savory dishes.
Goat Milk Available in powdered and liquid form (also in low-fat liquid) by Meyenberg. Not for those with true milk allergies; may not work for lactose-intolerant.	1 cup. Most closely resembles cow's milk in color (pure white.)	In any recipe. Works especially well in ice cream, puddings and other milk-based dishes. Aseptic and powdered varieties have stronger flavor.
Oat Milk	Not recommended for those with gluten-intolerance.	
Coconut Milk	Very high in fat. Not tested with baked goods in this book. However, many people use coconut milk successfully.	

NOTE: Ask your health professional if these alternatives are safe for your diet.

If the recipe calls for Dry Milk Powder: Use same amount of non-dairy milk powder. Read labels to avoid problem ingredients such as casein. You may also use 3/4 as much goat's milk powder, if approved for your diet. Milk-allergic people should avoid goat's milk. Lactose-intolerant people should check with a physician. Or, omit dry milk powder and add same amount of sweet rice flour. Baked goods won't brown as much without dry milk powder. In yeast breads, rising and browning are diminished without milk powder.

Baking with Dairy Substitutes

(continued)

In place of 1 cup evaporated skim milk, use:

SUBSTITUTE	AMOUNT TO USE	WHEN TO USE/TIPS
Ener-G® NutQuik or SoyQuik or other non-dairy milk powder. Mix at double strength.	1 cup	Recipes using evaporated skim milk. Flavors will be stronger. Calories and nutrient values will double.

In place of 1 cup buttermilk, use:

SUBSTITUTE	AMOUNT TO USE	WHEN TO USE/TIPS
Use 1-2 Tbsp. fresh lemon juice or cider vinegar or reconstituted Ener-G® yeast-free/gluten-free vinegar and enough rice, soy, or nut milk to equal 1 cup.	1 cup. Some non-dairy milks produce a thinner buttermilk. If so, use 2 tablespoons less of non-dairy buttermilk per cup specified in recipe.	Any recipe calling for buttermilk

Density of Milk: Whether you're using liquid non-dairy milks or mix your own from powder, remember that the thinner the milk the less you'll need. For example, reduce the liquid by 1 tablespoon per cup if you use skim milk in place of whole milk, or a very thin rice milk instead of a thicker version. You may need to experiment a bit to achieve the desired results since liquid milk densities vary by brand and the ratio of powder to water will affect the density of milks made from non-dairy powders.

Also, when rice milk is used in a recipe that will be thickened such as pudding add 2 teaspoons unflavored gelatin powder dissolved in 1/4 cup of the recipe liquid for 10 minutes. This improves the thickening process.

Note that plain milk may contain one set of ingredients but flavored versions may contain different ingredients.

Lactose-Reduced Milk: You may use lactose-reduced milk in these recipes. However, make sure you can tolerate these milks before cooking with them and be certain to read the label to make sure they contain no other offending ingredients. Also, some recipes may not produce the same results as those with "regular" cow's milk or non-dairy milks.

Note: Ask your health professional if these alternatives are safe for your diet.

Baking with Dairy Substitutes

(continued)

In place of 1 cup yogurt, use:

SUBSTITUTE	AMOUNT TO USE	WHEN TO USE/TIPS
Goat Yogurt (Persons with true milk allergy should avoid all goat products. Lactose-intolerant persons should check with a physician.)	1 cup	Any recipe calling for yogurt. However, the tapioca in goat yogurt may make baked item "doughy".
Soy Yogurt	1 cup	Not well suited to heat, but works well in dips, ice cream, and other non-baked items. Won't drain.
Non-Dairy Milk Liquid	2/3 cup	Any recipe calling for yogurt. Best to add liquid in 1/3 cup increments, to avoid adding too much.

The suggestions offered in this section on dairy substitutes are primarily for baking. Bear in mind, however, that the same amount of milk substitute such as rice, soy, or nut milk can be used in non-baked items—like milkshakes, puddings, ice cream, or smoothies.

Cheese: Although there are several "non-dairy" cheeses such as Parmesan cheese made from rice, soy, or nuts, it is difficult to find one that doesn't have additional problem ingredients. For example, they may contain milk proteins called calcum caseinate, sodium caseinate, or casein. Others include oats (which is off-limits for celiacs) or texturized vegetable protein (which can have various sources, but is often soy).

Sour Cream and Cream Cheese: Soyco makes a rice-based version, however, check the label to make sure it's right for your diet—the milk protein, casein, is present in both items. Soymage makes a casein-free sour cream alternative.

Keep in touch with your natural food store. New, non-dairy cheeses are being developed.

Note: Ask your health professional if these alternatives are safe for your diet.

Baking with Egg Substitutes

Eggs are one of the hardest ingredients to exclude because they play such critical roles in baking. They can be used as binding agents (hold ingredients together), moisturizers (add moisture), or as leavening agents (make things rise) in baking. Generally speaking, egg-free baked goods rise less and have a denser texture than those made with eggs. Here are some general guidelines when modifying recipes to exclude eggs.

Eggs As Binders:
If the recipe has only one egg but contains a fair amount of baking powder or baking soda, then the egg is the binder.

In place of 1 egg as a binder, use:

SUBSTITUTE	AMOUNT TO USE	WHEN TO USE/TIPS
Tofu (soft silken) by Mori-Nu®	Use 1/4 cup for each egg and blend with recipe liquid in food processor until very smooth before using.	Cakes, cookies, breads. Baked goods won't brown as deeply. Makes very moist, heavy baked goods.
Puréed fruits/vegetables Apples, apricots, prunes, or pears. Puréed vegetables–– corn, carrots, potatoes. Baby food without fillers.	Use 3 Tbsp. to replace each egg. Increase liquid in recipe by 1 Tbsp.	Use in baked goods where the flavor of the fruit or vegetable purée complements or doesn't detract from dish's flavor.
Unflavored Gelatin Powder May use animal-based (Knox) or vegetable-based (kosher) gelatin powder (also called agar).	Mix 1 envelope of unflavored gelatin with 1 cup boiling water. Substitute 3 Tbsp. for each egg. Refrigerate. Microwave to liquefy.	Baked goods such as cookies, cakes, breads.
Arrowroot, Soy, Lecithin (may use liquid or granular lecithin)	Whisk together 1/4 cup warm water, 2 Tbsp. arrowroot, 1 tbsp. soy flour, and 1/4 tsp. lecithin.	Stronger flavored dishes since soy flour and lecithin may affect overall taste of dish.
Flaxseed (available as brown or golden seeds or as ground flaxmeal)	For each large egg, soak 1 tsp. flaxseed meal in 1/4 cup boiling water for 5 min. If using flaxseeds, pulverize in small coffee grinder first. 1 large egg equals 1/4 cup flax mix. Bake dish slightly longer; 25° lower. Reduce oil 1 to 2 Tbsp.	Cool mixture before using Best in "dark" color dishes. Mild flavor. Baked goods are heavy, dense. Best in cookies, bars. Slight laxative effect. Refrigerate to avoid rancidity.

Note: Ask your health professional if these alternatives are safe for your diet.

Baking with Egg Substitutes

Liquid Egg Substitutes: You may use liquid egg substitutes in place of real eggs. But please note that liquid egg substitutes actually contain eggs. The yolks have been removed to reduce the fat and cholesterol. *People with egg allergies cannot safely consume these products because they still contain eggs. Also, some egg substitutes contain other problem ingredients such as modified food starch—which may or may not be wheat-based.* Read the label.

Eggs as Leavening Agents:
If there are no other ingredients that make the baked item rise, then the egg is the leavening agent.

In place of 1 egg as a leavener, use:

SUBSTITUTE	AMOUNT TO USE	WHEN TO USE/TIPS
Ener-G ® Egg Replacer	Ener-G® recommends 1 1/2 tsp. Egg Replacer powder mixed in 2 Tbsp. water. In this book, I use 2-3 times as much powder for better results.	All baked goods. Flavorless, so won't affect taste of recipe. For added lightness, whip in food processor or blender for 30 seconds.
Buttermilk-Soda	Replace liquid in recipe with equivalent amount of buttermilk (or thinned yogurt if you're not dairy-sensitive.) Replace baking powder with same amount of baking soda, not exceeding 1 teaspoon per cup of flour.	All baked goods, but this technique works best in dishes that don't require a lot of "rising" to look good, such as cookies, bars and flatbreads.

Other Hints when Omitting Eggs (when eggs are leavening agents)

(1) Add air to lighten the recipe by creaming the fat and sweetener together with your electric mixer. Then add dry ingredients.

(2) Whip the liquid ingredients in a food processor or blender for 30 seconds as another way of incorporating air into the recipe.

(3) Add an extra 1/2 teaspoon baking powder per egg. Do not exceed 1 teaspoon baking powder per cup of flour or a bitter taste will develop. As an alternative to commercial baking powder (it contains corn), try the homemade version on page 211.

(4) Recipes with acidic liquids such as buttermilk, molasses, lemon juice, or vinegar tend to rise better than those with non-acidic liquids such as water or milk.

Note: Ask your health professional if these alternatives are safe for your diet.

Baking with Egg Substitutes

(continued)

Eggs as Moisture:
The egg's purpose is to add moisture if there are leavening agents in the recipe, but not much water or other liquid in the recipe.

Generally speaking, baked goods without eggs are somewhat heavier and more dense than those with eggs. For that reason, slightly increase the leavening agent in egg-free recipes to compensate for the egg's natural leavening effect. In addition, using liquid sweeteners such as honey or molasses for part of the sugar in a recipe helps compensate for the loss of the "binding" effect of eggs.

In place of 1 egg as a moisturizer, use:

SUBSTITUTE	AMOUNT TO USE	WHEN TO USE/TIPS
Fruit juice, milk, or water	Use 2 Tbsp. Increase leavening by 25-50%. May need to bake items slightly longer.	Baked goods such as cakes, cookies, bars
Puréed fruit: Bananas, applesauce, apricots, pears, prunes. (The natural pectin in fruits, especially prunes, traps air which helps "lighten" baked goods.)	Use 1/4 cup. Increase leavening agent by 25-50%. May need to bake items slightly longer.	Baked goods where the fruit's flavor complements the overall dish such as applesauce in spice cakes, bananas in banana bread, apricots and pears in mild-flavored items, and prunes in dark, heavily-flavored items such as chocolate or spice cakes.

Note: Ask your health professional if these alternatives are safe for your diet.

Baking with Wheat-Free Flours

This table presents a summary of the baking characteristics, color, flavor, and storage recommendations for wheat-free flours (and grains) used in this book. General comments are also offered.

FLOUR	CHARACTERISTICS
Arrowroot	
Baking	Good in baking because it adds no flavor of its own and lightens baked goods. If used as breading, produces golden brown crust. Twice the thickening power of wheat flour.
Color/Flavor	Snow white in color. Looks like cornstarch. Flavorless.
Comments	Silky, fine powder from West Indies root. Replaces cornstarch or tapioca flour in baking.
Storage	Air-tight containers in cool, dry, dark place.
Bean Flour	
Baking	Two kinds of bean flour: (1) pure garbanzo or chickpea flour, and (2) garbfava flour made from a mixture of garbanzo and broad (fava) beans (from Authentic Foods – See Mail Order Sources). Both flours provide beneficial protein for baking. May totally (or partially) replace rice flour.
Color/Flavor	Light tan or yellowish. Slight "beany" flavor, especially if flour is pure chickpeas or garbanzo beans—less so with garbanzo/fava bean combination. The latter imparts slightly sweeter taste to baked goods.
Comments	Adds important protein to otherwise "starchy" gluten-free flour blends. Not widely available in stores, but can be ordered. See Mail Order Sources.
Storage	Air-tight containers in cool, dry, dark place.
Cornmeal	
Baking	Excellent in corn bread, muffins, and waffles—especially when blended with corn flour. Blue cornmeal can be used in muffins and waffles.
Color/Flavor	White or yellow. Tastes like corn. Blue cornmeal is grayish-blue and has a somewhat stronger flavor.
Comments	Coarser than corn flour. Often used in Mexican dishes. Used in Polenta. Make sure cornmeal does not contain wheat. Not the same as masa harina which <u>may</u> contain wheat.
Storage	Air-tight container in cool, dry, dark place.

Note: Ask your health professional if these alternatives are safe for your diet.

Baking with Wheat-Free Flours

(continued)

FLOUR	CHARACTERISTICS
Cornstarch	
Baking	Helps lighten baked goods, but use only in combination with other flours—not alone. Commonly used as thickener in sauces and gravies.
Color/Flavor	Snow white color. Flavorless, although more noticeable than arrowroot.
Comments	Highly refined and contributes little nutritional value.
Storage	Air-tight container in cool, dry, dark place.
Potato Starch	
Baking	Excellent baking properties, especially when combined with eggs. Lumps easily, so stir before measuring.
Color/Flavor	Very white. Bland flavor.
Comments	Very fine, powdery texture. Made from starch in potatoes. Not the same as potato flour, which is made from dried, ground potatoes with skins. Potato flour is heavy and used very little in wheat-free cooking.
Storage	Air-tight container in cool, dry, dark place.
Rice–White	
Baking	Dry and gritty by itself; works fine when combined with other flours. Should be about 2/3 of total flour. The coarser the grind, the more liquid needed.
Color/Flavor	White color. Bland, pleasant-tasting flavor.
Comments	Milled from broken hulls of rice kernel. Among least "allergenic" of all flours. Mostly starch. Nutritionally inferior (bran layers milled away).
Storage	Air-tight container in cool, dry, dark place.
Rice–Brown	
Baking	Dry, gritty—but excellent in baked goods.
Color/Flavor	Off-white color. Mild flavor. Makes baked goods slightly ivory-colored.
Comments	Higher in nutrients than white rice since brown rice still contains bran.
Storage	Air-tight container in cool, dry, dark place. Somewhat shorter shelf life due to high oil content in bran. Refrigerate or freeze.

Note: Ask your health professional if these alternatives are safe for your diet.

Baking with Wheat-Free Flours

(continued)

FLOUR	CHARACTERISTICS
Sorghum	(milo) Available from Jowar Foods (See Mail-Order Sources.)
Baking	Somewhat dry—increase liquid and oil by 5-15%. Best used to replace rice flour. Works very well in egg-free recipes.
Color/Flavor	Light tan. Mild flavor.
Comments	Excellent way to introduce variety and more protein into gluten-free diet.
Storage	Air-tight container in cool, dry, dark place.
Soy	
Baking	Excellent. Works well in baked goods with nuts, fruits, or chocolate. Adds moisture to baked goods. Best combined with other flours such as rice.
Color/Flavor	Yellow in color. Bland, somewhat nutty flavor—somewhat "beany". Can be camouflaged by mixing with spices, fruit, nuts, or chocolate.
Comments	Makes crispy coating for breading. Higher in protein, fat than other flours. Short shelf life; buy small amounts to avoid spoilage.
Storage	Air-tight container in cool, dry, dark place. Best if refrigerated.
Sweet Rice	
Baking	Not the same as white rice flour. Manufacturers suggest using in muffins, breads, and cakes although some sources recommend using only small amounts. Helps bind baked goods because of its sticky nature.
Color/Flavor	White, bland in flavor. Easily confused with white rice flour.
Comments	Sometimes called sticky rice or glutinous rice—doesn't contain wheat gluten. Often used in Chinese cooking. Contains more starch than rice flours, making it an excellent thickener. Inhibits separation of sauces when chilled or frozen.
Storage	Air-tight container in cool, dark, dry place.
Tapioca	
Baking	Excellent in baked products as 25-50% of total flour. Lightens baked goods, adds "chewiness" to breads. Browns; makes crispy breading.
Color/Flavor	Snow-white, velvety powder. "Anonymous" flavor.
Comments	Sometimes called cassava or cassava starch. Use like arrowroot.
Storage	Air-tight container in cool, dark, dry place.

Note: Ask your health professional if these alternatives are safe for your diet.

Substitutes for Wheat as Thickener

In place of 1 tablespoon of wheat flour, use the following:

INGREDIENT/ AMOUNT	CHARACTERISTICS	SUGGESTED USES
Agar (Kanten) – 1 1/2 teaspoons	Follow package directions. Colorless and flavorless. Sets at room temperature. Gels acidic liquids. Thin sauces need less.	Puddings, pie fillings, gelatin desserts, ice cream, glazes, cheese. Holds moisture and improves texture in pastry products.
Arrowroot – 1 1/2 teaspoons	Mix with cold liquid before using. Thickens at lower temperature than wheat flour or cornstarch. Better for eggs or sauces that aren't boiled. Add during last 5 minutes of cooking. Serve immediately after thickening. Clear, shiny, Semi-soft when cool.	Any food requiring clear, shiny sauce, but good for egg or starch dishes where high heat is undesirable. Gives appearance of oil even if none used.
Bean Flour – 3 teaspoons	Produces yellowish, rich-looking sauce.	Soups, stews, gravies (Use garbfava for less "bean" flavor.)
Cornstarch – 1 1/2 teaspoons	Mix with cold liquid before using. Stir just until boiling. Makes transparent, shiny sauce. Slight starchy flavor. Thicker, rigid when cool.	Puddings, pie fillings, fruit sauces, soups. Gives appearance of oil if none used.
Gelatin Powder – 1 1/2 teaspoons	Dissolve in cold water, then heat until liquid is clear before using.	Jello puddings, aspics, cheesecakes. Won't gel acids such as fresh pineapple.
Guar Gum – 1 1/2 tsp.	Mix with liquid before using. **Caution to celiacs**: High fiber content; may act as laxative.	Good for rice flour recipes
Kudzu (kuzu) Powder – 3/4 tsp.	Dissolve in cold water first. Odorless, tasteless. Produces smooth, transparent, soft sauces.	Puddings, pie fillings, and other dishes that must have "gelatin-like" consistency
Sweet Rice Flour – 1 tbsp.	Excellent thickening agent. May be called "glutinous" rice.	Sauces such as vegetable sauces. (Has no gluten)
Rice Flour (brown or white) – 1 tbsp.	Mix with cold liquid before using. Somewhat grainy.	Soups, stews, or gravies or hearty, robust sauces

Note: Ask your health professional if these alternatives are safe for your diet.

Substitutes for Wheat as Thickener

(continued)

In place of 1 tablespoon of wheat flour:

INGREDIENT/ AMOUNT	CHARACTERISTICS	SUGGESTED USES
Tapioca Flour – 1 1/2 Tbsp.	Mix with cold or hot liquid first. Add during last 5 minutes of cooking. Produces transparent, shiny sauce. Thick, soft gel when cool.	Soups, stews, gravies, potato dishes
Quick-Cooking Tapioca – 2 tsp.	Mix with fruit, let stand 15 minutes before baking.	Fruit pies, cobblers, and tapioca pudding
Xanthan Gum – 1 tsp.	Mix with dry ingredients first, then add to recipe.	Puddings, salad dressings, and gravies

Wheat Flour Equivalents

Use the information in this table to convert your own recipes to wheat and gluten-free—or to modify recipes in this book. Each type of flour has unique characteristics that affect the texture, taste, and appearance of baked goods.

In place of 1 cup of wheat flour, use:

FLOUR	AMOUNT
Corn Flour	1 cup
Cornmeal	3/4 cup
Cornstarch	3/4 cup
Garbanzo (Chickpea) Flour	3/4 cup
Garbanzo (Chickpea) and Fava (Broad) Garbfava Flour from Authentic Foods	7/8 cup (use 1:1 ratio in dishes with <1 cup flour)
Nuts (ground fine)	1/2 cup
Potato Starch or Potato Starch Flour	3/4 cup
Rice Flour (Brown or White)	7/8 cup
Sorghum Flour (milo) from Jowar	7/8 cup
Soy Flour	1/2 cup + 1/2 cup potato starch flour
Sweet Rice Flour	7/8 cup
Tapioca Flour or Tapioca Starch	1 cup

Flours from reputable sources usually measure consistently time after time, although differences in flour milling processes may affect consistency and texture. As you become more experienced with these flours, you can judge if the dough is too dry, too moist, or just right.

NOTE: Ask your health professional if these alternatives are safe for your diet.

Hidden Sources of Wheat & Gluten

Wheat flour is present in many products, but it isn't always listed as such. Avoid products containing ingredients such as all-purpose flour, unbleached flour, bread flour, cake flour, whole-wheat flour, semolina, or durum because these are alternate terms for wheat flour and will contain gluten. And, yes—white bread contains wheat (and, therefore, gluten). Also, you must check to see whether your food is prepared in the same receptacle or manufacturing line as wheat-containing foods or somehow contaminated with wheat flour—even though it's not listed as an ingredient. Finally, this list may change over time so you must continually be careful and read labels.

• **Beverages:** Avoid beer and ale, gin, whisky (bourbon, scotch and rye), vodka (if it's grain-based; potato and grape-based vodka are wheat-free), Postum, and Ovaltine.

• **Breads:** Unless the label says "wheat-free", avoid any biscuits, breads, crackers, croutons, crumbs, doughnuts, tortillas, or wafers. (You should also avoid breads made of oats, spelt, kamut, barley and rye because they are similar to wheat and contain gluten.)

• **Candy:** Wheat may be an ingredient (for example, licorice contains wheat flour) or used in the shaping or handling of the candy.

• **Caramel Color:** Manufactured by only two companies in the U.S. and generally believed to be gluten-free, whether in liquid or powdered form. However, caramel color is not the same as caramel flavoring. See below.

• **Caramel Flavoring:** Because this is made by several different companies, processes may vary. Therefore, it <u>may</u> contain malt syrup or wheat starch.

• **Cereal:** Avoid those made from wheat, rye, oats, barley, spelt, and kamut or if they contain malt flavoring or malt syrup. Some associations also advise Celiac Sprue patients to avoid quinoa and amaranth, however, these grains are gluten-free. The possibility of cross-contamination is still an issue.

• **Coffee:** Some decaffeinated, flavored, and instant coffees may cause distress for persons who avoid wheat and gluten. Be sure to choose gluten-free versions.

• **Condiments and Baking Ingredients:** Check labels, especially on mixed spices, ketchup, some dried or prepared mustards, mayonnaise, salad dressings, and most soy sauces. Look for wheat-free or gluten-free versions of these ingredients.

• **Dairy Products:** Some flavored yogurts contain modified food starch (which could be wheat). Look for those with pectin (this is fruit). Malted milk, processed cheese spreads, and chocolate milk may contain wheat. Low-fat sour cream may contain wheat.

• **Desserts and Other Sweets:** You'll bake your own pies, cakes, and cookies—but also avoid commercial pudding mixes, marshmallow creme, cake decorations, and marzipan because they may contain wheat flour as a thickener or binder.

Hidden Sources of Wheat & Gluten

(continued)

• **Distilled Vinegar:** Vinegar made from wine, rice, or cider is usually safe for wheat-sensitive persons. Look for pure apple cider vinegar, not apple-flavored vinegar. Controversy exists over whether vinegar made from grain contains residues from wheat.

• **Hydrolyzed Plant Protein (HPP):** Can be made from wheat starch.

• **Hydrolyzed Vegetable Protein (HVP):** Labels should list the source of protein.

• **Flavorings and Extracts:** Grain alcohol is often an ingredient. Look for gluten-free flavorings and extracts.

• **Meat, Fish, and Eggs:** Avoid any meat that's been breaded or in which fillers might be used such as sausage, luncheon meats, or hot-dogs. Avoid self-basting turkeys. Buy low-salt tuna in spring water rather than oil. Egg-substitutes are not pure eggs but often contain many other additional ingredients—possibly wheat flour.

• **Modified Food Starch:** This could be corn or wheat or some other unidentified food starch. Unless the label specifically states the source, it's best to avoid altogether.

• **Pastas:** You can eat some Oriental rice noodles, bean threads, and commercial pasta made from rice, corn, tapioca, or potato starch flour. Be sure to read labels since some pasta is made from a mixture of flours which may also include wheat or a member of the wheat family.

• **Soups and Chowders:** Many canned soups, soup mixes, and bouillon cubes or granules contain hydrolyzed vegetable protein (HVP) which may contain wheat.

• **Texturized Vegetable Protein (TVP):** This protein can be made from wheat starch.

• **Vegetables:** Avoid vegetables that are breaded, creamed, or scalloped because this usually involves wheat flour or bread crumbs made from wheat flour. When you see "vegetable starch" or "vegetable protein" on a label, this could mean protein from corn, peanuts, rice, soy—or wheat.

An excellent resource to help you know which commercial products are gluten-free is the Celiac Sprue Association's Cooperative Gluten-Free Commercial Products Listing. See Associations & Resources in the Appendix.

Hidden Sources of Dairy Products

Milk and milk products can be hidden in a variety of foods. Your food choices should be guided by whether you are lactose-intolerant or allergic to milk proteins. And, when reading the ingredient list, remember that there are other words used to indicate milk. For example, casein is a milk protein and whey, another protein, is the liquid derived from drained yogurt. Other terms to avoid include: acidolphilus, caseinate, calcium caseinate, hydrolyzed milk protein or vegetable protein, lactalbumin, lactate, lactoglobulin, lactose, and potassium caseinate. Below is a partial list of hidden dairy in commercial goods.

Baked Goods and Cooking Ingredients
Bread
Biscuits
Cakes
Caramel Coloring or Flavoring
Chocolate
Cookies
Doughnuts
Hot Cakes
Malted Milk
Mixes for Cakes, Cookies, Doughnuts,
        Muffins, Pancakes, etc.
Ovaltine (and other cocoa drinks)
Pie Crust (made with milk products)
Soda Crackers
Zwieback

Casseroles and Side Dishes
Creamed Vegetables
Hash
Mashed Potatoes
Scalloped Dishes
Dishes in Au Gratin Style
Fritters
Rarebits

Dairy
Buttermilk	Ghee (clarified butter)
Cheese	Milk (all forms)
Condensed Milk	Non-Dairy Creamer
Cream	Skim Milk Powder
Cream Cheese	Sour Cream
Evaporated Milk	Yogurt
Ice Cream	Whey

Desserts
Bavarian Cream
Candies
Custard
Ice Cream
Sherbets
Sorbet (some versions)
Spumoni
Pudding

Egg Dishes
Omelets
Scrambled Eggs
Soufflés

Meats and Fish
Canned Tuna
Deli Turkey
Hamburgers
Meats Fried in Butter
Sausages

Sauces and Salad Dressings
Butter Sauces
Cream Sauces
Gravies
Hard Sauces
Mayonnaise (some brands)
Salad Dressings (especially boiled)

Soups
Bisques
Chowders

Hidden Sources of Eggs

Many commercially prepared foods—or ingredients you buy to prepare your own dishes—contain eggs. Here is a partial list of those items. Be sure to read labels and remember that the ingredient list may not specifically mention the word eggs, but instead use words such as albumin, livetin, ovaglubin egg albumin, ovamucin, ovumucoid, ovovitellin, lysozyme, or egg whites, egg yolks, egg solids, or egg powder.

Baked Goods and Baking Ingredients
Baking Powder
Batters for Deep-Frying
Breads
Breaded Foods
Cakes
Cake Flour
Cinnamon Rolls
Cookies
Donuts
French Toast
Fritters
Frostings
Icings
Malted Cocoa Drinks
Marshmallows
Muffins
Pancake Flour
Pancakes
Pancake Mixes
Pretzels
Waffles
Waffle Mixes

Condiments and Sauces
Hollandaise Sauce
Salad Dressings (especially boiled ones)
Sauces (may be thickened with eggs)
Tartar Sauce

Desserts
Bavarian Cream
Ice Cream
Ices
Macaroons
Meringues
Pies (Cream pie filling and some pie crusts)
Puddings
Sherbets
Soufflés

Meats, Meat-Related Dishes
Bouillon
Hamburger Mix
Meat Loaf
Meat Balls
Meat Jellies
Meat Molds
Pate (also called Fois Gras)
Patties
Sausages
Soups (e.g., consommés)
Spaghetti & Meatballs

Beverages
Eggnog
Malted Cocoa Drinks (e.g. Ovaltine)
Wines (may be "cleared" with egg whites)

Other
Pasta (and dishes containing pasta)
Tartar Sauce

Hidden Sources of Corn

Corn appears in many unsuspecting places as an emulsifier, sweetener, or main ingredient.

Baked Goods & Baking Ingredients
Baking Mixes for Biscuits, Doughnuts,
    Pancakes and Pies
Baking Powder
Batters and Deep-Frying Mixtures
Bleached Wheat Flour
Breads and Pastries
Cakes
Cookies
Cereals
Corn Syrup
Cream Pies
Glucose Products
Graham Crackers
Oleo
Powdered Sugar
Tortillas
Vanilla
Vinegar (distilled)
Xanthan gum

Beverages
Ales
Beer
Bourbon and Whisky
Carbonated Beverages
Instant Coffee
Milk (in paper cartons)
Fruit Juices
Grape Juice (look for pure grape juice)
Soy Milk
Tea (instant)
Wines (some contain corn)

Non-Food Items
Adhesives and Glue
Bath Powder
Envelopes
Plastic Food Wrappers
Stamps
Talcum Powder
Toothpaste

Condiments, Sauces & Snacks
Catsup
Cheese
Commercial Syrups (e.g., Karo)
Fritos
Peanut Butter
Popcorn
Salad Dressings (e.g., French)
Soups (cream-style)
Tortilla Chips

Desserts
Candy
Frosting
Gelatins or Jello
Ice Cream and Sherbet
Jams and Jellies
Puddings or Custards
Sauces for Cakes or Sundaes

Meats & Side Dishes
Bacon
Bologna
Canned Peas
Chili
Chop Suey
Gravies
Grits
Hams
Sandwich Spread
Sauces for Meats
Sausage
Vegetables (in cream sauces)

Pharmaceuticals, Drugs, Additives
Aspirin, Cough Syrup, and other tablets
Dextrin
Dextrose
Mannitol
MSG (Monosodium Glutamate)
Nutra-Sweet
Sorbitol
Vitamin C Preparations

Hidden Sources of Soy

Soy appears in a variety of commercially prepared foods, as well as many ingredients.

Baked Goods and Baking Ingredients
Breads
Cakes
Cereals
Cooking Spray
Crackers
Lecithin (derived from soy)
Oils
Oleo or Margarine
Pastries
Rolls
Shortening

Beverages
Coffee Substitutes
Lemonade Mix
Soy Milk

Condiments, Sauces, Snacks, and Soups
Butter Substitutes
Cheese
Soy Sauce (and other Oriental sauces)
Worcestershire Sauce
Salad Dressings
Soup

Desserts
Caramel
Candies
Candy Bars
Custards
Ice Cream
Nut Candies

Meats and Meat-Related Dishes
Luncheon Meats
Sausage (certain kinds)

Miscellaneous
Baby Foods
Bean Sprouts
Pasta from Soy Flour
Tempura
Tofu

Associations & Resources

The following is a partial list of resources for people who must live or choose to live on special diets. Ask your physician about local support groups for people with food allergies, celiac disease, diabetes, or other conditions where certain ingredients must be omitted from one's diet. This partial list is offered as a resource and is not intended as an endorsement of any kind.

Allergy & Asthma Network, Mothers of Asthmatics, Inc. 3554 Chain Ridge Road, Suite 200 Fairfax, VA 22030-2709 (800) 878-4403 (help line) (703) 385-4403	American Academy of Allergy, Asthma & Immunology 611 E. Wells Street Milwaukee, WI 53202 (800) 822-2762 (help line) (414) 272-6071
American Diabetes Association, Inc. 1660 Duke Street Alexandria, VA 22314 (800) DIABETES or (800) 232-3472 www.diabetes.org	American Dietetic Association 216 West Jackson Boulevard, Suite 800 Chicago, IL 60607 (312) 899-0040 (800) 366-1655 National Nutrition Hotline www.eatright.org
Asthma & Allergy Foundation of America 1125 15th Street, N.W., Suite 502 Washington, D.C. 20005 (800) 7ASTHMA (help line) (202) 466-7643 aafasupgr@aol.com (support groups) www.aafa.org	Celiac Disease Foundation 13251 Ventura Blvd., Suite 3 Studio City, CA 91604-1838 (818) 990-2354; (818) 990-2379 - FAX http://www.celiac.org/cdf
Celiac Sprue Association/USA PO Box 31700 Omaha, NE 68131-0700 (402) 558-0600; (402) 558-1347 - FAX csaceliacs.org celiacs@csaceliacs.org	Food Allergy Network (FAN) 10400 Eaton Place, Ste.107 Fairfax, VA 22030 (800) 929-4040 or (703) 691-3179 http://www.foodallergy.org fan@worldweb.net
Gluten-Free Living (newsletter) PO Box 105 Hastings-on-Hudson, NY 10706 (914) 969-2018 (914) 969-2018 - FAX	Gluten Intolerance Group of NA - (GIG) 15110 10th Ave. SW Suite A Seattle, WA 98166-1820 (206) 246-6652; (206) 246-6531 - FAX gig@accessone.com
Living Without (magazine): *A lifestyle guide for people with food and chemical sensitivities* 1202N 75th Street, Suite 294 Downers Grove, IL 60516 (630) 415-3378; (847) 816-6045 - FAX pwagener@livingwithout.com	National Jewish Center for Immunology & Respiratory Medicine 1400 Jackson Street Denver, CO 80206 (800) 222-5864 (LungLine) (303) 388-4461

Mail Order Sources
For Wheat-Free/Gluten-Free Ingredients & Products

If you don't have a natural food or specialty food store nearby, the following companies take phone or mail orders. Contact them for a catalog.

A & A Amazing Foods, Inc. (also called Absersold Foods) PO Box 3927 Citrus Heights, CA. 95611 (800) 497-4834 (gluten-free milk powder and liquid called Dari-Free))	Authentic Foods 1850 W. 169th Street, Suite B Gardena, CA 90247 (800) 806-4737; (310) 366-7612 (310) 366- 6938 - FAX http://pages.prodigy.com/AUTFOODS (garbfava flour, bean flour, mixes)
Bickford Flavors 19007 St. Clair Avenue Cleveland, OH 44117-1001 (800) 283-8322 (flavorings, extracts)	Bob's Red Mill Natural Foods 5209 S.E. International Way Milwaukie, OR 97222 (800) 553-2258 (503) 653-1339 - FAX www.Bobsredmill.com (flours, grains)
Cybros, Inc. PO Box 851 Waukasha, WI 53187-0851 (800) 876-2253 (flours, breads, cookies)	Dietary Specialties, Inc. PO Box 227 Rochester, NY 14601 (800) 544-0099 (716) 232-6168 - FAX www.colorwheel.com/DS (pasta, flours, cookies, mixes, crackers, ingredients, condiments)
Ener-G Foods, Inc. P.O. Box 84487 Seattle, WA 98124-5787 (800) 331-5222 (206) 764-3398 - FAX www.ener-g.com (flours, ingredients, mixes)	Gluten-Free Cookie Jar PO Box 52 Trevose, PA 19053 (215) 355-9403 (breads, cakes, muffins, mixes)

This list is offered as a convenience and is not intended as an endorsement of any particular company. Nor is it intended to be a complete list of mail-order sources. It was updated when this book was published. However, the names, addresses, phone (or fax) numbers, and e-mail addresses of these companies may have changed as well as the product lines they carry.

Mail Order Sources
For Wheat-Free/Gluten-Free Ingredients & Products

(continued)

Gluten-Free Pantry PO Box 881 Glastonbury, CT 06033 (203) 633-3826 (800) 291-8386 (orders) (860) 633-6853 - FAX http://www.glutenfree.com pantry@glutenfree.com (mixes, ingredients, appliances)	Jowar Foods, Inc. 113 Hickory St. Hereford, TX 79045 (806) 363-9070 (806) 364-1984 - FAX http/www.jowar.com
King Arthur Flour PO Box 876 Norwich, VT 05055 (800) 827-6836 (800) 343-3002 - FAX (flours, mixes, xanthan gum)	Miss Roben's PO Box 1434 Frederick, MD 21702 (800) 891-0083 (301) 898-42489 (301) 631-5954 - FAX http://www.jagunet.com/~msrobensmissroben @aol.com (baking mixes, ingredients)
Mr. Spice Healthy Foods 850 Aquidneck Avenue Newport, RI 02842 (401) 848-7700 (401) 848-7701 - FAX (gluten-free, salt-free, fat-free sauces)	Pamela's Products, Inc. 364 Littlefield Avenue South San Francisco, CA 94080 (415) 952-4546 (415) 742-6643 - FAX (mixes, cookies, biscotti)

Internet Support Lists
These Internet news groups provide discussions on important topics:

Celiac Disease and Wheat Sensitivities: To join, in the body of an e-mail to:
http://rdz.acor.org/lists/celiac/index.html send the following:
SUB CELIAC firstname lastname

Celiac-Diabetes: To join, in the body of an e-mail to:
http://listserv@maelstrom.stjohns.edu send the following:
SUB CELIAC-DIABETES firstname lastname

Dairy Sensitivities: To join, in the body of an e-mail to:
listserv@MAELSTROM.stjohns.edu send the following:
SUB NO-MILK firstname lastname

Food Exchanges

The food exchanges in this cookbook were calculated using Food Processor software from ESHA, a state-of-the-art program used by major food corporations. Further information is based on "Exchange Lists for Meal Planning", published jointly in 1995 by the American Diabetes Association and the American Dietetic Association.

Following these guidelines, exchanges are given for the major groups: Carbohydrate, Meat, and Fat. Exchanges are calculated to the nearest 1/2 in order to provide a high degree of precision; exchanges smaller than 1/4 are not reported. If your diet does not require this much precision, simply round the exchanges to the desired precision. Additional nutrient values are offered for each recipe including calories, fat, protein, carbohydrates, sodium, cholesterol, and fiber to further assist you in managing your diet.

The following chart shows the amount of nutrients in one serving from each list.

Groups/Lists	Carbohydrate (grams)	Protein (grams)	Fat (grams)	Calories
Carbohydrate				
Starch	15	3	1 or less	80
Fruit	15			60
Milk				
Skim	12	8	0-3	90
Low-Fat	12	8	5	120
Whole	12	8	8	150
Other Carbohydrates	15	varies	varies	varies
Vegetables	5	2	—	25
Meat & Meat Substitute				
Very Lean (VL)	—	7	0-1	35
Lean (L)	—	7	3	35
Medium-Fat (MF)	—	7	5	75
High-Fat (HF)	—	7	8	100
Fat	—	—	5	45

The nutrient values and corresponding food exchanges for each recipe are as accurate as possible, but will naturally vary due to preparation techniques, brands used, serving sizes, and various other factors. For best results, consult your physician, dietitian, or other health professional for guidance in using this information.

Cooking Oils

Use this chart to determine which oil is best for you. It's best to consult with your health professional about this decision. The lower the smoking point, the more quickly oil burns.

Oil	% Saturated	% Poly-unsaturated	% Mono-unsaturated	Smoking Point
Canola oil	6	32	62	400°
Safflower oil (refined)	10	77	13	450°
Sunflower oil	11	69	20	450°
Corn oil (unrefined)	13	62	25	320°
Olive oil	14	9	77	350°
Soy oil	15	61	24	450°

Source: *Compositions of Foods*, United States Department of Agriculture.

Raw & Cooked Food Equivalents

Use this handy chart to figure out how much raw food you'll need to have a certain amount of cooked food.

Amount	Measure	Amount	Measure
Berries 1 pint	2 3/4 cups	Flour 1 pound	4 cups
Butter or Margarine 1 stick 1 pound	1/2 cup (8 Tbsp.) 4 sticks or 2 cups	Herbs 1 Tbsp. fresh	1 tsp. dried
Cheese 8 oz. cream cheese 8 oz. cottage cheese 4 oz. Parmesan, grated	1 cup 1 cup 1 1/4 cups	Pasta 8 oz elbow macaroni 8 oz. wide noodles 8 oz. angelhair pasta 8 oz. spaghetti	4 cups cooked 3 3/4 cups cooked 5 1/2 cups cooked 4 cups cooked
Chocolate 1 square 1 square	1 ounce 3 Tbsp. cocoa + 1 Tbsp. oil	Rice 1 cup white 1 cup brown 1 cup instant	3 cups cooked 3-4 cups cooked 1 1/2 cups cooked
Cream 1 cup heavy cream	2 cups whipped	Sugar 1 lb. granulated 1 lb. brown 1 lb. confectioners'	2 cups 2 1/4 cups 4 1/2 cups
Dried Beans or Peas 1 cup	2 1/4 cups cooked		

Appliances, Pans, & Utensils

Appliances

People often ask me what type of appliances I use when developing recipes for my cookbooks. I use a Welbilt 2200T bread machine (there are more recent models with more features available), a very simple version that bakes perfect bread every time. When mixing extremely heavy bread doughs by hand, I use an Oster Kitchen Center (which has a heavy-duty mixer). And, I use regular beaters—not dough hooks—for mixing bread dough.

For cake, cookie batters and cooking class demonstrations, I use a hand-held Hamilton Beach mixer. It has a fairly powerful motor, which is essential for heavier dough. A Hamilton food processor (using knife blade) is indispensable for blending batter and dough because it is very fast and does a better job of distributing the moisture throughout the ingredients than an electric mixer. In fact, I wouldn't be without this indispensable appliance (which costs about $40 on sale at discount stores.) There are, however, much more expensive versions available.

My range is an electric Jenn-Aire and I have two ovens: a Jenn-Aire and a Kitchen Aid. Remember that different brands and types may produce slightly different outcomes. Follow the directions exactly the first time you make any recipe, then make changes as needed—such as longer or shorter baking times.

One of the handiest appliances in my kitchen is a small, handheld coffee grinder. Ranging in cost from $10 to $30, these devices are wonderful for grinding fresh lemon or orange peel. I use a potato peeler to remove all the peel (leaving behind the white pith), tear the peel into bite-size pieces, and then let the coffee grinder turn the peel into the consistency of grated citrus peel. You'll get far more peel from an orange or lemon than the conventional method of using a grater. To clean the coffee grinder, pulverize a tablespoon of white rice kernels in it, discard the rice, and then wipe clean with a damp paper towel. Avoid using the same grinder for grinding both coffee and citrus peel (unless you like the flavor of coffee-flavored citrus!)

Pans

I bake almost exclusively in nonstick pans because gluten-free batters tend to stick. The darker finish on nonstick pans also helps the browning process. In-sulated baking pans tend to make baked goods somewhat soggy (except for some cookies). Be sure to use utensils specially designed for nonstick pans so you don't scratch the specially treated surfaces. Generally speaking, using several smaller pans in place of one large pan assures that the finished product will rise and bake thoroughly. However, for your convenience I usually offer directions for using both large and small pan sizes.

Pan Substitutions

When substituting one size pan for another, this chart will help you choose. When measuring bake ware, measure across top of pan, from inside edge to inside edge. For fluted baking molds, measure from inside edge of outward curve to inside of exact opposite curve. Measure depth on inside vertical from the bottom of dish or pan to top edge. If you're not sure about volume of particular pan or dish, fill with water. Then, pour water into measuring cup.

Pan or Dish	Equivalent in Cups
13 x 9-inch baking dish	12 - 15 cups
10 x 4-inch tube pan	12 cups
10 x 3 1/2-inch Bundt pan	12 cups
9 x 3-inch tube pan	9 cup
9 x 3-inch Bundt pan	9 cups
11 x 7-inch baking dish	8 cups
8-inch square baking dish	8 cups
9 x 5-inch loafpan	8 cups
9-inch deep-dish pie plate	6 - 8 cups
9 x 1 1/2-inch cake pan	6 cups
7 1/2 x 3-inch Bundt pan	6 cups
9 x 1 1/2-inch cake pan	5 cups
8 x 1 1/2-inch cake pan	4 - 5 cups
8 x 4-inch loaf pan	4 cups

Here are the most common sizes for various pots and pans so you'll know what the recipe intended when it says "small" saucepan or "medium" skillet.

Dutch Ovens
Small = 2 quarts
Medium = 6 quarts
Large = 8 quarts

Roasting Pans
Small = 13 x 9 x 2 inches
Medium = 14 x 11 x 2 inches
Large = 16 x 13 x 3 inches

Saucepans
Small = 1 quart
Medium = 1 1/2 - 2 quarts
Large = 4 quarts

Shallow Baking Dishes
Small = 1 quart
Medium = 2 quarts
Large = 3 quarts

Skillets
Small = 7 or 8- inch diameter
Medium = 9 or 10-inch diameter
Large = 11 or 12-inch diameter

Stockpots
Small = 6-8 quarts
Medium = 12 quarts
Large = 16-20 quarts

Utensils & Other Helpers

Serrated knives or electric knives are especially helpful in cutting breads. You can find electric knives in discount stores for around $15. They are also great for cutting a pie crust. I use waxed paper or parchment paper for baked goods that must be removed from the pan whole, rather than sliced. The new teflon liners, available at kitchen stores or by mail-order, are also great for baking.

ABOUT THE AUTHOR

A former university professor and marketing executive with a Fortune 500 corporation, Dr. Fenster graduated from the University of Nebraska with a degree in Home Economics and was a home economics specialist with the Cooperative Extension Service at North Dakota State University. Her graduate degree in Organizational Sociology helps her understand the symbolic role that food plays in our lives and how special diets can affect that symbolism.

After discovering her own food sensitivities several years ago, Dr. Fenster studied extensively to find flavorful alternatives for problem ingredients. She understands the importance of a healthy diet and the desire for fine dining— all the more challenging when one has to avoid certain ingredients.

She serves as vice-president of her local asthma and allergy support group (affiliated with the Asthma and Allergy Foundation of America) and is a member of the Celiac Sprue Association/USA, the Gluten Intolerance Group of North America, and the Celiac Disease Foundation.

Committed to helping others eat the dishes they want (without the ingredients they don't want) Dr. Fenster makes radio and TV appearances, publishes books and articles in newspapers and magazines, and consults with health profession- als, natural food stores, and corporations serving those on special diets. She is associate food editor at Sully's LIVING WITHOUT magazine, an on-line advisor for Veggie Life magazine, and a frequent guest speaker at associations and organizations across the country.

If you would like Dr. Fenster to speak to your organization, please contact:

Savory Palate, Inc.
8174 South Holly, Suite 404
Littleton, CO 80122-4004
(303) 741-5408   (303) 741-0339 - FAX
savorypala@aol.com

If you have comments, suggestions, or success stories please send them to Dr. Fenster at the above address.

SPECIAL DIET SERIES ORDER FORM

Name_____

Address_____

City/State/Zip_____

Telephone (   ) _____

Please send the following items to the address above:

Money-back guarantee!	QUANTITY	PRICE (Canada & UK add $5)	TAX (Colorado Residents only)	TOTAL
Wheat-Free Recipes & Menus *(275 recipes for breads, desserts, entrees – 2nd edition is dairy-free)*		$19.95	$.76 per book	
Special Diet Solutions: *healthy cooking without wheat, gluten, dairy, eggs, yeast, or refined sugar*		$15.95	$.61 per book	
Special Diet Celebrations: *without wheat, gluten, dairy, eggs, or sugar. Nearly 300 recipes for special events.*		$18.95	$.72 per book	
Bookmarks (handy, laminated summaries at your fingertips) Baking With Wheat-Free Flours Baking With Alternative Sweeteners Baking With Dairy Substitutes Baking With Egg Substitutes	_____ _____ _____ _____	$1.50 each $1.50 each $1.50 each $1.50 each	$.06 $.06 $.06 $.06	_____ _____ _____ _____
Buy 2 books–get bookmarks free!			SUB-TOTAL	
		Shipping & handling ($3 per book)		
		(Canada: $5)		
		Total Amount Enclosed		

Please allow 2 weeks for delivery

☐ Check
(payable to
Savory Palate, Inc.)

☐ Visa, MasterCard, Discover
Account
Number_____
Expiration
Date_____
Customer
Signature_____

SAVORY PALATE, INC.
8174 South Holly, Suite 404, Littleton, CO 80122-4004
You may also order from our WEB site at www.ReadersNdex.com/specialdiet

In Colorado	FAX (303) 741-0339	**Outside Colorado**
(303) 741-5408	e-mail: savorypala@aol.com	(800) 741-5418 (orders only)

Also available at bookstores, natural food stores, BarnesandNoble.com, and Amazon.com